This book

CURE AND
NAIL TECHNIQUES

RELATED MACMILLAN TITLES

The Nail File by Leo Palladino and June Hunt

Science and The Beauty Business: Volume 1, *The Science of Cosmetics*, and Volume 2, *The Beauty Salon and its Equipment*, both by John V. Simmons

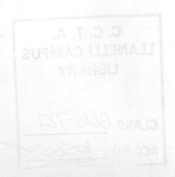

Manicure, pedicure and advanced nail techniques

ELAINE ALMOND

B.Sc.(Hons), Cert.Ed., C.Biol., M.I.Biol., LCSP(B.Th.), BABTAC

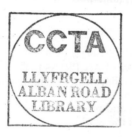
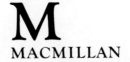

MACMILLAN

First published 1992 by
THE MACMILLAN PRESS LTD
Houndmills, Basingstoke, Hampshire RG21 2XS
and London
Companies and representatives
throughout the world

ISBN 0–333–56313–1 hardcover
ISBN 0–333–63007–6 paperback

A catalogue record for this book is available
from the British Library.

Printed in Hong Kong

10 9 8 7 6 5 4 3 2
01 00 99 98 97 96 95 94

CONTENTS

ACKNOWLEDGEMENTS

The author wishes to thank personally the following people and organisations for their assistance in producing this book.

Dr Andrew L. Wright, Consultant Dermatologist, Bradford Royal Infirmary, for his time and encouragement, and for providing his unique nail disease/disorder photographs.

For providing scientific and general information: Rosemary Barnes (Toriess Limited); Dr G. D. S. Beechey; Anthony G. Broughton (Protecto PLC & Atom Chemicals Limited); Tony Coomber (Light Concept Nails Limited); Russell Leach (Star Nails); Claudette J. Noe (Backscratchers); and Dr Peter D. Samman.

For a superb job on the many technique photographs taken for this book, many thanks to the photographer, Darren Smith, of Chorley, Lancashire.

Stanley Thornes, Russell Leach and Kevin Quinn (Willen Limited) for their help, encouragement and support at a very crucial time during the preparation of this book.

Gareth and Pat Hardwick, of Grafton International Limited, whose ongoing encouragement, support, help and advice was much appreciated.

For photographs supplied: Dr P. K. Buxton and The Medical Photography Department (Victoria Hospital, Kirkaldy, Fife); Cereal Partners UK; Tony Coomber (Light Concept Nails Limited); Ellisons; European Touch Limited; Valerie Foote (Salon System); and the Hairdressing & Beauty Equipment Centre.

Last but by no means least, many thanks to Suzannah Tipple, Andrew Nash and Isobel Munday of my publishers.

This book is dedicated to my mother, Doris Ramsbottom, and my husband, Michael Almond, for their loyal support and understanding.

Note about pronouns

There are male and female nail technicians, just as there are male and female clients. However, to use 'he or she' and 'him or her' throughout the text becomes cumbersome in a book such as this: for simplicity and ease of reading, therefore, we have used simply 'she', 'her' and so on throughout.

INTRODUCTION

The easiest and best way for people to achieve and keep beautiful fingernails and toenails is by making regular visits to a professional manicurist and pedicurist. Here their nails will be trimmed and filed to their proper length and shape, the cuticles will be softened, pushed back and trimmed if necessary, and a protective coat of nail varnish will be applied to guard against splitting, peeling and other damage.

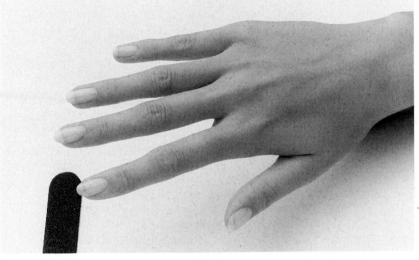

Light Concept Nails

The work of the professional manicurist no longer stops there, however – never before in history has such a variety of artificial nail products been available to extend, repair or simply strengthen the nail plate; never before has the colouring of the nail plate reached such heights of artistic achievement. To fulfil the demands of present-day clients, the modern manicurist and pedicurist needs to be conversant with more than simply the basic knowledge of her trade. Her status has rapidly changed from that of a person who simply cared for the appearance of the natural nails and their immediate surroundings, to that of a nail technician, capable of drawing on advances in modern technology to allow her clients to enjoy the luxury of long, matching, beautiful nails at all times.

As a reflection of these trends, this book encompasses all the information that the modern manicurist, pedicurist and nail technician will need during the course of her training and career.

PART I Manicuring and pedicuring as a career

1 The MANICURIST

Manicuring is a service industry and as such is similar in its demands to other service industries, such as nursing or waitressing. Being in a service industry means that the person is paid to do a service for other people.

As with all jobs, a person is good at their work only if they take pride in what they do, and it takes a particular kind of special person to make a success in the service industries. For example, a nurse should take just as much pride in keeping the bedpans clean as she does in giving painless injections. These are both parts of her job, her chosen vocation, and her pride in her work should not let her lower her standards or carry out any aspect of her work with less than a good heart. In a similar way, a manicurist should be able to take as much pride in sculpting and airbrushing a complete set of nails as she does in performing a first manicure on a ten-year-old child or helping a departing client to put her coat on.

A manicurist is there to serve the public. If she does not serve them well, in all aspects of her work, her clients will go elsewhere.

Personality

Bearing these thoughts in mind, it is clear that a manicurist should have an outgoing personality and a caring nature, and should really like people. These traits will express themselves in many ways in her job – for instance, liking people will give her genuine compassion for them: she will be able to hold 'trivial' conversations about each client's day-to-day life and to remember those conversations and her clients so that she can continue the chat the next time the client comes into the salon. Because she cares, little things like remembering what shade of varnish the client wore to a special occasion earlier in the year will come automatically to her. In this way, the client begins to feel special and wanted, simply because she *is* special and wanted to that manicurist who takes pride in her job and gets enjoyment from her clients.

Being outgoing will lead to the manicurist having outside interests apart from her work. This in turn will mean that she will be able to relate to people and to hold conversations with them on a variety of everyday topics, instead of being 'blinkered' by her job.

Clients obviously want a top-class job doing; given a choice, though, most would rather have a 98 per cent perfect job done by a caring person than a 100 per cent job done by a surly or uncaring person.

A manicurist must also be able to control her feelings. Any pressures and worries outside work, such as a row with a boyfriend or illness in the family, must be put aside when she is at work. The client is paying for the attention and skills of the manicurist: she isn't paying to listen to the problems of the manicurist, or to have a poor manicure because the manicurist can't concentrate on her work.

A manicurist must also have good health and a positive outlook. Clients often prefer to book all their appointments with one manicurist whose work they trust. They usually do not like to be moved around to alternative people when their normal manicurist is absent. If this happens frequently, clients may settle with another manicurist in the same salon, or even go elsewhere. The employee who is often absent may therefore find it difficult to build up her own regular clientele.

When dealing with clients on a one-to-one basis, as the manicurist does, there is often no one else available to take over bookings if the manicurist is ill. This causes innumerable problems when it happens unavoidably, and so uncalled-for absenteeism is fair neither to the other staff nor to clients who are left trying to deal with these problems. A manicurist must not be prone to absenteeism, nor to giving in to minor illnesses like headaches or period pains. The ethic of 'working yourself better' must apply.

A person who is introverted, moody, a complainer, self-centred, prone to absenteeism or illness, or selfish, with no real affinity or liking for people, should not consider becoming a manicurist. Any one of these character traits should warn the person (or a potential employer!) that she is not right for the job.

Conduct

A manicurist should take care to be punctual, both in arriving for her work and in keeping to her appointment times. Often clients have busy schedules to keep to – they may have a follow-on appointment somewhere else, or be on their lunch break. If they have taken the trouble to come on time, they will not appreciate having to wait for the manicurist. A manicurist who is often behind in her work is encouraging the client herself to be late for her appointments – or even encouraging her to go elsewhere.

A manicurist spends long periods in close proximity to her clients, so particular attention should be paid to aspects of oral and bodily hygiene.

A manicurist should pay special attention to her own appearance. She is a professional person who needs to present a professional image which will gain the respect of her clients (Figure 1.1). Points to

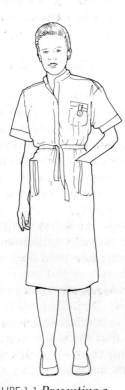

FIGURE 1.1 *Presenting a professional image*

remember could include these. She should wear smart, well-fitted overalls, always clean and pressed. Shoes should be low-heeled and sensible. Make-up should be basic, pleasant and not overdone. Hair should be worn in a style taken back from the face so it does not fall forward as the manicurist is working. Jewellery should be simple and kept to a minimum, so that it does not interfere with work.

The manicurist should also be aware of her posture, for the sake of her health as well as her appearance. She should make an effort to stand or sit correctly at all times.

The nails of a manicurist can be a walking advertisement: as such, they should be kept nicely manicured and varnished in an artistic design or a colour that can be bought from the salon. Many clients will choose their colour or nail art from the appearance of the manicurist's nails.

Client care

A manicurist should at all times be aware of and look after the needs of her clients. For example, a simple thoughtful act like greeting them with their name as they enter the salon can be very important in making the client feel welcome. There is something especially welcoming about being greeted by name and clients are usually impressed that they have been remembered. If the manicurist is not very good at remembering names, a useful tip is to check the appointment book, reminding herself of the name just prior to the client's arrival. Using the name a few times during the course of conversation, whilst also noting what the client looks like, will soon enable her to remember the name.

On arrival, the manicurist could also help the client off with her coat and show her to her seat.

She should be able to make light conversation, taking care to avoid 'unsafe' topics – politics, religion, debatable current issues or morbid topics. The client is there to enjoy herself, not argue or be depressed! With practice, the manicurist will develop the ability to concentrate on her work even when talking. If she cultivates the art of being a good listener, leading the client to talk simply by the occasional use of a few well-chosen words, her work will be much easier. She must also recognise when her client simply wishes to sit quietly.

The manicurist should not encourage gossip, divulge secrets, or talk about other clients during conversations with clients or friends. The manicurist needs to be discreet, knowing when to change the conversation and not showing favouritism.

The manicurist can and should look to the needs of the clients in many other ways, such as making sure that the client does not leave her rings behind, and that she pays, buys any items she requires, gets her car keys out and is helped on with her coat *before* her varnish application, to minimise the hazard of smudging the nail varnish. She should check to see whether the client wants a drink or magazine during her stay in the salon, and that her varnish is dry before she leaves. In other words, she must try to be courteous, kind and considerate to the client, from entry to exit.

PROFESSIONAL ETHICS

Professional ethics is about right and wrong. Good professional behaviour is best explained by examples such as the two below.

Example 1

Imagine a quiet salon in which the manicurist is sitting doing nothing. A potential client comes in, requesting a full set of permanent false nails. On inspection, the lady's nails prove to be unsuitable for the application of this type of nail: they are extremely short and bitten, with 'bulbs' of flesh protruding beyond the edge of the nail plate. It would be professional to carry out a cheaper, temporary treatment and allow the client's nails time to grow a little before putting on the more expensive permanent nails.

Suppose, however, that the manicurist has not taken much money that day, the appointment book is empty, the temptation to increase the takings is too great, and the manicurist does apply the permanent false nails, disregarding the long-term interests of her client. What would be the result of this unethical behaviour?

The client would go away temporarily happy. However, her new extensions would not last very long, so she would rapidly become unhappy. One of two things would then happen. She might come back and complain, in which case it would cost the manicurist time and money to rectify the situation. The manicurist would also have to work hard to regain the client's trust and confidence in the product, herself and the salon. Or she might not come back to complain, but she might tell everyone she knew not to go to that manicurist or salon because the standards were so bad. Perhaps this suggests why the manicurist wasn't busy in the first place.

Example 2

The manicurist is offered a job with a new salon just setting up. Ignoring her contract of work with her employer – standard terms of which are are usually at least one week's notice and an agreement not to work for at least one year within one mile of her previous salon – she leaves immediately to go to the new job. What would be the result of this unethical behaviour?

Firstly, she would of course risk her former boss suing for breach of contract. Secondly, a salon that poaches staff is not being ethical either, so the chances are that the manicurist would not like the new employment, or that the new business would close down fairly quickly. The manicurist would then have to look for another job. The only reference that she could get from her previous employment would include the fact that she had broken her terms of contract and left without notice. This is not a good reference with which to go job-hunting. All she had to do to avoid this situation was go to her boss, discuss the matter with her, hand in her notice and work it out properly. Who knows – doing the right thing initially might even have won her an incentive to stay, in the form of promotion within her original firm!

Ethics, in fact, can be summed up by that one short phrase – *doing the right thing*. There are seven basic ethical guidelines. The professional manicurist should:

1 *Know her subject well* She should keep up to date with new advances by reading around, attending courses and visiting exhibitions whenever possible.

2 *Take pride in her career and her job of work* This pride means that she is unable knowingly to do a bad job of work because she recognises that all jobs reflect her overall professionalism.

3 *Keep her word and fulfil her obligations* If a client asks her to get in a special item for the client to buy and she agrees to do this, then she must follow this through and not just forget. If she advises that a set of nails will last at least two weeks, then they must do so, or she must replace them free of charge. She must never make empty promises and wild claims: this undermines her own reputation and that of the profession as a whole.

4 *Look to her own reputation, both inside and outside work* The new professional starts with no reputation: with care she can build a good one. Unethical behaviour can destroy it, however, and once destroyed, a good reputation takes an awfully long time to build up again. The manicurist must cherish and maintain her reputation, behaving well in all aspects of her life.

5 *Never criticise other salons, manicurists, or their work* The manicurist doesn't know the true story behind any gossip, or behind any job of work that comes to her from another salon. She must keep her opinions to herself and never lower herself by criticising others.

6 *Be loyal to her employer* Employers have a lot of responsibilities, worries and overheads that employees cannot begin to comprehend unless they themselves have been self-employed. It should be remembered that without employers employment opportunities, especially for the trainee, would be limited.

It is the manicurist's responsibility to be open and honest with her employer. If she is unhappy, she must discuss this with her boss – how can her employer help if she does not know of any problems? Most employers are fair; if an employee is fulfilling her part of the job bargain, then no reasonable request will be denied. The employer will wish her workforce to be happy and to improve the workplace. After all, a happy salon is a successful salon.

7　*Be loyal to her workmates*　How much nicer it is to work in an atmosphere of teamwork, where all the staff help one another instead of falling out all the time! Everyone has their moods, up and down, but a good workmate remains consistent in her attitudes, and is loyal and supportive of her friends during their downs as well as their ups. As part of the team, each manicurist is a key contributor to the atmosphere at work.

By following these seven guidelines to professional ethics, the manicurist will find that she is automatically 'doing the right thing'.

DIET AND FITNESS

Being drawn to and a part of the beauty industry, most manicurists take great pride in their appearance, and wish to have a slim and fit body, clear skin and shining hair, as well as to be nicely made-up and dressed. The demands of the job also ask that the manicurist be healthy and not prone to illness.

By following a few simple rules of living, the manicurist can go a long way to creating inner vitality, good health and stamina. She owes it to herself and her chosen profession to do so.

Diet

Diet simply means what we eat every day of our lives. In order to survive, our bodies need vitamins, minerals, water, proteins, carbohydrates, roughage and fats (Figure 1.2). Vitamins and minerals have been placed first: if we looked at each food that we are about to eat and asked 'What vitamins and minerals are there in this food that will do me any good?' before we ate it, and refused to eat foods which did not contain many of these vitamins and minerals so essential to our health, we would be going a long way towards creating a good diet for ourselves. Gone would be the crisps, chocolate bars, cakes and biscuits, for a start, along with so much of the overprocessed and under-nourishing foods which are an accepted part of our eating patterns today. Each person should make every mouthful of food count in the quest for health.

The *minimum daily requirements* of a good diet for an averaged-sized woman are as follows:

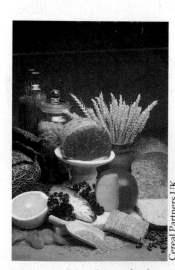

FIGURE 1.2 *Nutritious foods for a healthy diet*

Cereal Partners UK

- [ ] 150–200 g (6–10 oz.) of protein, chosen from fish, low-fat cheeses, eggs, chicken, liver and lean meat.
- [ ] 300 g (12 oz.) of fresh vegetables, preferably those which grow above ground (e.g. green leafy vegetables).
- [ ] 300 g (12 oz. – around three items) of fresh fruit.
- [ ] 150 g (6 oz.) of unrefined carbohydrate (e.g. baked potatoes, wholemeal bread, breakfast cereals, cooked rice or pasta).
- [ ] 0.25–0.5 litre ($\frac{1}{2}$–1 pt.) of semi-skimmed or skimmed milk.

This is quite a lot of food, but if this and nothing more was eaten and the lower protein and milk levels chosen, a person would quickly but safely lose weight.

Our food should be centred around fresh, whole produce which provides lots of vitamins and minerals. As many vegetables as possible should be eaten raw. The best way to do this is to eat a large salad every day. Food should not be fried.

Only when the above foods have been eaten and drunk should we eat anything else – for example, it is not good practice to skip the salad lunch (full of vitamins and minerals) and have a nutrient-depleted and high-fat pie instead!

When more food is required, simply eat more of the foods named above. A greater variety of this type of 'whole food' can be introduced into the diet, such as yogurt, nuts, dried fruits, grains and pulses.

Drinking

Fluids are vital for the correct functioning of our bodies. Around 70 per cent of the body is composed of water.

Under normal circumstances, an average of 2 litres ($3\frac{1}{2}$ pints) of water per day is lost from our bodies by evaporation and excretion: this has to be replaced by drinking and eating. The manicurist, however, spends a lot of her time inside in a warm environment, which encourages perspiration. She also talks a lot during her work, so she will lose a lot of body fluids through her lungs. Because of this, she will need to drink more than average and quite frequently throughout the day to replenish her body fluids and maintain health.

The ideal fluid to drink is the one that the body needs: water, with no additives. When we drink other fluids, such as coffee or cola, the additives in the drinks start to build up in our bodies and can cause problems. For example, the toxins contained within twenty cups of strong coffee, if they were to be absorbed all at once, could even prove fatal. In reality, the cups of coffee we drink are spread out through the day, and the body's mechanisms work hard to remove these toxins from our system, so we do not in fact die. The end result, though, is that the body uses a lot of energy to rid itself of toxins and is never truly free of them. The body therefore functions at a lower level of efficiency than it could. Headaches, tiredness, disturbed sleep patterns and skin eruptions can all be attributed to an overload of toxins in the body.

Ideally, therefore, water should be drunk, and plenty of it. If a change is desired, then drink a variety of beverages to avoid toxin build-up – herb and normal teas, diluted fruit juices, coffee substitutes, yeast extract drinks and so on. The old adage of 'moderation in all things' applies to drinking as well as to eating.

(One good tip for cleansing the body of toxins and getting some of our all-important water intake is to drink up to half a litre (a pint) of warm water first thing in the morning, thirty minutes before anything else is eaten or drunk.)

Exercise

Manicuring is a sedentary job: the manicurist sits down for most of the day and does not get any exercise at work.

Exercise is essential to maintain muscular tone, and this is essential if the figure is to be maintained. On a less visible level, exercise is necessary to maintain heart and lung capacity (related to stamina), boost the blood circulation (taking food and oxygen to the tissues and removing their waste products) and assist with the correct functioning of all the body organs and systems. In other words, exercise is essential to maintain the general health of the body.

Exercise does not have to mean enforced jogging at six in the morning or immensely vigorous aerobics sessions. Exercise should be something involving movement which the person finds enjoyable and therefore easy to maintain on a regular basis. Ideally, this exercise should exert the body – make it have to breathe really hard to keep up – for three twenty-minute periods a week. Examples of this could be a brisk walk, a dance at a disco, a cycling session or a swim.

In addition to this, the manicurist should spend thirty minutes daily in natural light. This might be achieved whilst walking to work, or during a walk at lunchtime, or playing in the garden with the children after work.

The manicurist works inside under artificial lighting all the time. Studies have shown that this can be detrimental to health in many small ways, usually linked with hormone production and the emotions. These studies, however, have proved that exposure of the eyes to natural light for as little as thirty minutes every day will overcome this problem and have a beneficial effect on the emotions, moods and general health.

After this essential basic routine, any extra exercise is a bonus.

POSTURE

A manicurist spends long hours at her manicure station working with her arms forwards and her head inclined downwards. This position places a strain on the trapezius muscles across the back of the shoulders. As a result, these muscles have a tendency to tighten up. In doing so, they exert pressure on the nerves leading away from that part of the spine to the arms.

If this situation is left to progress, this pressure can start to irritate these nerves, ultimately leading to headaches, or pins and needles, pains, or loss of sensation in the hands and arms. This situation can be avoided if the manicurist pays proper attention to the way that she sits whilst working, and also if she stretches and flexes the shoulders at convenient times throughout the day to prevent tension build-up.

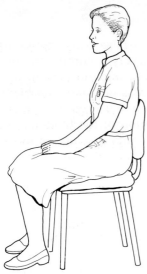

FIGURE 1.3 *Correct posture when sitting*

Sitting

The manicurist should have a properly designed stool with a back support. She should sit erect with her weight evenly distributed on the stool and both feet flat on the floor. She should have her bottom back against the stool, her lower back slightly hollowed, and her shoulders held back and down (Figure 1.3).

When not working on a client her head should be erect, with her chin tucked in and her ears directly over her shoulders. It is best to imagine a string pulling up from the crown of the head. If this is tried, by getting hold of some hair at the crown and pulling upwards, it can be seen how the head and back fall into alignment along a straight spine. When rising from a seat and when sitting down, the movement should be as if this string is pulling up and releasing so that the body is rising and falling straight – not by poking the chin forwards to stand up, and the bottom out to sit down!

When working, the manicurist can lean slightly forward from this position. The client's hands should be held at an easy distance for working so that the elbows are not sharply angled.

The manicurist should check frequently for tension in her shoulders, especially on a busy day. A common fault is to lean on one elbow whilst working (the left one, if right-handed), thereby pushing up the left shoulder and causing problems in this area.

It is equally important that the manicurist does not go home and slouch in a chair with her shoulders rounded over while watching television or relaxing. This is adding to her postural problems of the day. An ideal chair for relaxing will allow her shoulders and head to drop back a little, thus releasing the tension from the trapezius muscles along the top and back of the shoulders.

Shoulder stretching

To release tension in the shoulders:

1 Rotate the shoulders backwards three times, then forwards three times, in large circles.
2 Let the head drop onto the chest, then slowly rotate it on the shoulders by keeping the face forwards, but rolling the head around onto one shoulder, to the back, to the other shoulder and to the chest again. Do this three times one way, then three times the other way.
3 If there is space, rotate both arms in full circles three times forwards and three times backwards.

These two or three exercises, repeated two or three times throughout the day, should keep the neck and shoulders free from any aches and pains.

Hands and wrists

A manicurist, especially if she specialises in false nail techniques, constantly uses her hands and wrists in a very vigorous manner. Over the years, filing movements and supporting and pulling people's fingers around can take their toll. If care is not taken, problems can occur, causing time off work or even enforced retirement. Tenosynovitis, for example, is an inflammation of the tendons and synovial capsules of the wrists and finger joints that makes movement of the hands and wrists extremely painful. Carpal tunnel syndrome gives pain, 'pins and needles' or partial paralysis in the hand; it results from a narrowing of the carpal tunnels, the passages through which nerves pass between the arms and the hands. These are two examples of repetitive strain injuries: problems caused by the over-use of the hands, wrists and fingers in small, strenuous, repeated movements, such as occur in filing.

In order to avoid these problems, the manicurist should vary the work that she does – for instance, manicures and re-varnishes should be interspersed with nail extensions. The work station should be at the right height and comfortable to work at. She should also make sure that she does not work for too many hours at any one time, that she gets sufficient rest periods, and that she takes sufficient holidays. If any pain is felt in the hands, the manicurist should take a rest to allow her injury to heal.

PART II   # Hygiene

2 MICRO-ORGANISMS

Micro-organisms are small, single-celled organisms, which cannot be seen except through a microscope. A group of them together may be visible with the naked eye – the grey-white mould sometimes found on fruit or bread, for instance, is actually a colony of the microscopic fungus belonging to the genus *Mucor*.

Micro-organisms fall into three distinct categories: bacteria, viruses and fungi. It is because of these organisms and their ability to cause disease that sterilisation procedure must be rigorously followed in the salon. An understanding of the life cycles of bacteria, viruses and fungi, and the ways in which these micro-organisms are transmitted from one host to another, is vital if the reasons for sterilisation procedure are to be understood.

Basic cell structure

Each cell is bounded by a membrane known as the cell wall. The functioning of the cell, and the synthesis of proteins (including enzymes), is controlled by nucleic acids – deoxyribonucleic (DNA) or ribonucleic acid (RNA). The DNA is contained within another membrane, making a so-called nucleus. The living material within the cell is called protoplasm: protoplasm within the nucleus may instead be called nucleoplasm, and protoplasm outside the nucleus may be called cytoplasm.

BACTERIA

Bacteria are micro-organisms which are to be found in one of three distinct forms (Figure 2.1):

- □ rod-shaped (bacillus);
- □ round (coccus);
- □ spiral (spirillum).

Each bacterium consists of a cell wall, cytoplasm and DNA, but there is no nuclear membrane, hence no distinct nucleus (Figure 2.2). Many bacteria, mainly belonging to the bacilli and spirilli, can move by whip-like movements of the flagella.

Bacterial reproduction is usually 'asexual': it requires no sexual partner occurring instead by simple cell division – the cell simply splits into two daughter cells. This is a quick and efficient method for

SPHERICAL BACTERIA (COCCI)

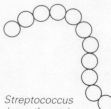

Diplococcus
(pneumonia)

Staphylococcus
(pustules, boils, etc.)

Streptococcus
(sore throats)

ROD-LIKE BACTERIA (BACILLI)

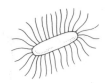

Bacillus tuberculosis
(tuberculosis)

Clostridium tetani
(tetanus)

Bacillus typhosus
(typhoid fever)

SPIRAL FORMS

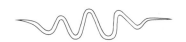

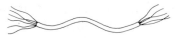

Spirillum

Treponema pallida
(syphilis)

Vibrio
(cholera)

FIGURE 2.1 *Forms of bacteria*

such organisms. From one cell, if it could divide once every 30 minutes, there would be 64 bacteria after 3 hours, over a million bacteria after 10 hours, and over one thousand million bacteria after 15 hours. They would over-run the Earth in a few days, were it not that their death rate balances this increase. However, these figures perhaps indicate how quickly a disease could establish itself from a single bacterium.

Bacteria can also reproduce sexually, leading to a sharing of the genetic characteristics of two partners and the evolution of new types.

Most bacteria can survive, reproduce and grow, at a reduced level, outside their preferred hosts or habitats – provided that they have moisture, an organic food source, some warmth (around body

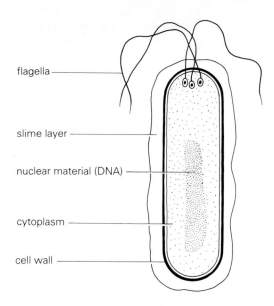

flagella

slime layer

nuclear material (DNA)

cytoplasm

cell wall

FIGURE 2.2 *A typical bacterial cell*

temperature), carbon dioxide, and a neutral pH. When their preferred host is again available they will colonise it and grow and reproduce at normal speed again.

In very unfavourable conditions, bacteria secrete a hard shell around themselves, thereby forming spores. In the spore the living material is held dormant (alive but not functioning) inside the shell, which protects it from most external conditions, such as drought, heat and cold. When the danger has passed and conditions are more favourable, the spore breaks open to release the bacterium which then proceeds to multiply and colonise again by simple cell division (Figure 2.3).

Bacterial spores are remarkably resilient. Most live bacteria are killed within minutes when the temperature rises above 60 °C, yet spores can survive boiling water (100 °C) for six hours or more. Growing bacteria are killed by normal household antiseptics and disinfectants either instantly or within 30 minutes: spores remain unaffected by these solutions after several hours, and need special compounds for their destruction.

Bacteria of one form or another are adapted to, and found in, remarkably diverse environmental conditions. They are found in the bodies of *all* living organisms, and in all parts of the Earth, including on land, in the ocean depths, in arctic ice and glaciers, in hot springs, and even in the upper atmosphere. There are more bacteria than any other type of living organism. One gram of fertile soil contains approximately 100 million mixed bacteria. Even the bowel of an adult human contains between 1300–2200 g (3–5 lb.) of micro-organisms, most of which are bacteria.

Fortunately, most bacteria are non-pathogenic (they do not cause disease) and many types are actually beneficial and necessary to life. Bacteria are responsible for the nitrogen cycle in soils, which traps nitrogen from the atmosphere and makes it available for plant growth; for the fermentation used in producing cheeses, yogurt and

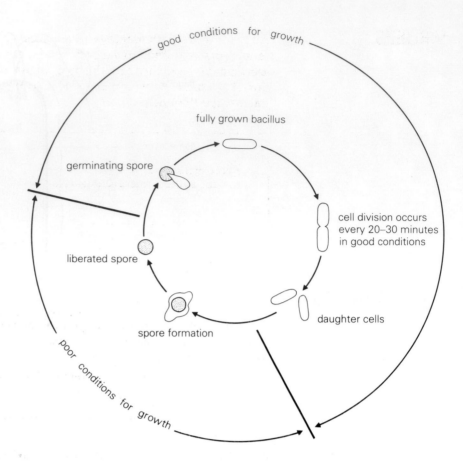

good conditions for growth

fully grown bacillus

germinating spore

cell division occurs
every 20–30 minutes
in good conditions

liberated spore

daughter cells

spore formation

poor conditions for growth

FIGURE 2.3 *The life cycle of a spore-forming bacterium*

the like; for decomposition and soil enrichment; and for the functioning of septic tanks. They form a part of many industrial processes, and they are invaluable in genetic research.

However, there are a good many varieties of bacteria which are pathogenic (disease-causing). Such bacteria are responsible for tuberculosis, whooping cough, salmonella, pneumonia, blood poisoning, diphtheria, meningitis, cholera, syphilis, typhoid fever and tetanus, to name just a few. Others cause sore throats, tonsillitis, scarlet fever, boils, abscesses, pustules and minor infections. Some bacteria attack the tissues directly, while others produce toxins (poisons) which inflict damage on the host. One kind of bacteria that every nail technician will encounter at some stage in her work is the *Pseudomonas* species (see pages 224–5).

A human body can have natural defences against bacteria, in the form of antibodies in the bloodstream, or immunity can be medically induced through vaccination. Certain diseases can be prevented or treated by injections of anti-toxins or of serum (the liquid part of blood) which already contains antibodies. Antibiotics are medicines which kill bacteria: they form the basis of modern medical treatment of bacterial infections. Bacteria can, through their capacity for genetic recombination and rapid evolution, develop resistance to antibiotics.

VIRUSES

All viruses are pathogenic – all are capable of causing disease. The term 'virus' is applied to a group of infective agents so small that they are able to pass through the tiny pores of a collodion (unglazed porcelain) filter. They can be seen only with the help of an electron microscope (Figure 2.4).

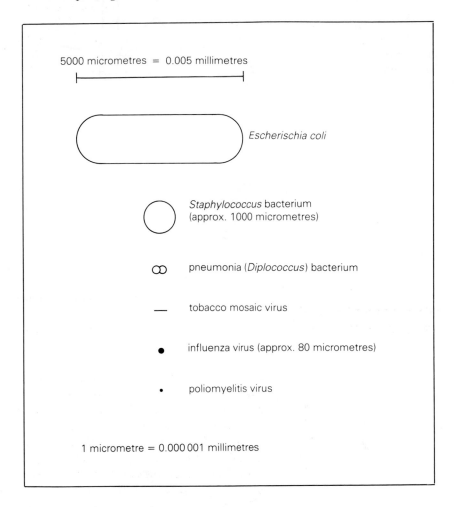

5000 micrometres = 0.005 millimetres

Escherischia coli

Staphylococcus bacterium
(approx. 1000 micrometres)

pneumonia (*Diplococcus*) bacterium

tobacco mosaic virus

influenza virus (approx. 80 micrometres)

poliomyelitis virus

1 micrometre = 0.000 001 millimetres

FIGURE 2.4 *A comparison of the sizes of bacteria and viruses*

A free virus particle is best thought of as a little packet of nucleic acid material, which can be of either DNA or RNA, inside a protein coat (Figure 2.5). It cannot be considered to be alive when it is in this free and infectious form, as it does not grow, multiply, feed or respire. Hence it cannot be 'killed' in the strict sense of the word.

The purpose of the protein coating is to protect the enclosed nucleic acid material and permit its transfer from inside one host cell into the next potential host cell. The viral nucleic acid material contains all the information necessary for the takeover of the reproductive and manufacturing functions of the new host cell. More virus particles can then be made using the host cell's chemical energy, proteins and nucleic-acid synthesising ability. After replication, the virus particles leave the cell – sometimes killing it, sometimes not, depending on the

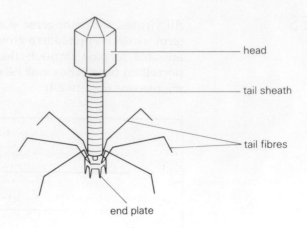

FIGURE 2.5 *A typical bacteriophage virus: the end plate attaches itself to a bacterium; then the tail sheath contracts, injecting the nucleic acid from the head into the bacterial host*

virus involved – and go on to infect other cells (Figure 2.6).

Polio, hepatitis, measles, mumps, smallpox, rabies, influenza, herpes simplex and the common cold are all examples of diseases caused by virus particles. Because of their non-living nature, viruses cannot be killed by drugs. Treatment is aimed primarily at prevention: vaccination gives protection by stimulating the production of antibodies in the body, which can then resist the virus.

Outside the body, some viruses (such as the human immunodeficiency virus, HIV) cannot live at all: transmission in such cases requires direct contact between the blood or other body fluids of the people concerned. Other viruses are far more hardy than bacteria: to destroy them you must treat them in the same way as the equally resilient bacterial spores.

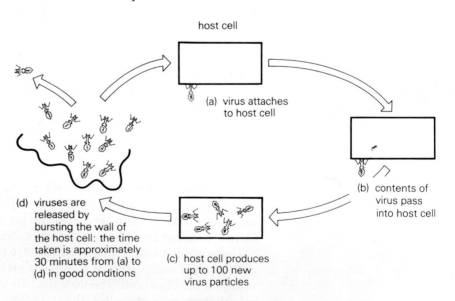

FIGURE 2.6 *The reproduction of a bacteriophage virus*

FUNGI

Fungi are related to plants but they lack chlorophyll, the green pigment that enables plants to trap the energy of sunlight and so synthesise materials such as sugars, starches and proteins. Because they lack chlorophyll fungi cannot make their own food but must live as parasites, obtaining their food from a live host, or saprophytes, obtaining their food from dead organic matter. They range in size from the microscopic, unicellular yeasts to much larger, multicellular organisms such as mushrooms and toadstools.

The fungi form a large group of organisms which contains pathogenic as well as non-pathogenic varieties. Many of the functions they perform can be both beneficial and harmful – for example, decomposition is essential for the renewal of soil but is also responsible for food spoilage. Fermentation is used in the manufacture of alcoholic drinks, vinegar, cheeses and bread dough. It also spoils food. Industrially, fungi are used in the manufacture of antibiotics, vitamins, and some chemicals, including acetone, alcohol and enzymes. The only fungi that concern the manicurist are as follows.

The yeasts of the genus *Saccharomyces* belong to the class Ascomycetes (sac fungi). These can reproduce by a form of simple cell division known as budding, in which the daughter cell forms a small bud at the side of the main cell and breaks away when it is complete (Figure 2.7). Yeasts do not form mycelia. Yeasts can also reproduce sexually. Spore formation results in short-lived spores which need to find a place favourable to growth (one offering moisture and warmth) quickly in order to survive. Yeasts are spread in the salon by direct contact or by contact with contaminated manicure equipment.

Some species of the fungus *Candida*, growing in a yeast-like form, can become parasitic, often attacking the skin in damp, warm areas of the body, such as a lifted nail plate, to cause secondary infections. *Candida* is more commonly known as the organism responsible for the infection of mucous membranes termed 'thrush'.

Athlete's foot (tinea pedis) and ringworm (tinea unguium) are skin diseases caused by fungi. (These fungi belong to the class Deuteromycetes. Deuteromycetes are known as the 'imperfect fungi' as they are the only class which have never been seen to reproduce sexually.) This class is responsible for most of the fungal diseases in plants and animals. All the varieties of tinea are caused by species from three

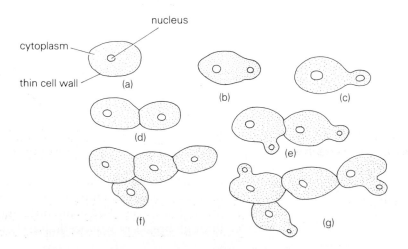

FIGURE 2.7 *The reproduction of yeast cells by budding*

genera, *Microsporum, Trichophyton* and *Epidermophyton*, all of which are mycelial in their method of growth (Figure 2.8). They reproduce by spore formation, and these spores are spread when an infected person walks barefooted on the floor. The spores will remain viable for relatively short periods if conditions allow – they need moisture and average temperatures, as found around swimming baths and on cubicle floors. They need to find a host quickly in order to survive. They are picked up by other feet simply by being stepped upon; they will then grow, making a limited mycelial growth in the epidermis of the skin of the foot. These species obtain their food by digesting and using keratin, the protein of the horny outer layers of the skin, hair and nails. They are spread in the salon by direct contact or by contact with contaminated manicure and pedicure equipment.

Fungal infections, also called mycoses (singular: mycosis), usually only infect the outer layers of the skin and the nails. They are frequently unsightly and very difficult to cure once established, but are not considered dangerous.

There are other, internal, fungal infections, some of which can be fatal (aspergillosis or farmer's lung, for example, sometimes contracted from mouldy hay, is caused by fungi of the *Aspergillus* genus), others of which are mild (thrush, for instance, is caused by the fungus *Candida albicans*). These are of no concern to the manicurist in her work as they cannot be transmitted through professional contact.

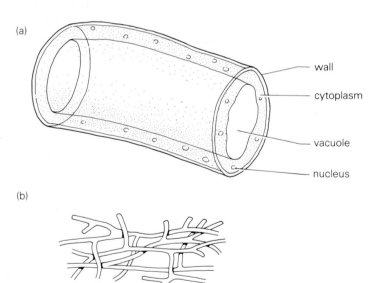

FIGURE 2.8 *Part of a fungal hypha, and several hyphae together forming a mycelium*

TRANSMISSION OF INFECTION

Diseases can be passed into the body in the following ways:

1   through the mouth, via food, water and the air that we breathe;
2   through the nose, in the air that we breathe;
3   through the eyes, if dust and dirt should enter them;
4   through breaks or wounds in the skin.

In addition,

5 viruses and bacteria can also be transmitted via body-fluid contact.

The human body has defence mechanisms to enable it to combat attacks through the first three of these areas: the antiseptic properties of the tears in the eyes, the mucous membranes and cilia in the respiratory system, and the digestive enzymes and hydrochloric acid in the digestive tract. It also has secondary defences internally, including the white blood cells and the potential to form antibodies and antitoxins.

Breaches in the body's primary defence mechanism, the skin, present a different problem. They should not happen in the course of a manicurist's work, but occasionally they do.

The manicurist needs to keep a high level of general hygiene in the salon to combat transmission of general infection. She also needs to maintain a high level of sanitation specific to her work in order to minimise transmission of infection through the skin or via body fluids. In doing so, not only is she preventing the spread of infections between her clients, she is also protecting herself from contracting infections from them.

3 SALON HYGIENE

Terms used

☐ *Sterilisation* The process of rendering harmless any equipment or articles which are liable to communicate disease through the spread of micro-organisms or their spores. To *sterilise* is to make something sterile by killing or destroying all micro-organisms and their spores. *Sterile* means free from living disease micro-organisms and their spores.

☐ *Sanitation* Cleanliness, and the following of correct procedure to prevent the spread of disease. *Sanitary* means clean, with particular regard to being free from disease-causing micro-organisms.

☐ *Hygiene* The principles of good health; the science of sanitation. *Hygienic* means clean, with particular regard to being free from disease-causing micro-organisms.

☐ *Disinfection* The process of rendering harmless any people, articles, rooms, equipment and so on which are liable to communicate disease through the spread of micro-organisms. To *disinfect* is to reduce the incidence of micro-organisms in an environment to an acceptably low level. A *disinfectant* is a toxic chemical or a procedure which will kill most micro-organisms, thus reducing their incidence in the environment to such a level. Disinfectants do not necessarily destroy spores, and they are too strong to be used on living tissue.

☐ *Antiseptic* A substance, usually a chemical, which will kill, limit or prevent the growth of micro-organisms. Antiseptics can be safely used on living tissue, including the skin.

Some disinfectants can also be used as antiseptics provided they are diluted to the right strength. Care must be taken always to follow the manufacturers' instructions regarding the dilution of disinfectants and antiseptics. If excessively diluted, they can actually *feed* the bacteria instead of killing them. Using an incorrect dilution can also stimulate the development of strains which are resistant to the disinfectant being used, thus causing problems in the future. If antiseptics are used at a strength greater than that recommended, they can cause chemical burning of the skin. The correct dilution of disinfectants and antiseptics is therefore very important.

When to sterilise, disinfect or use antiseptic

Sterilisation procedure kills *all* micro-organisms – bacterial, viral and fungal – *and* their spores. Disinfection and antiseptics kill a large percentage of bacteria, fungi and fungal spores, reducing their presence to a level acceptable to hygienic practice.

From this it follows that if the manicurist is guarding against bacteria, fungi and fungal spores, then the use of disinfection procedures and antiseptics is sufficient. If there is a possibility that viruses or bacterial spores are present and thus needing to be destroyed, then sterilisation procedures must be followed.

The only viruses which the manicurist will have to guard against in her work are those which are spread by accidental blood-to-blood contact, in particular hepatitis B (HBV) and human immunodeficiency virus (HIV). Sterilisation procedures are therefore only necessary for items which may have come into contact with blood or blood serum (the clear, liquid part of blood), such as cuticle clippers, cuticle knives, chiropody sponges and chiropody blades. It is necessary to keep two or more sets of all these items so that one set can be undergoing sterilisation whilst the other set is in use. Other items which could become contaminated through their use on damaged tissue are cuticle sticks, files, cottonwool and tissues, all of which are disposables and must be dispensed with in the correct way after use or suspected contamination (see page 38).

The incidence of bacterial spores in a correctly run salon environment is so low as to be negligible. Sterilisation of towels and other articles used on and around clients is therefore unnecessary as long as a rigorous and regular routine of disinfection is practised in the salon.

Pre-cleaning

Whether items are to be sterilised or disinfected, they should be pre-cleaned by scrubbing in hot, soapy water (itself a method of disinfection). A liquid soap should be used: hard soaps can leave deposits, which may prevent follow-up processes from working properly.

STERILISATION

The two methods of sterilisation which are most practicable for the small salon environment are:

1 the use of an autoclave;
2 the use of chemical sterilising agents.

The autoclave

Water, under normal atmospheric pressure, boils at 100 °C. If pressure is applied to the water, its boiling point rises. It can be made to rise to temperatures which will kill all micro-organisms, their spores and viruses. An autoclave (Figure 3.1) is a metal 'pan' which is specially designed to create and withstand the heat and pressures necessary for sterilisation.

The only type of autoclave which can be used with total safety in a salon environment is an electrical one which has a fully automatic cycle. A measured amount of water is placed into the autoclave, and the pre-washed tools are placed on a rack above the water so that the steam can circulate freely around them. The lid is closed and the autoclave switched on. During use the water boils, creating steam which forces the air out of the pan through a valve. When all the air has been expelled, this valve closes. The pressure builds up inside the pan, which causes the temperature to rise. When the sterilising temperature has been reached, the automatic programme maintains the temperature and pressure for the required length of time and then switches off the autoclave.

When the pressure returns to normal the lid can be removed and the sterile articles taken out.

Articles taken from an autoclave are sterile only until they come into contact with the air or some other item. If sterility has to be maintained, it is therefore necessary to transfer them to a sterilising cabinet. In the salon, however, the purpose of sterilisation is to

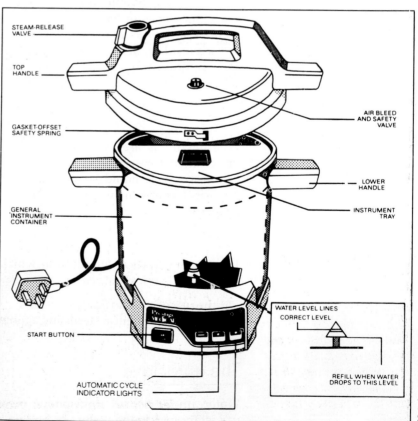

FIGURE 3.1 *An automatic electronic autoclave steriliser*

Hairdressing Beauty Equipment Centre

protect against hepatitis B virus; and to a lesser extent against the much weaker HIV, which would normally be destroyed by less severe methods anyway. As long as the tools are kept in hygienic surroundings after sterilisation, and wiped with surgical spirit before use on a client, their level of cleanliness is sufficient.

The temperatures and pressures necessary to achieve sterilisation are 15 minutes at 121 °C (this is obtained at a pressure of 15 pounds per square inch, or p.s.i.), or 3 minutes at 134 °C (obtained at a pressure of 32 p.s.i.).

It is possible to double-check that the autoclave is achieving sterilisation conditions. Special 'TST control strips' are available which can be placed in the autoclave at the start of its cycle. These strips have a yellow dot on them which turns purple when sterilisation is complete.

Chemical sterilising agents

The aldehydes

The aldehyde group is the only group of chemical sterilising agents suitable for use in the salon. Formaldehyde is used in vapour sterilisers. This type of steriliser is not ideal, as to be effective the vapour needs to touch all parts of the equipment. The fumes are also toxic to the manicurist. The use of formaldehyde is actually banned in some countries, including Germany. These sterilisers used to be a useful supplement to the general hygiene of the salon, for example as a place to keep tools after sterilisation or overnight, and to store buffers, files, cottonwool, cuticle sticks, and the like. Because of the recently recognised toxicity of formaldehyde, these functions are perhaps now best served by an ultraviolet 'sterilising' cabinet.

The glutaraldehydes have emerged as the favoured group for chemical sterilisation in the salon (Figure 3.2). However, some people

FIGURE 3.2 *Activated or balanced glutaraldehyde solutions are used in a deep container with a close-fitting lid: the container includes a perforated tray with handles which can be lowered into the solution, then lifted out and the tools rinsed with water while still in the tray, thereby avoiding any body contact with the corrosive solutions used*

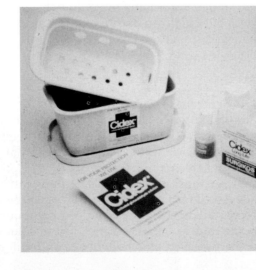

Cidex

believe that the glutaraldehydes are not so much sterilising agents as high-class disinfectants: their performance can be erratic unless the instructions for use are rigidly adhered to. However, the glutaraldehydes are invaluable in a small salon where an autoclave is not available, so the manicurist must be scrupulous in treating her solutions with care at all times so that they remain effective.

Glutaraldehydes can be obtained as a 2 per cent solution with an acid pH: in this form they are stable but inactive. The addition of a buffer compound activates the glutaraldehyde solution by making it slightly alkaline. Once activated, the effective sterilising life of the solution varies from 14 to 30 days, depending on the product. The active product will kill all micro-organisms and the HIV and HBV viruses in 10 minutes, whilst spores require a three-hour (although some people would say a ten-hour) immersion.

A strong chemical such as this requires certain precautions in its use. It must never be used on, or come into contact with, the skin – it is a strong irritant.

☐ Equipment must be thoroughly rinsed after soaking.
☐ If the solution is accidentally splashed into the eye, it must be rinsed out quickly with quantities of clear water. Medical attention should be sought immediately as it can endanger the sight of the eye.
☐ Most glutaraldehydes have extremely unpleasant fumes. New varieties are trying to avoid this problem.
☐ Glutaraldehyde solutions can strip the plating off plated tools.

Finally, it must be mentioned that the glutaraldehydes can be expensive to buy and use on a regular basis.

This form, termed activated glutaraldehydes, used to be the only way of obtaining and using glutaraldehydes. Recent developments have produced acid-balanced glutaraldehydes with added surfactants: these will undoubtedly supersede the earlier compounds. These new products are already activated and do not require the addition of a buffer. They are stable and have an indefinite shelf life. The added surfactants not only help to dissolve the outer coat of the virus but cut down on fumes and help to stop the plating from being removed from the soaking tools.

The halogens

Chlorine (used in bleach) and iodine belong to the group of chemicals known as halogens. Bleach is a good sterilising fluid, but it is slightly corrosive. Used in the salon, a dilution of 10 per cent is effective for most disinfection purposes.

Iodine too is a good sterilising fluid, but has the disadvantage that it will discolour fabrics. However, it can be used to disinfect surfaces. Recent advances have produced compounds containing complexed iodine and 2-phenoxyethanol. These solutions are equal in efficiency to the balanced glutaraldehydes and will destroy the HBV and HIV viruses in 10 minutes (spores require longer). Unlike the glutaral-dehydes, though, they are not corrosive and do not have toxic fumes.

Ultraviolet sterilising cabinets

These deserve a mention simply because they do not sterilise efficiently enough to be the sole method of sterilisation in the salon. They sterilise only those surfaces that are actually bathed in the ultraviolet (UV) light: in the case of irregularly-shaped objects such as cuticle clippers, they do not effect efficient sterilisation. They are useful for storing autoclaved sterile implements until these are needed for use on the client.

Care must be taken to replace the ultraviolet bulb regularly, following the recommended length of time of use specified by the manufacturer. This is because the ultraviolet output, and therefore the effectiveness of the lamp, decreases with usage. It is not uncommon to see these bulbs being changed only when they have failed completely, which is usually long after they have become totally ineffective.

There is a link between UV light and the formation of eye cataracts. It is important that these units remain sealed to prevent the escape of UV light.

Heat sterilising cabinets

These are small ovens which reach high temperatures. A temperature of 160 °C needs to be held for one hour, or 190 °C for 2 minutes, in order to effect sterilisation. The problem here is that the repeated use of these high temperatures affects the hardness of the metal implements, causing them to lose their sharp edges. Such cabinets are therefore not really suitable for salon use.

Glass bead sterilisers

These are small sterilising appliances normally used by electrologists. They reach high temperatures and the heat is transmitted to the immersed tools via the tiny glass beads they contain. Only the parts of the tool actually in contact with the glass beads are sterilised, however, so irregularly-shaped objects like cuticle clippers cannot be considered to have been sterilised completely. The high temperatures reached will cause the metal to lose its hardness, gradually causing blades to lose their sharp edges.

DISINFECTION

The two methods of disinfection which are most practicable for the small salon environment involve the use of heat or the use of chemicals.

Heat

Boiling water

Quite simply, this means immersing the pre-washed metal implements in a pan of rapidly boiling water for 10 minutes. (Sodium carbonate can be added to the water as a precaution against rusting.) After this time, the tools are tipped out onto a clean disposable towel where they will dry rapidly due to their heat. (The rapid drying will counteract rusting.) This is a quick and efficient method of disinfection which should be employed as part of the general salon hygiene *at least once a week*, if only to effect a thorough cleansing of the implements prior to sterilisation. This cleansing is more thorough than simply scrubbing with liquid soaps and water.

Steam

This involves suspending the pre-washed implements in circulating steam for 10 minutes. The easiest way to do this is in a special automatic steaming appliance. These appliances simply require the addition of a measured amount of water before they are switched on: they then run through their disinfecting cycle. Although a useful addition to salon hygiene, they achieve no more than the copious use of surgical spirit and occasional immersion in boiling water.

Alcohol

Alcohols are a class of chemical compounds in which carbon (C) and hydrogen (H) are attached to a hydroxyl group (OH). The variations in their proportions give rise to the many varieties of alcohols, methyl alcohol (CH_3OH), ethyl alcohol (C_2H_5OH) and isopropyl alcohol ($(CH_3)_2CHOH$) being the three most commonly used in the work of the manicurist.

Methyl alcohol (methanol)

Methyl alcohol is sometimes called wood alcohol as it can be made from the distillation of wood; it can alternatively be made from methane. In many of its properties it is similar to ethyl alcohol: both are colourless and inflammable; both will mix with water. Methyl alcohol, though, is a stronger solvent, more highly volatile and more toxic than ethyl alcohol. Methyl alcohol is metabolised in the body to form highly poisonous products, to the extent that as little as 10 ml of pure methyl alcohol, if drunk, can produce permanent blindness. 100 ml can be fatal. Methyl alcohol and methylated spirits, which contains methyl alcohol, must *never* be drunk.

Methyl alcohol is used commercially in the making of formaldehyde, and in the manufacture of spirit varnishes and polishes. Crude methyl alcohol is used, with ethyl alcohol, to make methylated spirits.

Ethyl alcohol (ethanol)

Ethyl alcohol is ordinary alcoholic spirit, produced by the action of yeast (fermentation) on sugars and starches such as cereals, potatoes, molasses and paper-mill waste. It is the substance in beer, wines and spirits that makes them intoxicating. It is a colourless, volatile, inflammable liquid which mixes easily with water. It is used as a solvent in the manufacture of perfumes and lacquers, and would be used more extensively were it not for legal restrictions on its use. (It is necessary to have a permit from the Customs and Excise before industrial methylated spirit, which is almost pure ethyl alcohol, can be bought and kept on the premises.) These restrictions on its use have led to the development and use of alternative solvents for many purposes.

Isopropyl alcohol (isopropanol)

Isopropyl alcohol is an alcohol made out of by-products of the petroleum industry. Like the other alcohols, it is a colourless, volatile, inflammable liquid which mixes with water. It is one of the cheapest alcohols and is poisonous if swallowed. For many uses it has replaced ethyl alcohol because of its similar solvent properties as well as its cheapness.

Acetone is produced from isopropyl alcohol.

Methylated spirit (70 per cent alcohol)

Methylated spirit is ethyl alcohol combined with other substances. There are different grades of methylated spirits available, the grade depending on the use to which the spirits are to be put. The common purple one which the manicurist will use in her work is called mineralised methylated spirit: it consists of 90 volumes of ethyl alcohol (95 per cent), 9.5 volumes of methyl alcohol, and 0.5 volumes of crude pyridine (a solvent extracted from coal tar which has an extremely unpleasant taste and smell which discourage people from drinking the methylated spirit). In addition, a tiny quantity of petroleum oil and a small amount of methyl violet colouring agent are added to indicate that the liquid is dangerous and unfit to drink.

Methylated spirit is used industrially as a solvent, a cleaning fluid and a fuel. It is a good disinfectant which, because of its hygroscopic (water-attracting) properties, will rapidly dehydrate bacteria. It will also dissolve fats and oils, hence its use in degreasing the surface of the natural nail plate before the application of artificial nails. It makes a good cleaning and disinfecting agent for glass and tiled surfaces in the salon, and for wiping over the work area.

Methylated spirit is not a good antiseptic as its frequent use will harden the skin.

Surgical spirit

Surgical spirit is methylated spirit without the methyl violet colouring and with the addition of small amounts of castor oil and oil of wintergreen. The last two are both soluble in alcohol and are lubricants, so surgical spirit has all the disinfectant and solvent properties of methylated spirit but can also be used as a good antiseptic: it will not harden the skin. The oils leave a slight film of moisturising lubrication on the surface of the skin and nails, which means that surgical spirit cannot be used to wipe over the surface of the natural nail plate before the application of nail varnish or artificial nails – the oil film left behind would prevent the efficient adhesion of the varnish or glue to the nail plate.

Surgical spirit is used in the health service to cleanse and decontaminate the skin before surgery, injections and so on. Because it can safely be used on the skin, it is classed as an antiseptic as well as a disinfectant. In manicuring it is invaluable for wiping tools between clients if disinfection only, and not sterilisation, is required. It is advisable to keep in the manicure tray a small glass jar containing surgical spirit, cushioned at the base with cottonwool so that tools are

TABLE 3.1 *Sterilisers, disinfectants and antiseptics*

Sterilisers	Disinfectants	Antiseptics
1st choice Autoclave: 15 minutes at 121 °C *or* 3 minutes at 134 °C	70 per cent alcohol (methylated spirit)	Surgical spirits
	Surgical spirits	Isopropyl alcohol with or without Hibitane (chlorhexidine)
2nd choice Chemical agents (e.g. activated or balanced glutaraldehydes)	Isopropyl alcohol with or without Hibitane (chlorhexidine)	Brand-name antiseptic soaps, creams and liquids
3rd choice Hot oven cabinet: 160 °C for 1 hour	Quaternary ammonium compounds	Soap and water
	Brand-name disinfectants	
	Bleach (10 per cent dilution)	
Not as good as prime sterilisers glass bead sterilisers; ultraviolet cabinets; chemical cabinets	Soap and water (min. 60 °C)	
	Boiling water (10 minutes)	
	Steam suspension (10 minutes)	
	Iodine	

Note If using chemical sterilisers or disinfectants on metal tools, ensure that they contain a rust-inhibiting formulation (e.g. sodium nitrite). This is not necessary for the alcohols.

not damaged; the clippers and knife can be placed in this when not in use. There should be enough surgical spirit in the container to cover the ends of the tools. The cottonwool and surgical spirit must be discarded and replaced for each new client, or at least at regular intervals, such as at lunchtime and at the end of the day.

Because of its oil content, surgical spirit is not as good as methylated spirits for wiping over surfaces.

ANTISEPSIS

All suitable antiseptics are chemicals. They include surgical spirit; isopropyl alcohol, with or without added chlorhexidine gluconate (Hibitane); and a large number of brand-name antiseptic liquids, soaps and creams containing a wide variety of antiseptic formulations such as chlorhexidine, Hexachlorophane, Triclosan, and Cetrimide.

Antiseptic procedures

☐ The manicurist should wash her hands with an antiseptic soap, preferably a liquid soap from a pump dispenser, before and after each client. She should dry her hands with disposable paper towels or with a hot-air dryer. For added protection, an antiseptic cream containing for example chlorhexidine can be applied to the hands after drying.

☐ The client also should be encouraged to wash her hands with an antiseptic soap, preferably from a pump dispenser, before the treatment is commenced. She should dry her hands on disposable paper towels or with a hot-air dryer. It is advantageous if the salon has a small basin in the main working area for this purpose.

☐ If there is no basin available to the client, her hands should be wiped over with a soapy antiseptic solution prior to the start of the treatment.

☐ When carrying out a pedicure, an antiseptic solution should be added to the soak water and the feet allowed to soak for a few minutes before the start of the treatment.

☐ If the client is cut during a treatment, then an antiseptic should be applied immediately in the form of solution on clean cottonwool or a disposable surgical wipe from a sealed package. A pad of dry cottonwool should always be placed between the wipe and the manicurist's hands to protect the manicurist from possible blood contact. All these items should be disposed of correctly and carefully (page 38).

GENERAL SALON HYGIENE

The salon

The salon should be kept clean and dry, as it is bacteria which are the main source of infection within the salon and most of these will dehydrate (dry up) and die in a clean dry atmosphere. As far as possible, the salon should be light and airy, as sunshine inhibits the growth of micro-organisms, and the circulation of air will prevent the development of the warm, moist conditions which encourage bacterial growth.

Floors and chairs

Floors should be kept clean, and vacuumed or mopped regularly. Chairs should be washed down regularly with household detergent and hot water. Hot soapy water is in itself a good disinfectant and antiseptic and should be used liberally.

Surfaces

All surfaces in the salon should be washed down regularly with household detergent and hot water. Cream cleansers can be used, but abrasive cleansers should be avoided as these leave scour marks which can harbour bacteria. Surfaces being used for manicure should be wiped down and disinfected between clients, using 70 per cent alcohol, isopropyl alcohol plus chlorhexidine, or any other purpose-made formulation. Glass surfaces are the easiest to clean.

Equipment

Overalls

The manicurist's overall must be clean and pressed every day. It should be washed in soapy water in a minimum 60 °C wash as most bacteria are killed at a 60 °C temperature.

Towels

Each client should have a clean towel and the towels should be laundered in hot (60 °C) soapy water to kill bacteria. However, there are special cool-wash powders now available which will disinfect and clean at only 30 °C, thus saving a little wear on the salon equipment.

Plastic manicure bowls

These should be washed between clients, using hot (minimum 60 °C) soapy water or a cream cleanser. The use of abrasive cleaners should be avoided as the scratches caused provide an excellent breeding ground for bacteria.

Emery boards and cuticle sticks

These need to be disposed of after use if the client has any damage to, or infection of, her skin or nail. However, cost dictates their use on three or four clients before disposal provided that the clients do not exhibit any problems.

Chamois leather buffers

The chamois leather should be removed from the buffer, washed in warm (60 °C) soapy water, rinsed and dried. It can then be replaced on the buffer, which has itself been disinfected by the use of surgical spirit or by boiling, depending on its composition. The buffer should be kept in a dry steriliser until its next use.

The difficulty in cleaning this type of buffer adequately has led to it being largely superseded by disposable buffers made of fine-grade emery papers or fabrics mounted onto sponge pads.

Implements

These must never be used on a subsequent client without first disinfecting or sterilising them. It is reasonable to use disinfection alone where there has been no contact with cuts or abrasions. This can be achieved by wiping the tools with surgical spirit, or placing them in a small jar of surgical spirit on the manicure or pedicure desk. (Isopropyl alcohol, with or without chlorhexidine or any other brand-name antiseptic solution containing a rust inhibitor such as sodium nitrite, could be used instead of surgical spirit.)

Where there has been contact with infection or an abrasion, however, sterilisation is needed and must be carried out, preferably using an autoclave or, if this is not available, by means of a suitable sterilising chemical such as activated or acid-balanced glutaraldehyde. Contaminated items must not be placed directly onto work surfaces but must be wrapped in a tissue until they can be sterilised. If tools are dropped onto the floor, they must not be used until they have been wiped over and cleansed with surgical spirit or a similar antiseptic. It is advisable to scrub the tools in hot soapy water and then boil them in water for 10 minutes, at least once every week, as a thorough cleansing and disinfection procedure. Sodium carbonate can be added to the water to prevent rusting.

Small tools must also be scrubbed clean with liquid detergents and water and then dried prior to their immersion in sterilising solutions. (Grime deposits can prevent the penetration of chemicals or steam.) Liquid detergents should be used for this purpose as soaps can form insoluble deposits with hard water, which would hinder the sterilisation procedure.

TABLE 3.2 *Hygiene in the salon*

Sterilise	Disinfect	Dispose	Use antiseptic	Use hygienic procedure
Cuticle knives	Surfaces	Chiropody blades	Client's hands	Dish dispenser: nail varnish remover; antiseptic solution; surgical spirit; methylated spirit
Cuticle clippers	Floors	Emery boards	Manicurist's hands	
Chiropody sponges	Chairs	Cuticle sticks	Client's feet (soak)	
Chiropody knives	Walls	Cottonwool		
Scissors	Overalls	Tissues		Pump dispenser: hand cream; massage oil or cream; liquid soap; antiseptic creams; foot cream
	Towels	Paper towels		
	Manicure bowls			
	Pedicure bowls			
	Toe separators			Tube dispenser: cuticle cream; nail buffing cream; antiseptic cream
	Tools at the manicure station			
	Any equipment and implements (e.g. bottles, trays dispensers, jars)			Care must be taken with all other cosmetics to avoid cross-contamination (e.g. varnishes, cuticle remover)
	Chamois leather buffer			

Because of the sterilisation procedures needed for these items, each manicurist must have at least two sets of tools so that one set can be in use whilst the other is undergoing sterilisation. When tools have been sterilised or disinfected, they should be kept in a dry 'sterilising' cabinet until needed for use.

Disposal of items

Used disposable sharp blades must be placed in a suitable screw-topped container which can be disposed of when full using the facilities available in each area. To find out about disposal of these containers, contact the environmental health officer at the local town hall.

All other disposable items should be placed in a lidded waste bin containing a bin liner. When full, the liner should be sealed and disposed of using available facilities.

Disinfectants, antiseptics and alcohols should be flushed down the sink with large quantities of running water.

Cosmetic materials

Cosmetic materials, such as hand and cuticle creams, obviously cannot be sterilised or disinfected in any of the previous ways.

When cosmetics are made, great care is taken to maintain hygienic surroundings and hence an infection-free product. Preservatives are also included in most products to prevent the growth of bacteria and fungi once the products are open to the air. In the salon, the most that can be done is to follow routines which maintain the cleanliness and hence the sanitation of the products being used.

☐ Wherever possible, pump dispensers (Figure 3.3) or dish dispensers (Figure 3.4) should be used to dispense measured amounts of cosmetic without the main body of the cosmetic being touched. This is possible with hand cream, massage oil, liquid soap and antiseptic creams.

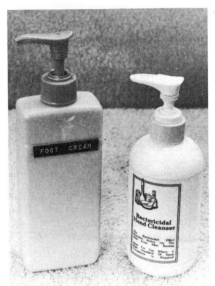
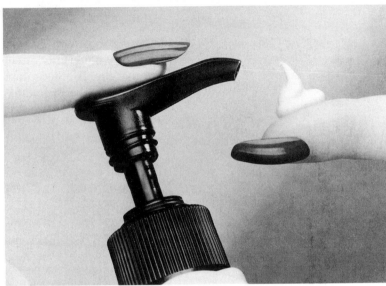

FIGURE 3.3 *Pump dispensers*

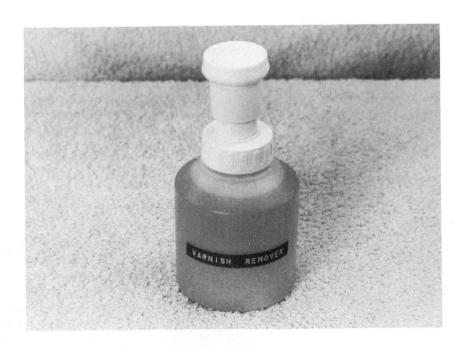

FIGURE 3.4 *A dish dispenser*

☐ Tube dispensers should be used where the cosmetic is too thick to be dispensed through a pump, as with cuticle creams.

☐ Where pump or tube dispensers are unavailable and the cosmetic is kept in a jar, a clean spatula or cuticle stick should be used to take sufficient product out of the jar for a single application on a client. The spatula should not be re-dipped into the jar to obtain more product. If only clean spatulas are used to remove product, and if the jar is kept tightly covered between uses, then the hygiene of the product is maintained.

☐ For cuticle remover solutions and nail varnishes, if these solutions are used on obviously infected clients, then the whole bottle, brush and solution must be discarded after use. Provided the clients are not visibly infected, then the use of these items on consecutive clients is acceptable. Each bottle should be used until empty, and then discarded: to maintain cleanliness, bottles should not be topped up from fresh, bulk supplies.

General hygiene: a checklist

1   Set up a sensible and hygienic cleaning routine for the salon. Make regular checks to be sure that it is being followed.
2   Keep the salon light and airy, clean and dry.
3   Pay special attention to personal hygiene, especially washing hands before and after each client.
4   Always disinfect or sterilise implements as necessary before their use on the next client.
5   Always follow carefully the instructions for the use of disinfectants and sterilising solutions. Never top up a solution or exceed the recommended dilution or soaking time. Always rinse and dry chemically sterilised implements before handling.
6   Wherever possible, use disposable items, for example client's and manicurist's hand towels and hand- and armrest covers.
7   Remember that all procedures are vital for the protection of the manicurist as well as for the protection of the clients.

AIDS AND HEPATITIS B

AIDS (acquired immune deficiency syndrome) is the most serious result of infection by a virus now known as the human immunodeficiency virus (HIV). People with this virus in their bloodstream are said to be HIV-positive. Not all HIV-positive people develop AIDS: some stay well, with no indication that they are carrying HIV; some become slightly ill, and others will go on to die from AIDS. However, *all* HIV-positive people are carriers of the virus.

HIV can disrupt the body's normal defences against disease. This causes the body to become open to infections which would not otherwise have occurred, including particular forms of cancer or serious infections, for example types of pneumonia. When these occur as a result of the disruption of the immune system caused by infection with HIV, then the person is said to have AIDS. She or he will eventually die from these illnesses.

The AIDS virus (HIV) is in fact easily destroyed outside the human body. Once any blood has dried, which can take a matter of seconds, the virus particles cannot survive. That is why HIV is spread exclusively by contact involving the direct transfer of blood or serum from an infected person to another person as can occur in sexual intercourse, the shared use of needles for injection, and so on. No one is known to have caught HIV from having a manicure or a pedicure treatment and no one ever should if simple sanitary procedures such as the ones outlined in this book are always followed.

Hepatitis B virus (HBV) is a virus which causes inflammation of the liver with resultant severe illness and jaundice. The disease can sometimes be fatal. Like HIV, HBV is transmitted by the transfer of blood or serum between an infected and an uninfected person. When a person recovers from hepatitis B, the virus remains in the bloodstream for many years, making her or him a carrier of the disease. HBV is far more common and is a much more resistant virus than HIV. There are an estimated 175 million carriers worldwide, which means that possibly one or two carriers a week are numbered amongst the clients in a busy salon. If adequate precautions are taken to prevent the possible transmission of the hepatitis B virus in the salon, then client and manicurist can both rest assured that neither HIV or any other viral or bacterial infection can be transmitted during the course of the treatment. The manicurist can be vaccinated against HBV.

It is because HIV and HBV particles are carried in blood that it is important that any equipment which has been contaminated with blood or serum is disposed of or sterilised before it is used again on another client.

Preventing transmission of HIV and hepatitis B

1 The manicurist must cover any exposed cuts, grazes or abrasions which she may have with waterproof dressings or rubber finger covers whilst she is working. If she has areas of skin breakage, such as a dermatitis or allergy rash, then she must wear disposable rubber (surgical) gloves for her work in order to protect herself. If the AIDS epidemic continues to spread with increasing speed, it will only be a matter of time before all manicurists are required to wear these surgical gloves for their own protection all the time they are at work.
2 The manicurist must wash her hands in hot soapy water, or an antiseptic cleaner and hot water, before and after each client.

3   If cutting blades are being used on a client during a pedicure, a fresh disposable blade must be used for each client and soiled blades must be stored carefully – in a suitable screw-topped bottle, for instance – ready for later disposal. The local environmental health officer should be contacted for information as to local facilities for disposing of the full container of sharp blades.

4   If styptic is in use in the salon, styptic pencil should not be applied directly to the client. It should be applied onto a piece of damp cottonwool and then the cottonwool applied to the cut. Alternatively, powder or aerosol forms of styptic are available: these are preferable for salon use.

5   If the client is accidentally cut during the course of a manicure or pedicure, a pad of dry cottonwool should be applied to the top of the cut before applying pressure to stop any bleeding.

6   If soothing antiseptic creams are to be applied to an area with a cut, the cream should first be put onto a square of clean gauze or cottonwool before being applied. Never apply creams to wounds directly with the fingers. Creams for use in this way should also be bought and used from tubes, not jars, again to prevent any risk of cross-contamination.

7   Do not use sharp or pointed instruments on or near areas of the client's skin that are obviously inflamed or infected.

8   If the manicurist cuts herself, she must wash the area and encourage bleeding under the flow of a cold water tap. After this, she must apply a waterproof plaster or dressing before returning to work.

9   If the manicurist has direct contact with another person's blood or body fluids, she must wash the area with soap and hot water as soon as possible.

10 In the event of an accident, such as a client falling and cutting herself badly, if there is a spillage of blood or other body fluids the manicurist will need to clean these up. She must wear disposable gloves and an apron, and use paper towels to mop up the spillage. The area must be disinfected with one part bleach to ten parts water. (Bleach destroys the AIDS virus, but care must be taken as bleach is corrosive and can damage the skin.) The gloves, apron and soiled towels should be placed in a plastic bag and later burnt. The manicurist's clothes can then be washed in the normal way in a washer on a hot cycle.

PART III Basic cosmetic science

4 COSMETICS

(See the section on skin disorders, page 306.)

TERMS USED

Allergy

An abnormal sensitivity (hypersensitivity) to a substance or food which would not provoke a reaction in, or prove completely harmless to, most people. (See the section on skin disorders, page 306.)

The substance causing the allergic reaction is known as an allergen or sensitiser. The most common sensitisers in the cosmetic industry are perfumes and colourants, although the widening range of chemical compounds used in making various products can cause skin irritations which affect only certain individuals. Even hypoallergenic (supposedly non-allergy causing) products will cause a reaction in some people.

The European Community (EC) is constantly reviewing the ingredients used by the cosmetic, medical and food trades in order to eliminate potential sensitisers and harmful ingredients. Proven harmful ingredients are then banned from use throughout the EC. One example of this was the ban placed on certain nail varnish colourants proved to be potent sensitisers. Manufacturers were forced to find alternatives and for quite a while popular colours were changing subtly with every batch of product made! Because of this care being taken, our cosmetics are becoming safer and less allergenic as time goes on.

Detergent

A substance which is able to mix with both oil and and water. Because of this ability, some detergents can act as emulsifiers or emulsifying agents. For example, in their usual states, oil and water will not mix but will form two separate layers in a container, one floating above the other. By bridging the oil and water states, the detergent breaks the oil into tiny droplets. These become suspended evenly in the water, forming an emulsion. Because they emulsify the oily films which trap dirt in the fibres of a fabric, allowing the dirt to become wet and float away, detergents are used as cleaning agents.

Emollient

An emollient is a substance which softens living tissue. Examples are spermaceti substitute, beeswax, petroleum jelly, lanolin, mineral oil, almond oil, castor oil and most vegetable oils. Hand creams usually contain emollients. When oil is used, a film of oil is left behind on the skin surface to replace that taken away by household detergents and the like: this leaves the hands feeling soft but not greasy.

Emulsion

An emulsion is a mixture of two liquids in which one liquid, such as an oil, is divided into minute particles and mixed evenly throughout a second liquid, such as water. Cosmetic emulsions are usually oil-in-water mixtures with a cream consistency.

An *emulsifying agent* is a substance which will cause two liquids which would not normally mix together, such as oil and water, to mix together evenly to form an emulsion. Examples of emulsifying agents are some detergents, soap, and beeswax.

To *emulsify* is to divide one liquid (such as oil) into small particles in

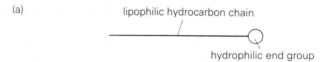

(a)

lipophilic hydrocarbon chain

hydrophilic end group

(lipophilic = oil-loving; hydrophilic = water-loving)

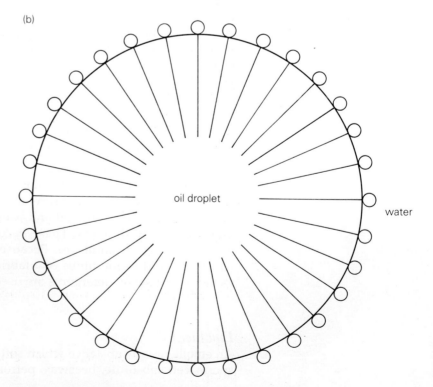

(b)

oil droplet

water

FIGURE 4.1 *(a) A molecule of an emulsifying agent. (b) An oil droplet in an oil-in-water emulsion: the molecules of the emulsifying agent form a film around the oil droplet, isolating it from other oil droplets and suspending it in the water*

suspension in another liquid (such as water) with which the first liquid would not normally mix.

An *oil-in-water emulsion* is one in which the oil phase is dispersed (mixed) in the water phase (Figure 4.1). This type of emulsion is less greasy than a water-in-oil emulsion because water is on the outside of the tiny, suspended oil droplets. Because of this, the oil-in-water emulsion will easily mix with water. The proportion of water in a stable oil-in-water emulsion should not fall below 50 per cent. Most cosmetic creams are oil-in-water emulsions.

A *water-in-oil emulsion* is one in which the water is dispersed in the oil. This type of emulsion is greasy, because oil is on the outside of the tiny suspended water droplets. Water-in-oil emulsions will not mix with water.

Homogeneous

(Of a mixture) Having uniform composition throughout. Emulsions are homogeneous.

Humectant

A substance which can absorb water from the atmosphere (that is, one which is hygroscopic). Glycerine is a humectant and is often used in hand cream formulations for its property of attracting water from the atmosphere and holding it next to, and thus moisturising, the skin.

Hydrophilic

'Hydrophilia' is love of water. Hydrophilic substances mix readily with water.

Hydrophobic

'Hydrophobia' is a fear of water. Hydrophobic substances are insoluble in (do not mix with), and actively repel, water. Oils and lanolin are examples. Protective, waterproof barrier creams for use on the hands are hydrophobic.

Hygroscopic

(Of a substance) Able to absorb water from the atmosphere. A substance that can do this is known as a humectant.

Lipophilic

(Of a substance) Soluble in oil. Lipophilic substances are 'oil-loving'.

Lipophobic

(Of a substance) Insoluble in oil. Lipophobic substances are 'oil-hating'.

pH
A measure of hydrogen ion concentration (acidity or alkalinity) in a solution (Figure 4.2). The scale of measurement runs from 1 to 14, with 1–6.9 being acid, 7 being neutral, and 7.1–14 being alkaline. 1 signifies the strongest acid, 14 the strongest alkali.

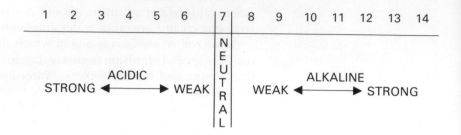

FIGURE 4.2 *The pH scale*

Palliative
A substance which will temporarily relieve symptoms without effecting a cure. For example, a foot cream or spray could temporarily relieve burning sensations in the feet without affecting the cause, which might for instance be ill-fitting shoes or overweight.

Sensitiser or sensitising agent
A substance which causes an allergic reaction.

Solution
A homogeneous mixture of two or more substances: the molecules of each substance are completely dispersed. The substance dissolved is the *solute*; the substance in which it is dissolved is the *solvent*. In an *aqueous solution* the solvent is water. ('Aqueous' means 'watery'.) In an *alcohol-based solution* the solvent is alcohol.

Toxic
Poisonous: able to kill or injure when introduced into a living organism.

Viscosity
The resistance of a fluid to flow. A thick fluid, such as set honey, does not flow easily and is said to be viscous. The thicker the fluid, the greater its viscosity. A hand cream is more viscous than a hand lotion.

Volatile
Able to evaporate very quickly.

Waxes, fats and oils

Waxes, fats and oils are all less dense than water and so will float on the surface of water. They are soluble in both alcohol and ether but not in water.

Waxes are lustrous and can be solid or viscous. They tend to be less greasy than fats and oils. They can be obtained from the surfaces of plants, such as carnauba wax from the palm tree; from animals, such as lanolin (woolwax) from the wool of sheep and spermaceti from the sperm whale; and from mineral sources, such as paraffin wax from petroleum.

Fats are usually soft, greasy solids. They are obtained from animal sources such as lard and suet from beef cattle.

Oils are often referred to as fats which are liquid at room temperature. They are obtained from animal sources, such as cod liver oil from fish; from plant sources, such as almond oil from almond nuts and olive oil from olives; and from mineral sources such as petroleum jelly and mineral oil, both extracts of petroleum.

The oils and fats which have been extracted from animal and plant sources are described as organic. Like other things that were once alive, they will decompose and become foul-smelling as time passes. Preservatives can be added to delay this decomposition, but in order to avoid this problem as far as possible, the majority of cosmetic products are based on mineral oils in preference to plant oils.

RAW MATERIALS

Each of the ingredients listed below, except the essential oils and colourants, can be obtained from any good dispensing chemist. The essential oils can be obtained from health food shops and the colourants are food colourants obtainable from grocery shops.

Acetone (dimethyl ketone, CH_3COCH_3)

A colourless, clear, volatile, highly inflammable liquid, which has the characteristic sweet odour of pear drops. It mixes with both water and fats. It is widely used in industry as a solvent for numerous organic substances and is a component of most paint, varnish and lacquer removers. It is often used as the base for nail varnish remover and as the solvent in some of the cheaper nail varnishes. Used in isolation, it has a very drying action on the skin and nails. For this reason, its use in nail products is gradually being superseded by other, more gentle solvents such as methyl ethyl ketone or dimethyl ketone. Acetone is prepared from isopropyl alcohol. It is found naturally in blood and urine as it is a waste product of some chemical reactions in the body.

Almond oil and other plant oils

These oils help to nourish and protect the skin, and to retain its suppleness. They are emollient and form the basic constituent for oily preparations and anti-wrinkle creams. Almond oil is a light-textured, pale-yellow oil extracted from almond kernels.

Beeswax

A wax which is secreted by the abdominal glands of bees to make waterproof and secure chambers in their hives. They use these chambers to store their honey (honey comb) and rear their young. Beeswax is naturally pale yellow unless bleached. It is an emulsifying agent, used as an ingredient in many cleansing and moisturising creams. It can be bought as granules or, more commonly, as a disc-shaped block, each block weighing approximately 25 g (1 oz.).

Citric acid

This is found naturally in citrus fruits such as lemons and limes. It can be bought as colourless, translucent crystals or as a white powder. It has a bleaching action and astringent properties. It is used in bath salts, nail bleaches, astringent lotions and creams.

Coconut oil

A white, solid, greasy substance which is squeezed from the white flesh of the coconut (copra). Coconut oil is liquid in the tropics, its place of origin. It solidifies in our more temperate climate. It is a nourishing conditioning oil, used in sun-tanning lotions, lip salves, soaps and moisturising creams.

Colourants

Of natural or artificial origin, colourants are used to make a product more appealing to the consumer. For amateur use, simple, natural food colourings available from grocery shops are harmless and suffice. In the past, some artificial colourings have proved to be potent sensitising agents: advances in cosmetic science have produced safer colouring agents.

Distilled water

This is extremely pure water (H_2O), which has been purified by distillation.

Essential oils

Oils extracted from plants. They differ from the fixed or fatty oils, such as coconut oil, in that they are volatile – they evaporate very quickly. In general, each gives the plant in which it is found its characteristic odour or flavour, or other properties peculiar to it. Many essential oils are reputed to have therapeutic properties when used externally during massage techniques or when taken as medicines.

Formaldehyde (methanal, HCHO)

Formaldehyde is highly volatile (it boils at −21 °C) and is soluble in water, alcohol and ether. It is an inflammable, poisonous and colourless gas with a suffocating odour, often used to fumigate rooms. Formaldehyde is used in the production of Bakelite and other plastics and synthetic resins. It is also used in many beauty and other products as an antiseptic, disinfectant and preservative.

Why is such a poisonous chemical used in cosmetics and other products? Current testing has shown that at concentrations of less than 3.6 per cent it is safe to the human body; in fact, it is found in very low levels *in* the body, where it is needed as a constituent of some of the chemical processes in the body that support life. Most cosmetic products use a concentration of less than 1 per cent. It is so effective as a fungicide, bactericide and preservative, and at such low concentrations, that it is the preferred preservative in most mascara formulations.

As long as the dangers of a chemical like this are known, toxicity can be avoided. Fortunately, the pungent odour of formaldehyde serves as a warning if too much is present in items. A susceptible individual will suffer symptoms such as headaches, watering eyes, dizziness, or nose and throat irritations, warning her that the product in use is not suitable or safe.

In nail varnish, it is used in three ways: as a preservative, bactericide and fungicide, thus prolonging the shelf life of the product; as a nail hardener (although in some nails it causes brittleness and flaking); when condensed with aryl sulfonamide to form formaldehyde resin, to give a higher gloss and more adhesive power.

Recent publicity about formaldehyde has led to its discontinuance in many products, simply to allay the fears of the public. In formaldehyde-free products, synthetic resins called alkyds may be substituted, but these do not work as preservatives.

Commercially, formaldehyde is made by the oxidation of methanol.

Glycerine (glycerol, C$_3$H$_8$O$_3$)

Glycerine is a by-product of soap manufacture, the petroleum industry, and the fermentation of sugars. It is found naturally as a constituent of all animal and vegetable fats and oils. It will mix with both water and ethanol, but not with oil. It is an odourless, colourless, sweet-tasting, syrupy, hygroscopic liquid.

Being hygroscopic, glycerine attracts and holds moisture from the air, making it valuable as a moisturiser in cosmetics. Other qualities which make it invaluable for cosmetic use are its properties as a bactericide, solvent, softener and lubricant. It also improves the spreading properties of creams and thus is used in most commercial cream preparations, including aftershave creams, cleansing creams, vanishing creams, hair creams, and hand and body creams and lotions.

Glycerine is also used as a sweetener and in the manufacture of dynamite, liquid soaps, liqueurs, candies, inks, lubricants, antifreeze mixtures, medicines, as a source of nutrients for fermentation procedures, and to keep fabrics pliable. All in all, a very versatile chemical!

Gum tragacanth

This is a gum-like resin collected from the thorny bush shrub, *Astragalus gummifer*, which grows mainly in Iran, Turkey, Greece and southern and eastern parts of Europe. Stored dry, it is yellowish, brittle and usually powdered. Tasteless and odourless, it will only dissolve partially in water and needs an alkaline solution to dissolve fully. It is used as a thickening agent and as an oil-in-water emulsifier in toothpastes, hand gels and creams. It is also a stabilising agent.

Hydrogen peroxide (H_2O_2)

This is prepared by the action of a dilute acid upon a metallic peroxide. It is a colourless liquid which acts as a bleaching agent. Once mixed to a cream, it needs a stabiliser or preservative to maintain its bleaching properties.

Lanolin (wool wax)

A purified fat-like substance obtained from the wool of sheep. It is pale yellow, very greasy, and thick. It is used as an emollient and moisturiser in skin foods, hand and baby creams, and lipsticks. It will stabilise a water-in-oil emulsion. It is used in creams for dermatitis.

Mineral oil (liquid paraffin)

Belonging to the same hydrocarbon group as kerosene and medicinal paraffins, mineral or white oil is specially refined for cosmetic purposes. It is a nearly colourless, highly refined distillate of petroleum. It is used as a lubricant and as a base oil for cosmetics. Because it is a mineral derivative, it is slow to go rancid: it is often used in preference to the plant oils as the chosen emollient and skin lubricant.

Perfumes

Lemon oil is a volatile oil obtained from the peel of fresh lemons. It is used to give a lemon odour to creams. Other perfumes – synthetic and natural, oil- and water-soluble – are used simply to make the cosmetic smell appealing. Care must be taken that the perfumes used are not sensitising agents.

Petroleum jelly

A mixture of semi-solid hydrocarbons, petroleum jelly is a colourless to yellow-white, jelly-like semi-solid, obtained from the fractional distillation of petroleum, the process whereby the various substances that together constitute petroleum are separated from each other. Petroleum jelly is obtained earlier in the process than mineral oil. The more refined, white varieties are used in cosmetics as a lubricant and as a healing base in cold creams, lip salves and sticks, hand jellies, creams and cuticle creams.

Potassium hydroxide (KOH)

An alkali, used in a weak form (2–5 per cent) to manufacture cuticle remover. It is also often used as the alkali for soap making. It can be used as an emulsifying agent in vanishing creams.

Preservatives

These are essential to prevent the growth of bacteria and fungi in cosmetic preparations. A common one for amateur use is Nipagin M (methyl-*p*-hydroxybenzoate): a microspatula measure added to any of the home recipes given in the next chapter would extend their shelf life by a few weeks.

Rose-water

A distillation of rose petals and alcohol. It is slightly perfumed, clear and colourless. Its mild tonic action makes it suitable for all skin types and it is the main ingredient of skin-softening cream, astringents, lotions and many other cosmetics.

Spermaceti substitute

This is used in creams to improve gloss; it is also a stabiliser for oil-in-water emulsions. It is a wax and is a synthetic substitute for real spermaceti, which used to be obtained from the sperm whale.

5 RECIPES for HOME USE

SAFETY PRECAUTIONS

Before making any of the following recipes, please read and follow the safety guidelines given below.

Safety precautions: a checklist

1 *Overalls* An overall must be worn to protect the skin and clothes from the spillage of potentially harmful or hot substances. (An old shirt would suffice.)

2 *Hygiene* All equipment should be scrupulously clean, to avoid contamination of the finished products.

3 *Gloves* Rubber gloves should be worn if the substances being handled are potentially harmful, as for example is potassium hydroxide.

4 *Fire hazards* Inflammable substances such as acetone should be kept well away from naked flames.

5 *Spillages* If anything is spilled, either on the skin or on the table or floor, it must be immediately washed clean and the area dried.

6 *Eye care* If anything splashes into the eyes, it must be rinsed out immediately with a wash bottle of distilled water and the accident reported to the person in charge.

Warning

Home-made products, such as the ones included in this book, must *never* be used on or sold to clients. This is because they are not insured. If such a product were used on a client and resulted in an adverse reaction, she might make a legal claim against the salon. Product liability law automatically assumes that the product used is at fault: the practitioner then has the task of proving that it was not.

Products bought from manufacturers are normally protected by the manufacturer's product liability cover. Simply re-bottling the product, or even re-labelling an existing bottle and selling or giving that product to a client, immediately invalidates the manufacturer's insurance. The practitioner will be liable in the event of any claim.

Home-made products are uninsured, and are therefore usable only at the practitioner's own risk.

RECIPES

In AD 200, the Greek physician Galen mixed water, beeswax and olive oil into a cream. When rubbed onto the face, the water evaporated, cooling the skin – hence the name 'cold cream'. An emollient, oily layer was left behind on the surface of the skin, sealing in the body moisture. This fine oily layer replaced the oils lost through washing and so helped to retain the suppleness of the skin. It also provided a protective layer against the elements. Modern cold cream consists of virtually the same mixture of ingredients.

Vanishing creams are an elaboration on the basic cold cream formula. They seem to 'disappear' when rubbed into the skin, yet give the same beneficial effects. Most hand creams and modern moisturisers fall into this category.

None of the recipes given below contain any preservatives: they will keep for only two or three weeks before going mouldy (succumbing to the growth of fungi), going 'off' and starting to smell unpleasantly (succumbing to bacterial infection), or becoming rancid (oxidising). Preservatives can be added to increase the shelf life. Nipagin M is an example of a preservative which is available at chemists (see page 53). For personal home use, the following cosmetics are so easy to make that it is probably best to make the small quantities given on a frequent basis.

Moulds need oxygen to grow, so keep the finished products in airtight containers. Keep them cool also, to help retard fungal growth.

Signs of bacterial growth would be the separation and liquefaction of the emulsions or the appearance of small lumps in the creams, or both.

Rancidity is due to the oxidation of the oils. Plant oils become rancid more quickly than mineral oils.

Galen's original cold cream

Equipment
- ☐ Double boiler: a bowl snugly fitted into a pan of hot water over a heating element is ideal (Figure 5.1).
- ☐ Standard spoon measures (1 tablespoon = 15 ml).
- ☐ Grater.
- ☐ Stirring spoon.
- ☐ 150–200 g ($\frac{1}{2}$ lb.) jam jar and label.

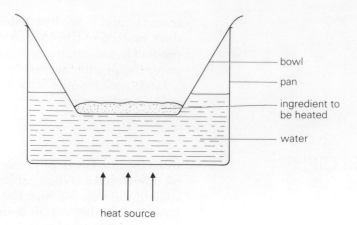

FIGURE 5.1 *A double boiler*

Ingredients
- ☐ 4 tablespoons olive oil.
- ☐ 1 level tablespoon grated beeswax, pressed very firmly into the measure (approx. 7 g, or $\frac{1}{4}$ oz.).
- ☐ 4 tablespoons rainwater (rose-water makes an excellent substitute).

Method
1. Place the beeswax and the olive oil into the double boiler and heat gently, stirring all the time, until the beeswax has melted.
2. Still stirring, slowly add the water. Some of the beeswax may solidify again, but keep stirring until it has all melted.
3. Remove from the heat and keep stirring until the cream has cooled and thickened.
4. Bottle and label.

The olive oil replaces necessary body oils and is an emollient; rose-water is a gentle astringent and moisturiser, returning liquid to the skin and tightening the pores; beeswax is the necessary emulsifier.

Lemon hand cream

Equipment
- ☐ Lemon squeezer and strainer.
- ☐ Double boiler.
- ☐ Standard spoon measures (1 tablespoon = 15 ml).
- ☐ Grater.
- ☐ Wooden stirring spoon.
- ☐ 200–250 g ($\frac{1}{2}$ lb.) jam jar and label.

Materials

- ☐ 4 tablespoons lemon juice (the juice of one large lemon), fresh or bottled.
- ☐ 4 tablespoons almond oil.
- ☐ 1 level tablespoon grated beeswax, pressed very firmly into the measure (approx. 7 g or $\frac{1}{4}$ oz.).
- ☐ 6 drops lemon oil.

Method

1 If using a fresh lemon, squeeze and strain the lemon juice.
2 Place the beeswax and almond oil into the double boiler. Heat gently until melted, stirring all the time.
3 Still stirring, add the lemon juice slowly (some of the wax may solidify again). When all the wax has melted, remove from the heat.
4 Stir until cool.
5 Add the lemon oil and stir.
6 Bottle and label.

Almond oil is an emollient and nutritive ingredient. The lemon juice is a protectant and texturiser which also helps to replace the skin's natural acid mantle, tightens the skin, and has a slight bleaching effect. Beeswax is the necessary emulsifier. This cream will soften and smooth rough hands and also protect them from work still to be done.

Coconut hand cream

Equipment

- ☐ Double boiler.
- ☐ Standard spoon measures (1 tablespoon = 15 ml).
- ☐ Grater.
- ☐ Stirring spoon.
- ☐ 200–250 g ($\frac{1}{2}$ lb.) jam jar and label.

Ingredients

- ☐ 1 level tablespoon grated beeswax, pressed very firmly into the measure (approx. 7 g or $\frac{1}{4}$ oz.).
- ☐ 2 tablespoons sweet almond oil.
- ☐ 2 level tablespoons coconut oil (approx. 25 g).
- ☐ 1 tablespoon glycerine.
- ☐ 3 tablespoons distilled water or rose-water.

Method

1 Place the beeswax, almond oil and coconut oil into a double boiler and heat gently until melted, stirring all the time.

2 Mix the water and glycerine together and add to the melted oils and waxes a drop at a time, stirring constantly, until all the liquid has been added. If some of the wax solidifies out at this stage, wait before adding more liquid and keep stirring until it has melted again. (This solidification can be avoided if the water and glycerine, before being added to the oils, are heated in a separate container until lukewarm, but this is not essential if the mixing is done slowly whilst still over the double boiler.)

3 Remove the mixture from the heat and stir constantly until it has cooled and forms a smooth cream. (On the way to this stage, it may look separated and as if it will never make a cream: just continue to stir and it will come together in the end.)

4 Bottle and label.

The almond oil is an emollient and nutritive ingredient. The beeswax is the necessary emulsifying agent. Coconut oil is added for its nourishing and conditioning properties. Glycerine is a bactericide, softener and lubricant, which also acts as a humectant. Further, it helps to improve the spreading properties of the cream. Rose-water is a gentle astringent and moisturiser, helping to add moisture to the skin surface.

Coconut hand cream makes a really good sun-tanning cream which intensifies the tan (due to the coconut oil content) and prevents the skin from drying and flaking. However, it contains no factor of sun protection, so care must be taken in its use.

Lanolin cuticle cream

Equipment
- □ Double boiler.
- □ Standard spoon measures (1 tablespoon = 15 ml).
- □ Grater.
- □ Stirring spoon.
- □ 125–150 g ($\frac{1}{2}$ lb.) jam jar and label.

Ingredients
- □ 8 level tablespoons white petroleum jelly (approx. 125 g) – buy a 125 g size and reuse the container for the finished cuticle cream.
- □ 1 level tablespoon lanolin (approx. 15 g).
- □ $\frac{1}{2}$ level teaspoon grated beeswax, pressed very firmly into the measure (approx. 1–2 g).

Method
1 Place all the ingredients into a double boiler and heat gently, stirring all the time, until they have melted.

2 Remove from the heat and continue stirring until the mixture has cooled a little and is beginning to thicken.
3 Bottle and label.

If it is desired to perfume the cuticle cream, then three drops of lemon oil can be added to the cooled cream prior to bottling.

The lanolin is an emollient. It is also very similar to human oils and will replenish these oils in the cuticle and nail plate, thus helping to prevent dryness. The beeswax is included as a nutritive and texturising agent to soften, nourish and protect the cuticle. The petroleum jelly is an emollient and skin lubricant. It is an ideal carrying medium for the lanolin and beeswax.

Oily nail varnish remover

Equipment
- Standard spoon measures (1 teaspoon = 5 ml, 1 tablespoon = 15 ml) – see below.
- Glass dish with a pouring lip.
- 250 ml glass bottle and label.

Ingredients
- 15 tablespoons acetone (225 ml).
- 1 teaspoon distilled water or rose-water (5 ml).
- $\frac{1}{4}$ teaspoon glycerine (approx. 1.5 ml).

Method
1 Mix all the ingredients together in a glass bowl.
2 Bottle and label.

The acetone is the solvent but, on its own, it is extremely drying to living tissue. Glycerine is a softener and lubricant, helping to counteract the drying effect of the acetone. However, glycerine will not naturally mix with acetone, so the distilled water has to be added as an emulsifying agent.

Warning
Acetone will dissolve plastic: be careful that the measures you use are of a type that will not be affected, and that neither the acetone nor the completed product comes into contact with anything plastic (such as a plastic sink).

Nail bleach

Equipment
- ☐ A small glass dish.
- ☐ A standard teaspoon (5 ml).
- ☐ A small brush (such as an eyeshadow applicator), to mix and apply the bleach.

Ingredients
- ☐ 2 teaspoons 20-volume peroxide (10 ml).
- ☐ 1 drop household ammonia (1 ml).

Method
1 The bleach must be made immediately prior to use by mixing the two ingredients together in the glass dish.
2 If a thicker consistency is desired – for use on stains on the skin or for body hair, for example – pure soap flakes or fuller's earth can be added to bind the ingredients into a paste form.
3 Leave the bleach on the stains for only 15 minutes before removing with warm water. The bleach will have lost its bleaching power after this time and, if it is necessary to apply more because of the stubborn nature of the stains, a fresh mixture must be made.

The peroxide is a bleaching agent. The ammonia speeds up and intensifies the process.

Cuticle oil

Equipment
- ☐ An empty 15 ml nail varnish bottle – the bottle and brush should be cleaned thoroughly with acetone (note the warning on page 59), then washed in hot soapy water, rinsed out and dried.

Ingredients
- ☐ 1 × 1000 mg capsule of vitamin E.
- ☐ 14 ml sweet almond oil.

Method
1 Combine the two oils in the empty bottle: they are then ready for use, complete with an applicator.

This oil can be used nightly at home to keep the cuticles back off the nail surface and prevent dryness in both the cuticle and the nail plate. Simply paint a thin film around the cuticle and nail wall, over the nail plate and under the nail tip. Do this last thing at night and leave on overnight.

Nail varnish drying oil

Equipment
- [ ] As for cuticle oil.

Ingredients
- [ ] 1 drop (1 ml) of pure essential oil of jojoba.
- [ ] 14 ml grapeseed oil.

Method
1 Combine the two oils in the empty bottle: they are then ready for use.

Paint a thin layer over the top of wet nail varnish to speed the drying and help to prevent smudging of the nail varnish. It does the latter by putting a slippery film on the surface of the nail varnish.

Massage oil

Equipment
- [ ] A standard teaspoon (5 ml).

Ingredients
- [ ] 1 × 500 ml glass bottle of sunflower seed or grapeseed oil (available from any supermarket).
- [ ] 1 teaspoon each of the essential oils of rosemary, lavender and sage.

Method
1 Add the essential oils to the bottle of carrier oil.
2 Stopper the mixture and fragrances, and leave them to blend for two or three days. Keep the blended oil in a cool, dark place in order to maintain the therapeutic properties of the oils for as long as possible.
3 The above oil will only keep for 2–3 months before losing its

properties and going rancid. To keep the oil for longer than this, replace 50 ml (10 per cent) of the carrier oil with wheatgerm oil, a natural anti-oxidant which will help to maintain the therapeutic properties of the essential oils and stop the carrier oil from going rancid. The addition of wheatgerm oil will increase the shelf life to approximately six months. It also makes the oil more nourishing, and ideal for drier skins.

The plant seed oil is a carrier oil. It absorbs at a rate compatible with the time taken to carry out a massage, thus providing lubrication for the treatment so that the skin is not pulled, dragged or nipped in any way. It also has nutritive properties. The rosemary oil acts to dispel tiredness and stimulate the blood circulation, helping to eliminate any fluid retention as well as relieving muscular aches and pains. The lavender oil acts to relax and harmonise the nervous system, as well as having powerful healing properties. Sage is a tonic oil which will stimulate a sluggish skin and help eliminate any fluid retention as well as relieving muscular and joint aches and pains.

Cuticle remover

Equipment
□   A standard teaspoon (5 ml).
□   A standard dessertspoon (10 ml).

Ingredients
□   1 dessertspoon (10 ml) of a 20 per cent solution of potassium hydroxide (available to order from any chemist in 500 ml bottles).
□   1 teaspoon (5 ml) glycerine.
□   2 dessertspoons and 1 teaspoon (25 ml in total) of distilled water or rose-water.

Method
1   Mix all the ingredients together and bottle the product. This will make a 5 per cent solution of potassium hydroxide. The glycerine is a humectant and will help to prevent the potassium hydroxide from drying out the cuticle area.

Warning
Potassium hydroxide (KOH) is a caustic (burning) substance. If it comes into contact with the skin or eyes, the area should be washed immediately with plenty of cold water. Replace the lid on the bottle of 20 per cent KOH solution immediately after use and do not allow the finished 5 per cent solution to remain on the skin for longer than 10 minutes before removal.

PART IV

Manicuring and pedicuring

6 TOOLS of the TRADE

Terms used

- *Equipment* Any large, durable or permanent apparatus necessary for the manicure or pedicure procedure, such as a stool.

- *Implements* Any small but durable item or tool used in the manicure or pedicure sequence, such as cuticle clippers.

- *Materials* Any disposable item which is used on the client as part of the treatment and then discarded, such as cottonwool.

- *Cosmetics* or *cosmetic materials* Products which are intended to cleanse, beautify or in general impart a sense of well-being to the user, such as hand cream. Cosmetics are used up during a manicure and must therefore be replaced.

EQUIPMENT

The client's chair

This must be comfortable, as the client will be sitting in this chair for up to two hours, depending on the treatment. Chair arms, a straight, padded back and a padded base aid in the provision of this comfort. There must also be room to place the pedicure bowl at the foot of the chair so that both manicure and pedicure may be carried out at the same station.

The client's chair must be positioned far enough away from the manicure table to allow the client's arms and the arms of the manicurist to be easily extended. If the client is too close to the manicure table, the manicurist will have to work with her elbows sharply bent and her shoulders raised, leading to unnecessary tiredness and muscle strain. If the client is too far away from the manicure table, the manicurist will have to lean forward a long way, leading to back strain.

The manicurist's or pedicurist's stool

A manicurist who is sitting at a manicure station for most of the day needs a stool with a backrest in which she can sit with her lower back near the back of the chair and lean slightly forward whilst working on the client (Figure 6.1). This correct sitting posture helps to avoid backstrain and general tiredness. The full weight of the manicurist's body must be distributed evenly over the surface area of the stool. Crossed-leg positions and sitting to one side must be avoided as, over a period of time, they can cause backache, sciatica and circulatory problems such as varicose veins.

A pedicurist's stool must be lower than the manicurist's so that at various stages throughout the treatment the client can rest her feet comfortably upon the seated pedicurist's knees.

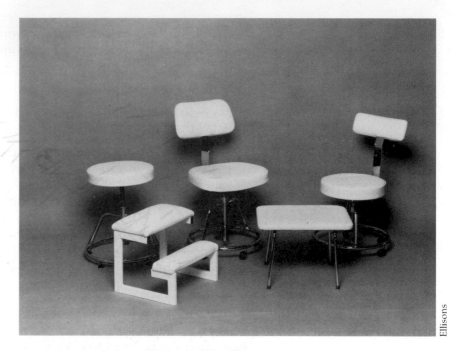

FIGURE 6.1 *Stools for manicurists and pedicurists*

The manicure table

This can be of many designs (Figure 6.2). At its simplest, a stable, overbed trolley makes a suitable, temporary manicure table. It is adjustable in height, easily moved around on castors and can be slid in front of and close to the client with a minimum of fuss. At its most complex, a more permanent manicure station is a low desk with knee-holes at both sides, two or three drawers for additional equipment on the working side of the manicurist, racks and trays to hold all the implements, materials and cosmetics, and an adjustable desk light or magnifying lamp to ensure adequate lighting. Electrical sockets, paper-towel roll holders, padded arm supports, and extractor fans to eliminate fumes and dust are included on many purpose-built tables.

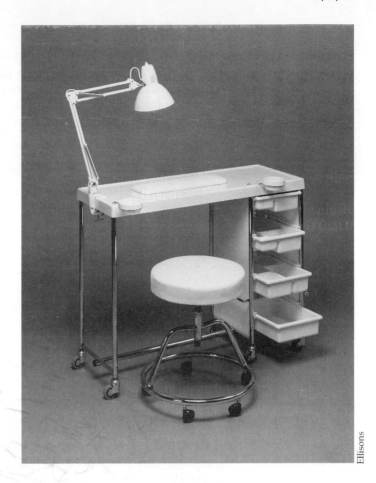

FIGURE 6.2 *A manicure table*

The hand and arm support

This consists of a 2–3 cm thick sponge pad, measuring about 20 cm × 30 cm, which is covered in a washable and clean slip or towel. Placed on the table, this provides support for the client's hands and arms during the manicure sequence. If a sponge pad is not available, a folded towel, covered with a smaller clean towel, will provide a suitable alternative. Many modern manicure tables already have a cushioned pad fixed in place: this simply needs covering with a towel for reasons of hygiene.

The manicure/pedicure (supply) tray

This is primarily for holding the cosmetics used in the treatment. An ideal tray should be easy to sterilise and should also contain or have room for receptacles for the materials and implements used in the treatment.

The waste bin

This should be of the covered, flip-top, floor-standing variety. If the treatment is not being carried out at a permanent station, then it is more practical for the supply tray to contain a glass receptacle for the disposal of waste cottonwool and tissues. This receptacle must be emptied and cleaned between clients.

The laundry bin

Simply a covered bin in which dirty linen can be placed until such time as it can be laundered.

Towels

For a manicure treatment two towels, approximately 30×60 cm in size, are required, one to cover the hand and arm support, and one for the manicurist to use during the treatment. For a pedicure, two larger towels are required, one to cover the floor area underneath and surrounding the pedicure bowl, and one for the pedicurist to work with.

All towels must be freshly laundered in hot (60 °C) water and completely dry for each client. It adds a nice touch if the clean towels can be kept in a warm cupboard so that they are brought out warmed for each new client.

To save on laundry, many manicurists cover the base towel with a fresh, disposable tissue towel for each new client and only launder the base towel at the end of every day. In this way, only the top towel needs to be fresh for each client.

Glass or pottery receptacles

These are to contain any cosmetics, materials or implements to be used in the treatment. One must contain a rust-inhibiting sterilising solution, such as surgical spirit, and be used for holding the metal implements (e.g. the cuticle knife) during the treatment. Another would hold the files and cuticle sticks. Glass or glazed pottery are preferable to plastic as they are easier to keep clean and germ-free.

Wherever possible, and for reasons of hygiene and speed of use, the containers for cosmetics should be of the pump dispenser type (e.g. for hand cream) or of the dish dispenser type (e.g. for nail varnish remover).

The manicure bowl

This is for holding warm soapy water in which to soak the client's fingers during the manicure sequence. Manicure bowls can be of many designs, from open bowls with or without disposable paper inserts, to closed-in, non-spill bowls with strategically placed finger and thumb holes (Figure 6.3). In practice, the closed-in bowls are preferable as they lead to fewer accidents and help to keep the water warm for a longer time. If this type of bowl is used, it must be of the type with a removable lid so that it can be cleaned and disinfected easily between clients.

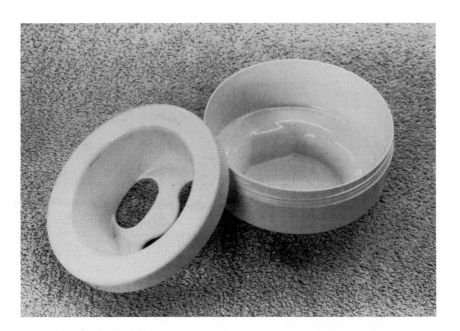

FIGURE 6.3 *A manicure bowl*

The pedicure bowl

This is for holding warm water, liquid soap and an antiseptic in which to soak the client's feet prior to and during a pedicure treatment. At its simplest, a plain washing-up bowl will suffice. More elaborate designs are available, with moulded foot cavities in which to soak the feet in a minimum of water. Unfortunately, neither of these types of bowl keep the water warm for long. However, there are electrically-operated foot-baths now available which keep the water warm and provide a relaxing, underwater, vibrating foot massage during the treatment (Figure 6.4). These are ideal, but care must be taken to ensure that the hands are not wet when connecting the appliance to, and disconnecting it from, the electricity supply. One solution is to place the bowl in position and connect it to the supply *before* filling the bowl with the antiseptic soap solution from another bowl. This also

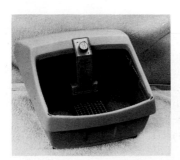

FIGURE 6.4 *An electrically-operated foot-bath*

makes the filling of the bowl easier as there is less weight to carry from the water supply to the pedicure station.

If a vibrating foot-bath is used, it is advantageous to place a firm sponge pad, approximately 10 cm thick, underneath the floor towel and foot-bath: this prevents the vibrations from being transmitted to the floor, and thus prevents excess noise during the treatment.

If a salon has the space, pedicures can be made even more luxurious by the use of a plumbed-in combined foot spa and client's seat (Figure 6.5).

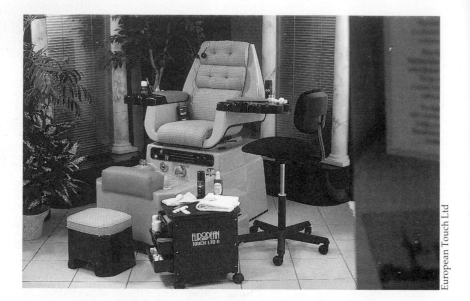

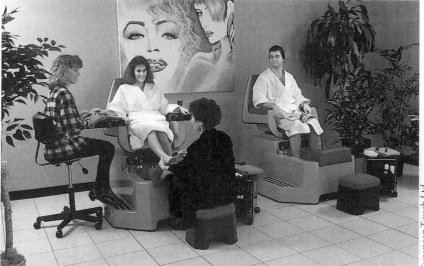

FIGURE 6.5 *Luxury whirlpool pedicure spas*

IMPLEMENTS

Cuticle sticks (orangewood sticks)

Made out of orangewood because it does not splinter and is non-absorbent, cuticle sticks are thin, cylindrical sticks of wood, pointed at one end and horseshoe-shaped at the other (Figure 6.6). Two of these are needed in the supply tray. They are used for the application of paste polish and cuticle cream to the surface of the nail. With the addition of an absorbent cottonwool tip, and using a suitable solvent or bleaching agent, they are used to clean and remove stubborn nail varnish, stains and grime from the nail wall and free edge of the nail.

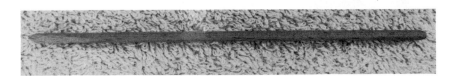

FIGURE 6.6 *A cuticle stick*

Cuticle sticks are also used to loosen the cuticle and skin debris from the surface of the nail, lifting and pushing it back in readiness for its being clipped away with the cuticle clippers. For this purpose, a small quantity of cottonwool must be added, both for its cushioning effect, so that the nail and nail wall are not damaged, and for hygiene, as the soiled cottonwool cover can be discarded straight away after use.

Emery boards

These should be 18–20 cm (7–8 in.) in length, thin, flexible and covered with a fine-graded emery (sand) paper on one side and a coarse-graded emery paper on the other side. The coarse side is used for reducing the length of the free edge of the nail. The fine side is used for bevelling and sealing this edge and obtaining a pleasing shape to the nail.

Emery boards are coated with a layer of aluminium oxide (Al_2O_3) crystals, commonly known as corundum. The mineral, aluminium oxide, can be mined or made synthetically, and can be a variety of colours, depending on the impurities contained in the crystals. The most common naturally-occurring colours are blue-grey to brown, hence this is the usual shade of natural emery boards.

Coloured, synthetic emery boards are also available: in these the emery paper is replaced by a more durable synthetic composite substance which can be scrubbed and sterilised. The synthetic coatings come in a variety of grades, from extremely coarse grades, reserved for reducing the length of false nails, to extremely fine grades, especially made for buffing out irregularities on the surface of natural and false nails. Because of the great variety of these files, each type must be individually assessed as to its suitability for use on the natural nail plate. (See page 216.)

Metal nail files

Frequently sold to the public for use on their nails, plain, rough, metal nail files should not be used in a professional treatment. Only a 'Diamond Deb', with its surface coated with industrial diamond chips, or a similar purpose-made synthetic variety, is acceptable (Figure 6.7). Even then, the file must be used only for reducing the length of the free edge of the nail, or on the more sturdy toenails. The harsh action of a metal file tends to tear apart the nail layers, and an emery board should always be used to bevel the nail edge after the use of such a nail file.

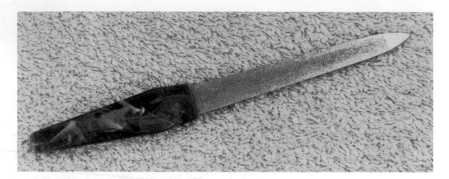

FIGURE 6.7 *A metal nail file (Diamond Deb) for shaping toenails*

Metal nail files are appropriate for use in a pedicure treatment: the dampness of the toes can ruin an emery board very quickly. The metal files are also thinner than emery boards, making it easier to file the shorter toenails. The pointed thin tip of a metal file is also ideal for cleaning under the free edge of the toenail.

The magnifying glass

This is for the close inspection of any suspected infections or nail conditions which may contra-indicate the treatment, and of any damage to the nail, to determine which type of nail repair would be most suitable. A magnifying glass can either be small and held in the hand, or form an integral part of the station lighting system.

The hoof stick or cuticle pusher

In appearance, this is like a thick cuticle stick with the rounded end shaped like a horse's hoof and made of rubber (Figure 6.8). It is used to loosen and push back the cuticle, but it is not as sensitive or accurate in its use as a cottonwool-covered cuticle stick. It is most suited for cuticle work prior to false nail application, or for use by the client at home, as the rubber cushioning will ensure that in any cuticle work she carries out she will not damage herself.

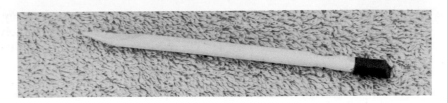

FIGURE 6.8 *A hoof stick*

The cuticle knife

This is a small knife, purpose-made to loosen and remove stubborn cuticle from the nail plate. Cuticle knives are available in various designs and choice depends a great deal on personal preference and familiarity in their use (Figure 6.9).

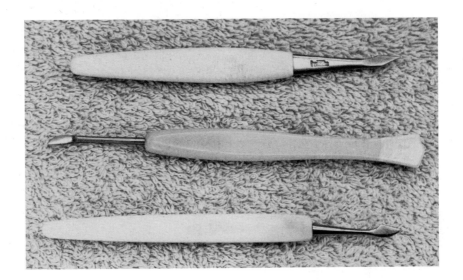

FIGURE 6.9 *Cuticle knives*

The cuticle knife must always be used with plenty of soapy water or cuticle remover liquid so that the knife does not scratch the surface of the nail. If the nails are adequately soaked and a reputable cuticle remover used in conjunction with a cottonwool-covered cuticle stick, use of the cuticle knife should be minimal.

It is often necessary to work around and neaten the margins of the nail with a cuticle stick after the cuticles have been worked on with a cuticle knife and clipped.

Cuticle clippers (cuticle pliers)

These are small, accurately-cutting clippers with a spring action, which are used to remove excess cuticle. Cuticle clippers must be sharpened regularly and carefully looked after to keep their blades in good cutting order. When not in use they should be protected from knocks, and they should be reserved solely for clipping cuticles.

Cuticle clippers are available with two types of spring (Figure 6.10):

1   a single spring, fastened to one handle and rubbing against the other: this type can 'squeak' when in use, and the springs suffer a great deal from metal fatigue, breaking frequently as a result;
2   a double spring, whereby each spring is fastened to a single handle and the springs interlock in the centre to provide the controlled cutting action needed, with no squeaking and very little metal fatigue.

The nipper heads of cuticle clippers also vary in size and style, personal preference dictating choice.

Care must be taken not to be over-zealous in the use of cuticle clippers, as damage can easily be caused to the skin at the base of the cuticle.

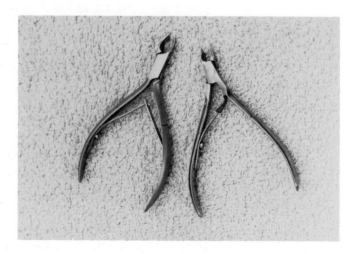

FIGURE 6.10 *Cuticle clippers, double-sprung and single-sprung*

The nailbrush

This is a small, soft brush which is used, with the aid of warm soapy water, to clean the nails and fingertips of any remaining debris, grease and cuticle remover.

Nail scissors

These are sometimes used to trim long nails prior to filing. Nail scissors for fingernails and toenails differ. For the hand, they are usually small and curved (Figure 6.11). For the toes, they need to be a lot sturdier and stronger, with shorter, thicker blades and longer, sprung handles to provide more controlled cutting power for the

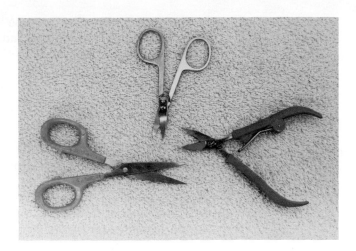

FIGURE 6.11 *Straight scissors (left), curved scissors (top), and acrylic tip nippers*

tougher toenails. In their extreme, they look like pliers, with cutting blades and a spring action (Figure 6.12).

To avoid possible snapping and shattering of the brittle nail plate, the nails should be softened in warm, soapy water prior to being cut with scissors.

Nail clippers

These provide an alternative way of reducing the length of the free edge of the nail prior to filing (Figure 6.12). They are ideal for cutting flat toe- and fingernails. However, they are difficult to use on a fingernail plate with a pronounced curve from one side to the other, as this curve can cause the nail to shatter if clipped. A nail should be clipped in two parts, first one side, then the other; the nail should have been pre-soaked in warm water to soften it to reduce the chance of breakage.

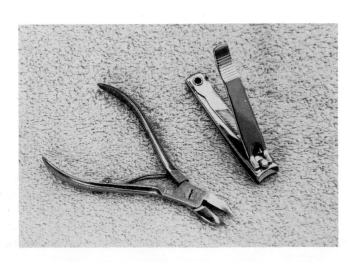

FIGURE 6.12 *Toenail scissors (left) and toenail clippers*

The choice between the use of nail clippers and scissors for reducing the length of toe- and fingernails is one of personal preference and experience.

Nail buffers

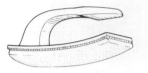

FIGURE 6.13 *A nail buffer*

Nail buffers fall into two distinct categories. The old type of buffer was designed to be used, with paste polish, to impart a natural shine to the nail surface as well as stimulate the blood circulation to the nail bed and matrix. This type (Figure 6.13) should have a removable frame to allow for the replacement and cleaning of the chamois leather or muslin cover. (It is difficult to sterilise the chamois leather covers effectively, hence the use of disposable muslin.) The newer type are synthetic, disposable buffers, designed solely to impart a shine to the nail plate or false nail surface. The most usual design of this type of buffer is the three- or four-sided buffer. Here, three or four grades of synthetic emery, from fine to extra fine, are used to cover and sandwich a thin sponge or plywood supporting pad. The coarsest emery should only be used at the first buffing, to buff away ridges or imperfections in the nail plate. Over-use of this quality of emery will thin and weaken the nail plate. This coarse emery is followed by the finer emeries in sequence, to impart a high gloss shine which will last for weeks. On subsequent buffings, only the finest emeries should be used.

These buffers are in turn being superseded by synthetic buffing fabrics of differing grades. These fabrics are inserted into holders of various designs, and prove sensitive and accurate in use.

Spatulas

If pump dispensers are not used for dispensing creams and the like, then spatulas are needed to remove creams from their jars to avoid contamination of the product. Spatulas should either be disposable or be made of materials which can easily be disinfected.

Toe separators

These are specially designed sponge pads which fit under and in between the toes to prevent them from touching and smudging wet nail varnish when it has just been applied (Figure 6.14). Toe separators should be washed in hot (60 °C) soapy water after every use.

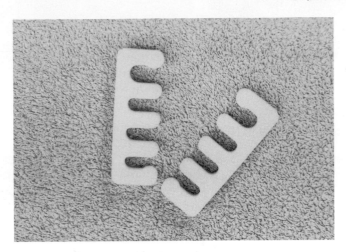

FIGURE 6.14 *Toe separators*

The corn plane

This implement, designed for the removal of hard skin, has a sharp, double-edged razor blade contained inside a safety holder so that only a thin paring of hard skin can be cut at each sweep of the blade (Figure 6.15). It must be used with great care, by experienced pedicurists only. The tool must be sterilised after every use and a new blade used for each client.

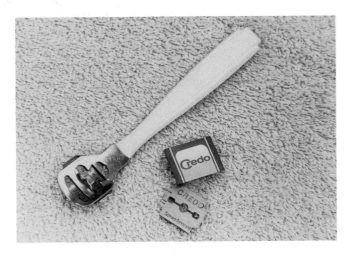

FIGURE 6.15 *A corn plane and a spare blade*

The hard skin rasp

This is a metal implement designed and used for grating hard skin away from calluses on the feet. It must be used with great care and sterilised after every use.

The chiropody sponge

These 'sponges' (Figure 6.16), often made out of reconstituted pumice or synthetic substitutes, are used for rubbing and wearing away the hard skin on foot calluses. They should be used with a lot of soap in order to prevent scratching, and should be sterilised after use.

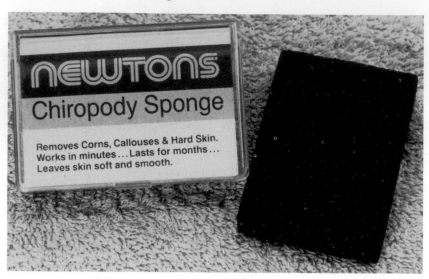

FIGURE 6.16 *A chiropody sponge*

MATERIALS

Absorbent cottonwool

To aid in the removal of nail varnish, cleansing the nail surface, covering cuticle sticks, applying cosmetics to the nails, and other general duties.

Nail Neats

Flat cottonwool pieces covered in loose muslin. An alternative similar product is viscose fibre tissue squares. These aid in the removal of nail varnish and the degreasing of the nail prior to varnish application. They are an improvement on plain cottonwool as they have a slight (but non-damaging) abrasive quality which eases the removal of products, and they do not shed fibres which could ruin a varnish application.

Small paper tissues

These are to assist in the cleaning of the nail and to prevent nail varnish from getting onto the towels if corrective work has to be done.

Paper towel

A sheet of paper towel is needed to cover the cotton towel on the sponge pad, thereby preventing any nail varnish or nail repairing substances from staining the towel.

COSMETIC MATERIALS

Nail varnish remover

Nail varnish remover is designed to dissolve nail varnish from the surface of the nails.

At its simplest, nail varnish remover is a mixture of solvents of nitrocellulose (e.g. acetone or ethyl acetate), to which may be added a small quantity of oil or an oily material such as glycerine. The oil is added to counteract the drying action that the solvent would otherwise have on the nail plate and surrounding tissues. Sometimes water is also added.

Modern professional removers use solvents that are less drying (e.g. ethyl acetate or methyl ethyl ketone), and non-greasy moisturising agents (e.g. Aloe Vera). Colourings, fragrances, alcohols, water and so on may all be added in the formulations of individual products.

Cuticle oil or cream

This is a mixture of waxes and nutritive oils (e.g. lanolin, white petroleum jelly, beeswax, and almond oil or cocoa butter). Vitamin E and jojoba oil are two popular nutritive ingredients.

The oil is designed to soften and nourish the cuticle and make the nail plate more flexible, by replacing the natural oils lost in daily life through exposure to detergents and other drying elements. In this way it helps to prevent or correct dry cuticle and brittle nail conditions. The cuticle cream or oil should be used within the manicure sequence and as a nightly home-care treatment.

Cuticle remover

This is a fluid-based alkaline lotion or liquid to which has been added a moisturising agent such as glycerine. The alkali usually used is potassium hydroxide, to which is added sufficient distilled water to make a 2–5 per cent solution. Although only mildly corrosive, cuticle remover should not be left on the skin for longer than 10 minutes.

Cuticle remover is used to soften the excess cuticle and the dead outer skin cells which collect around the nail groove. These can then be removed with the aid of a cuticle knife, cuticle stick and cuticle clippers to give a neat edge to the nail plate.

Paste polish (buffing cream)

This is a mildly abrasive cream or powder which is used in conjunction with a buffer to impart a shine to the surface of the nail. Tin oxide or pumice powder are the usual abrasive constituents of the cream. Paste polish does not contain any nutritive elements.

The friction that occurs during the buffing process draws the blood to the capillaries of the nail bed: this increase in the blood supply may have a slight stimulating effect on the health and growth of the nail.

If coloured nail varnish is not required, or if it is a male manicure, then the buffing procedure would be done last. (Often special buffing files, instead of paste polish and chamois leather buffers, are used to raise a high gloss shine.) If buffing is being carried out to remedy ridges, poor circulation, fragile nails and the like, it can be incorporated earlier in the manicure.

Nail varnish thinner

This is used to thin the nail varnish if it has thickened due to the evaporation of its solvent. Some types of nail varnish need to be thinned up to 20 minutes before use, to allow the pigments and other constituents to become equally distributed and blended throughout the varnish again. Nail varnish *remover* must never be used as a thinner because it contains oils and water and will prevent the nail varnish from drying properly. Only a pure solvent with no additives, such as amyl acetate or ethyl acetate, is suitable for thinning. Usually manufacturers produce thinners to match their own nail varnishes: because these use the same blend of solvents, they do not inhibit the setting of the varnishes.

Nail bleaches

These are used to remove stains from the surface of the nail, from underneath the free edge of the nail, and from the skin surrounding the nail. Nail bleaches usually contain diluted hydrogen peroxide, or organic acids such as lemon juice or citric acid, as their bleaching agents. Glycerine, a humectant, is often incorporated to counteract the drying effect of the bleach. Distilled water or rose-water is the usual dilutant, and the bleach can be left in a liquid form or mixed with other ingredients to form a cream.

Nail white pencil

This is a pencil with its central core mainly consisting of white pigments (e.g. titanium dioxide or zinc oxide) in a soap base. The application of its water-moistened tip to the undersurface of the nail produces an even white free edge to the nail. The whitener needs to be re-applied after washing. The use of nail white pencils and creams has been largely superseded by the technique of the 'French manicure'.

Nail strengtheners

These can be of many types. Plastic-based nail strengtheners help to prevent the nail from becoming fragile or over-brittle, as well as having a hardening effect on very soft nails. This type of preparation is usually applied over the nail plate instead of a base coat, or for client convenience may be incorporated by some manufacturers into a dual-purpose base coat/top coat. These formulations often use formaldehyde resins (e.g. toluenesulphonamide-formaldehyde resin) as well as formalin for their strengthening factors, although recent controversy over the use of formalin is leading to the development of alternative hardening ingredients.

Some liquid formulations contain up to 4–5 per cent formaldehyde. These types are best suited for use as a hardener on soft, flexible nails. Their over-use or their use on nails which are already hard will cause the nails to become brittle. Care must be taken not to let this type of formulation come into contact with the skin around the nail as it can cause it to become dry and hard and sometimes cause paronychia (inflammation, pus, and pain in and around the cuticle). Their use should be restricted to a frequency of no more than twice a week and to the tips of the nail only.

Other formulations are oil-based products containing strengthening ingredients and nutritive elements, including organic acids (oleic, palmitic, linolic and linoleic), vitamin oils (E, A, thiamin, riboflavin and niacin) and minerals (calcium and iron). These are ideal for flaky, brittle nails, and also serve to condition the cuticle and surrounding skin. They are applied, preferably at night-time, over the whole of the surface of the nail plate, around the nail wall and cuticle, and underneath the free edge of the nail plate.

Hand lotions and creams

Exposure of the hands to drying winds, central heating, and the frequent use of the soap and alkaline detergents used in 'housework', causes the hands and nails to lose their natural oils and become dry, chapped and irritated. Hand creams or lotions are used to replace the natural oils and to place a protective barrier on the surface of the skin.

A cream or lotion for use on the hands is required to perform some or all of the following functions:

1 it must provide a source of moisture which is readily available to the skin;
2 it must be able to give additional oils to the skin to replace those lost;
3 it must leave the hands feeling smooth, soft and supple, but not greasy;
4 it must be easy to apply in a controllable manner.

Hand creams range from those affording little more than slight emollience and a pleasant perfume, to the heavy treatment creams used in cases of severe damage to the skin. The latter are only available on medical prescription.

Within the manicure, if the cream is to be used for a hand and arm massage, it should have a slow absorption rate, allow free movement over the area of massage, and contain nutritive ingredients. For a quick hand massage or for nightly application, a faster-absorbing cream, also containing nutritive ingredients, should be selected.

Hand lotions and creams are always oil-in-water emulsions as these are less greasy than water-in-oil emulsions. They are usually of the same composition as 'vanishing creams' and have their property of seeming to disappear when being rubbed into the skin. They are basically mixtures of oils, water and emulsifying agents with the addition of nourishing, thickening, protective and texturising agents such as glycerine, gum tragacanth, jojoba oil, Aloe Vera gel, collagen, rice bran, beeswax, lanolin, cocoa butter, and lecithin. Perfumes, preservatives and colours are also added, and the main difference between a hand lotion and a cream is the amount of distilled water it contains.

Skin exfoliating creams

These are creams to which have been added abrasive ingredients such as oatmeal, or powdered organic or inorganic products. When the creams are worked into the skin, they gently abrade the dead skin cells away from the surface of the skin, leaving the skin smoother and cleaner. A gentle abrasive would be used on the hands; a coarser one would be needed for calluses on the feet.

Nail varnish quick-drying products

These can be of two kinds:

1 Quick-drying oils, which are painted over the surface of the wet varnish. These are often made of fine mineral oils and silicone. They put a film of slippery oil (the silicone provides the slip) on the surface of the varnish so that potentially damaging items slide off the nail surface instead of denting the varnish. Jojoba, palm or

avocado oils are often added to condition the cuticles. Care must be taken that the film of oil on the surface of the nail does not become transferred to clothing and stain it.

2 Quick-drying sprays, which are sprayed onto the surface of the wet nail varnish and surrounding nail wall. These contain lubricants or lubricating agents such as silicone which put a slippery film on the varnish surface. They also contain emollients such as jojoba, palm and avocado oils, which serve to condition the cuticle and nail wall. The sprays also contain a highly volatile propellant, usually one of the alcohols, which evaporates quickly and so helps to speed up the drying of the varnish. The sprays contain only a little oil and so are non-greasy in use.

Nail varnishes

First introduced into the USA in their present form in 1916, nail varnishes are used to add protection, colour or gloss (or all three) to the nail surface. They are solutions of nitrocellulose in very volatile solvents such as amyl acetate, ethyl acetate and acetone. They also contain pigment resins to colour them, and plasticisers (e.g. camphor) which prevent them drying too rapidly. Other constituents are diluents, resins, and pearlisers.

Nitrocellulose

A film-forming substance which makes up the bulk of the varnish. It gives durability, solubility and toughness. However, it does not adhere well, discolours as it ages (especially under UV light, which turns it yellow), lacks gloss, has a tendency to shrink, and, with age, loses its viscosity and ability to dry to a hard film. Other products can be added to counteract all these shortcomings.

Resins

Resins are used with nitrocellulose to reduce shrinkage, improve adhesion and flexibility, and provide gloss to the varnish. The most common resin to be used is toluenesulphonamide-formaldehyde resin. Others are maleic alkyd resins, acrylates, vinyls, some polyesters, and small amounts of nylon. Unfortunately, resins also tend to reduce the hardness of the varnish.

Plasticisers

These reduce shrinkage and improve flexibility in nail varnish. They also facilitate evaporation. Two common plasticisers are camphor and dibutyl phthalate. If too much plasticiser is added to the nail varnish, it will prevent the varnish from sticking to the nail.

Solvents

Solvents are used to wet the nitrocellulose and make the varnish of a suitable consistency to apply evenly with a brush. Butyl acetate and ethyl acetate are the most common solvents and they are usually mixed with toluene to stabilise them and regulate their evaporation. It is this evaporation which affects the drying time.

Diluents

Diluents help to stabilise the viscosity of the varnish and make the application easier. The most common diluents are three of the alcohols – ethyl, isopropyl and butyl alcohol.

Colourants

Creme varnishes contain insoluble colours mixed with small amounts of titanium dioxide. Iron oxide can also be added. *Pearlised varnishes* get their pearl effect from the addition of brilliant, reflective, transparent crystals of guanine; these are obtained from the skin and scales of small ocean fish such as herrings. *Synthetic pearlising* (e.g. titanium dioxide-coated mica flakes or bismuth oxychloride-coated mica flakes) is cheaper, but these particles tend to be larger than those of guanine and so settle out much more quickly.

Qualities

A nail varnish must have several qualities if it is to be successful.

1 It must have a quick drying time.
2 It must flow smoothly, making it easy to apply evenly with no streaks and little tendency to form air bubbles. (These are unavoidable if the product is vigorously shaken or overworked.)
3 It must dry to a high gloss.
4 Once dry, the surface must be hard and scratch-resistant, thus providing a protective coating to the surface of the nail.
5 The colour should be even in application and consistent between batches.
6 The product should adhere to the nail surface well, making it long-lasting in wear.
7 It must be flexible when dry, with no tendency to crack when bent.
8 It must not be allergenic, or harmful to the nails, or stain them with the pigment resins which it contains.
9 The pigment resins must not separate out of the product during storage.
10 Any pearlising should remain in suspension and not settle to the bottom of the bottle. (A little settling is inevitable, hence the ball bearings which help to redistribute it.)

Base coat

This is a primary nail varnish which seals the surface of the nail, thus helping to prevent discoloration of the surface of the nails by the coloured varnishes which may be applied later.

The use of a base coat also causes the nail varnish to adhere more readily to the surface of the nail. To achieve this, base coats contain a higher proportion of adhesive resins than normal varnishes. (It has been found that most allergies to nail varnish can be traced to the base coat used rather than to the coloured varnish: the problem will be due to the higher resin content.)

Base coat varnish dries more quickly and is harder than coloured varnishes and, used on its own, provides a low-gloss protective finish that resists chipping. It is often used for these qualities as a final finish over natural-looking false nails on which a coloured varnish is not desired.

Base coats have a lower non-volatile content and a lower viscosity than normal varnishes. This, as well as giving quick drying, results in a thinner application of the base coat to the nail plate. These are both desirable qualities in a good base coat. (A normal nail varnish cannot be this thin as it has to give a uniform colour film to the nail surface.)

Base coats are of two varieties, plain and ridge-filler base coats. The plain base coat is used on nails with no obvious irregularities. However, its use fills in any tiny flaws on the nail surface and this helps to give the follow-up coloured varnish a smoother and glossier finish. The ridge-filler base coats are thicker and are used on nails with irregular surfaces to help to minimise any ridges or pits present. This ensures a smoother application of the following coloured varnish than would have been possible over a normal base coat. Ridge-filler base coat is frequently the base coat used over false nails in order to minimise any irregularities.

The base coat must be thoroughly dry before the application of the next coat of varnish. Ridge-filler base coats take longer to dry than plain base coats.

Top coat

This is a final, clear, varnish sealer, which is applied over the top of the nail varnish. It imparts extra gloss and added strength, making the varnish more resistant to chipping.

Top coats are made using more nitrocellulose than plasticiser, and less resin and more diluent than normal varnishes. They tend to be fast-drying and tough when dry. Tricresyl phosphate is sometimes added to top coats to give a degree of flame retardance.

Between manicures top coats can be used daily to brighten up the coloured varnish, prevent chipping, give added strength to the nails (by increasing the film thickness) and make the salon manicure last longer. It is used daily over nail art creations to help them last longer.

PART V # The manicure

7 PRELIMINARIES

PREPARING THE MANICURE STATION

The manicure station (Figure 7.1) should have everything that the manicurist needs conveniently to hand so that the only reason she has to leave the area is to fetch hot water and to wash her hands.

The checklist on pages 90 and 91 lists the items needed; note, though, that not all of these are essential in carrying out a basic manicure. Some are needed when repairing or extending the nails, or when removing nail repairs or extensions. Others, for example the water spray and the nail-art items, are reflections of individual techniques.

The briefer checklist on page 92, 'Essentials for manicuring', is suited to the needs of a student in ensuring that she has gathered together all the equipment, implements, materials and cosmetic materials she will need in order to carry out the manicure procedure described in this book.

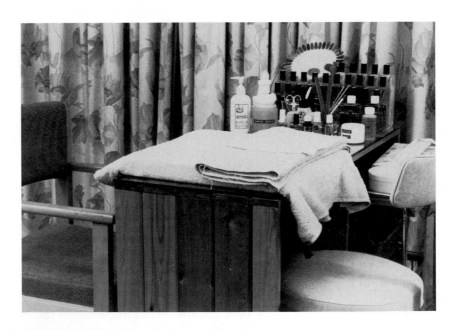

FIGURE 7.1 *A manicure station*

The manicure station: a checklist

1 A suitable table, with knee holes, drawers, power points and an angled desk lamp.
2 Tissue roll dispenser.
3 Two bins: one for waste, one for laundry.
4 A manicurist's stool, with back support.
5 A comfortable client's chair, with armrests.
6 A basin nearby for the client's use, with hot and cold running water, antiseptic soap in a dispenser, a nail brush in antiseptic solution, a paper towel dispenser or hot-air hand dryer, and a waste bin.
7 A manicurist's basin and preparation area set out as for the client (6), plus antiseptic or barrier creams for the manicurist's hands and a squeezy bottle dispenser of liquid soap for use in the manicure bowls.
8 A dry sterilising cabinet nearby in which to keep sterile tools and buffers.

In the desk drawers

9 Clean hand towels, new emery boards and cuticle sticks.
10 False nail systems; small, tightly stoppered bottles of acetone, methylated and surgical spirits; nail glues; two pottery dishes; nail mending systems (e.g. silk wraps); buffer files; heavy-duty files.
11 Small tissues; clean manicure bowl; unusual and extra varnish colours (e.g. black, white); nail white pencil; nail art items (e.g. tapes, diamante, transfers); nail bleach.

On the desk

12 A sponge pad covered with a clean towel and a length of clean tissue from the roll dispenser. This is for the client to rest her arms upon during treatment.
13 A clean hand towel, folded neatly on top of the sponge pad (12).
14 A pretty pottery dish in which the client may place her jewellery during the treatment.
15 A manicure tray.

In the manicure tray

16 Cottonwool in a dispenser or jar.
17 Surgical spirits, antiseptic solution and non-oily, non-acetone nail varnish remover, in either dish dispensers or bottles.
18 Hand cream (and massage oil or cream, if used as a separate item) in a pump dispenser, tube or squeezy dispenser, or in a covered container.

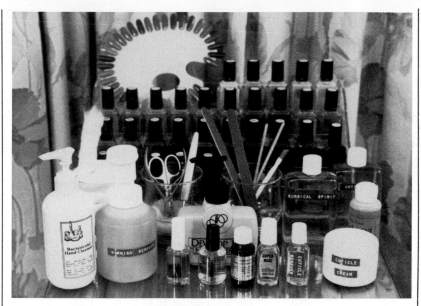

FIGURE 7.2 *The contents of the manicure tray*

19   Cuticle cream and buffing cream (paste polish), in either tube dispensers or covered containers.
20   A jar containing a spatula, for use in removing creams from their containers; two emery boards; two cuticle sticks.
21   A jar containing a small amount of cottonwool at the base and sufficient surgical spirit or antiseptic solution with rust inhibitor to cover the blades of a cuticle knife, cuticle clippers (pliers), nail scissors, and nail clippers if used.
22   Small brush bottles, containing cuticle remover, cuticle oil, nail dry oil, top coat, base coat, ridge-filler base coat, nail strengthener, and a good selection of coloured nail varnishes.
23   Nail dry spray.
24   Nail varnish thinner.
25   A water spray containing pure mineral or distilled water. The manicurist should carry a small magnifying glass with which to inspect anything unusual about the nails, such as suspected fungal infections.

An optional item for the desk top is a hot-air dryer for drying nail varnish and the like.

Essentials for manicuring: a checklist

Equipment

1 A manicure table, trolley or basket.
2 A client's chair and manicurist's stool.
3 A client's washable armrest.
4 A supply tray for holding cosmetics, implements and materials.
5 A manicure bowl for holding warm, soapy water.
6 A container for holding cottonwool.
7 A glass jar containing antiseptic solution or surgical spirits for holding implements.
8 A container for holding emery boards and cuticle sticks.
9 A receptacle for waste.
10 A hand towel.

Implements

11 Cuticle sticks (2).
12 18–20 cm (7–8 in.) emery boards (2).
13 A hoof stick (cuticle pusher) – optional.
14 Cuticle clippers.
15 A cuticle knife.
16 Nail clippers.
17 A nailbrush.
18 Nail scissors.
19 A chamois leather nail buffer.
20 A spatula.
21 A magnifying glass.

Cosmetics

22 Non-oily, non-acetone nail varnish remover.
23 Cuticle cream.
24 Cuticle remover.
25 Liquid soap.
26 Paste polish (buffing cream).
27 Hand cream.
28 Base coat, coloured nail varnishes, top coat.
29 Antiseptic solution.
30 A hot water supply.

Materials

31 Cottonwool.
32 Tissues.
33 Disposable paper towels.

CONTRA-INDICATIONS

Prior to the manicure, the client's hands are inspected to ensure that there are no conditions which would prevent or modify manicure treatment. Such conditions, or contra-indications, include the following:

☐ Never manicure a nail that shows any signs of disease, such as one where there is inflammation, pus or pain. Such a client must be referred to a doctor.

☐ Never manicure if the nail looks as though it could have been invaded by a bacterial or fungal infection. Signs of this could be a brownish-green or white discoloration, a change in the texture of the nail plate, crumbling of the nail plate and/or separation from the nail bed. Problems like these need to be treated by a doctor, otherwise they might lead to loss of the nail plate.

☐ Never manicure hands if there are any signs of a contagious condition, such as fungal infections of the nail area, ringworm or inflammation. These conditions could be transferred to the manicurist and to her other clients. The client must be asked to see a doctor for treatment, and the condition cleared up before manicuring is undertaken.

☐ Common and flat warts are caused by contagious viruses and thus should contra-indicate manicuring. However, warts are very common and in practice their position and numbers would be a guide as to whether a manicure can be carried out or not. A single wart on a finger can always be covered by a protective waterproof plaster before commencement of the treatment. A wart on the cuticle would be avoided during treatment.

There are many disorders of nails which would not contra-indicate a manicure. In fact, some disorders can benefit from a regular manicure, whilst others need to be attended to by a doctor. (See pages 299–331.)

Record-keeping and booking systems
This substantial topic is covered in its own right later in the book (pages 195–9).

SMOKING

Under no circumstances should the manicurist smoke whilst at work. Such behaviour is unprofessional. Ideally, the manicurist should not smoke at all because smoking leaves an unpleasant smell on the breath which is likely to offend clients.

The client should be discouraged from smoking while undergoing treatment for four reasons:

1 It is difficult to perform a treatment on a client who is using her hands to smoke when the manicurist needs these same hands to work on!

2 The manicurist may find it difficult to work if the client is blowing smoke into her face.

3   At the varnishing stage, ash in the air can land on and ruin the wet varnish application.

4   Most importantly, many of the products used in manicuring, especially for false nail application, are inflammable (e.g. acetone, methylated spirits, some nail varnish removers and varnishes). As such, it is positively dangerous for a lighted cigarette or naked flame to be in close proximity to these chemicals, so this must not be allowed.

The simplest way to prevent smoking during the manicure treatment is to put up a sign behind the manicure station stating:

> DUE TO THE INFLAMMABLE NATURE OF THE CHEMICALS USED IN MANICURING, WE REQUEST THAT CLIENTS DO NOT SMOKE IN THE MANICURE AREA.

If smoking is then allowed in a combined reception and 'waiting for varnish to dry' area, there should be no problems in preventing clients from smoking during their treatments.

Recent evidence regarding the hazards of passive smoking should eventually lead to the complete elimination of smoking in the salon: this is clearly the most sensible course for the salon owner.

SAFETY IN THE SALON

Safety rules: a checklist

At the manicure station

1   Keep all sharp implements out of the reach of children.
2   Always keep the tops on bottles (make a habit of replacing all tops immediately after use) so that if the bottles are knocked over they will not spill.
3   Keep all bottles and solutions out of the reach of children.
4   Do not allow smoking or naked flames near to any of the manicuring materials or chemicals.

In the store cupboard

1   All bottles and jars should be clearly labelled with their contents to guard against future confusion. Modern labelling includes instructions on what to do should swallowing, spillage or fire occur.
2   Labels should be used which will not be spoilt and made illegible by the contents of the bottles.
3   When pouring or handling liquids, always ensure that the label is facing the hand. In this way, if the contents trickle down the side of the bottle, they will not come into contact with the label and render it illegible.

4 No more than 2 litres of inflammable liquids (e.g. acetone, methylated and surgical spirits, or acrylic nail liquids) should be stored in any one place at any one time. This is important in case there is a fire on the premises: the fire would be fuelled by any inflammable materials present.

5 If it is necessary to store more than 2 litres of inflammable liquids on the premises, then these should be kept in a cool, fireproof outside lock-up cupboard, out of the sun, and labelled with a suitable clear sign, such as:

DANGER!

INFLAMMABLE LIQUIDS

Adequate labelling of storage cupboards is needed to allow emergency services such as fire-fighters to identify these chemicals. HAZCHEM signs are available for this purpose.

6 Volatile or inflammable liquids should ideally be stored in glass or metal containers, although modern fire-retardant plastics are now replacing these.

7 Other chemicals which are neither corrosive nor inflammable (e.g. liquid soap or disinfectant) should be kept in plastic or polythene containers, where possible, to reduce the dangers of breakage.

8 All inside storage areas or cupboards should be easily accessible to staff but inaccessible to clients and especially children. They should be labelled with a sign such as

---

DANGER!

POISONOUS AND INFLAMMABLE CHEMICALS

KEEP AWAY FROM CHILDREN

NO SMOKING ALLOWED

---

9 Inside storage areas should also be cool and dark, but brightly lit when necessary for ease of use. This is because heat and light contribute to bacterial growth and chemical degradation.

10 Heavy items, such as gallon containers, should be kept lower down than lighter items, such as extra nail varnishes, so that dangers from incorrect lifting or from the dropping of items can be avoided as far as possible.

11 Aerosols (e.g. nail dry sprays) must be stored in a cool place and must be disposed of in accordance with the manufacturers' instructions. Aerosols must never be disposed of in a fire – they would explode.

12 Any spillages must be cleaned up immediately, using plain water initially, followed by chemically neutral cleaning materials to avoid dangerous chemical reactions between the spilt liquid and the cleaners. The floor must be dried off thoroughly afterwards to avoid slipping.

8 The MANICURE

The procedure outlined in this text is one of several ways to give a manicure. Whatever procedure your instructor teaches you will be equally correct.

Before proceeding with the manicure, ensure that the client is warm, comfortable and relaxed. If she is wearing jewellery, this should be removed and placed in a visible receptacle for the duration of the manicure so that it does not get damaged or hinder the procedure in any way. If facilities are available, the client should be asked to wash her hands and scrub her nails with an antiseptic soap prior to the manicure.

Metal implements should be brought from the dry steriliser and placed into a wet steriliser – a jar containing a cottonwool cushion and a sterilising solution – for use during the manicure.

The manicurist should wash her hands and scrub her nails with an antiseptic soap prior to the manicure, and the client should be aware that she has done so.

PERFORMING THE MANICURE

1 Inspection

The hands and nails must be inspected closely for any signs which would contra-indicate proceeding with the manicure treatment (e.g. fungal infections), and for any areas which would need special care (e.g. hangnails).

If there is any doubt as to the perfect condition of the nail varnishes, the client should choose her colour at this stage (Figure 8.1): the manicurist can then check its consistency and thin it if necessary. This allows time for the pigments to blend properly.

2 Application of antiseptic

If client hand-washing facilities are not available, then, starting with the left hand and using a separate pad for each hand, both hands should be wiped over firmly and thoroughly with a cottonwool pad soaked in antiseptic liquid. This cleans the hands and lessens any risk of cross-infection from or infection of the client if accidents should occur. The hands should be dried and placed comfortably on the sponge support.

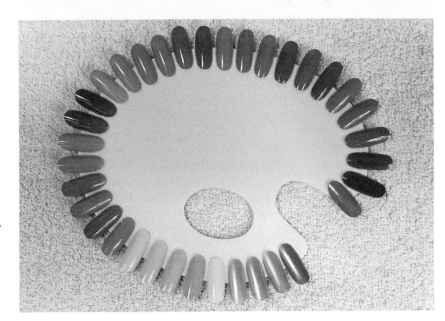

FIGURE 8.1 *A colour wheel, to assist clients in choosing their nail varnish: it is easily made from a make-up palette, some plastic nails, nail glue, and the salon's own range of nail varnish colours*

3 Removal of varnish

Next, the old varnish should be removed. By using a cottonwool pad soaked in remover and held between and beneath the first and second fingers of the right hand, the manicurist's own varnish is protected whilst achieving an efficient removal of the client's varnish (Figure 8.2).

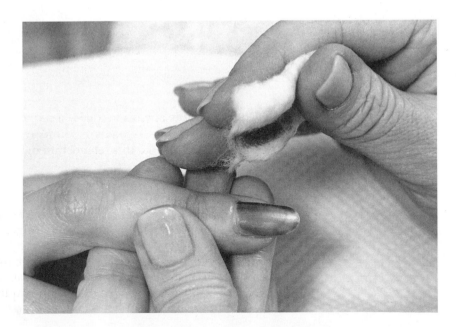

FIGURE 8.2 *Removing the old nail varnish after a thorough inspection of the hands and nails*

Holding the pad against the client's varnish for a few seconds softens the varnish and makes it easier to remove. Two or three firm strokes per nail should be sufficient for the removal of the varnish. A cottonwool-tipped cuticle stick, dipped in remover, should be used to remove any stubborn varnish which may still be adhering to the edges of the nail around the cuticle and nail wall (Figure 8.3).

Check for varnish stains on the surrounding skin and remove these with a clean pad.

The full removal may only require one pad for light colours, but three or four pads to remove a dark colour completely.

Check again for contra-indications or any possible problems, such as a split nail, which may have been hidden by the varnish.

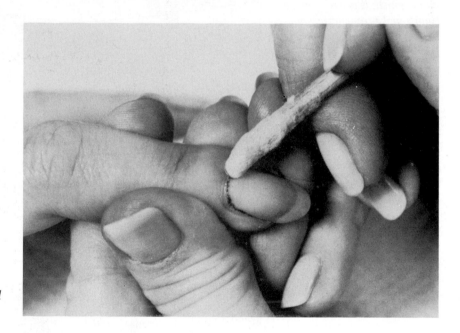

FIGURE 8.3 *A cottonwool-tipped cuticle stick being used to remove stubborn varnish*

It is advisable always to follow a sequence *throughout the whole of the manicure* so that it becomes a sound working routine. Keeping to a standard routine like this means that mistakes or omissions are much less likely to occur.

The right-handed manicurist should start with the left hand. Work first on the thumb, then the index finger, middle finger, ring finger and finally the little finger. Then work on the right hand, starting with the thumb, then the little finger, ring finger, middle finger and finally the index finger. This sequence, when followed during varnish application, will prevent the manicurist from smudging the newly applied varnish: each newly varnished nail is moved safely out of the way as the routine progresses. The sequence is reversed for left-handed manicurists.

4 Filing and bevelling

Placing the right hand comfortably on the sponge pad, the left hand should now be filed using an 18–20 cm (7–8 in.) emery board held at the widest end. The roughest edge of the emery board is drawn across the nail from the side of the middle, at an angle of 30° to the nail plate (Figure 8.4). This action reduces the length of the nail plate, shapes the nail and bevels the free edge, thus sealing the nail layers. A further sealing is effected by finally drawing the smooth side of the emery board across the nail with the same action, then drawing the smooth side downwards over the free edge, again at a 30° angle to the nail (Figure 8.5).

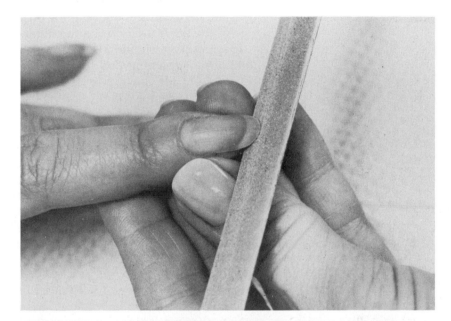

FIGURE 8.4 *Obtaining the desired length and shape: the emery board is held at 30° to the nail*

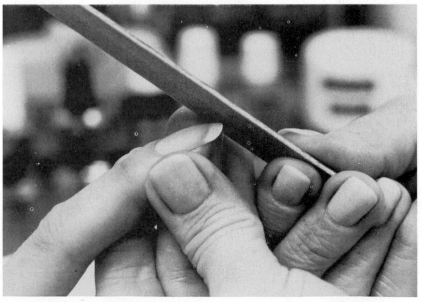

FIGURE 8.5 *Sealing and bevelling the edges: the smooth side of the emery board is drawn downwards at 30°*

The nail should *not* be filed backwards and forwards in a sawing manner, for three reasons:

1   sawing separates the layers of the nail, causing weakness and splits;
2   sawing causes friction heat which dries up the small amount of moisture between the layers of the nail plate at the edge of the nail and thereby gives rise to flaking at the tip of the nail plate;
3   sawing can be unpleasant for the client, 'grating' on her nerves like the sound of dry chalk on a blackboard.

Filing must be done at every manicure to strengthen and neaten the free edge and to help prevent splitting and flaking of the nail tip in between manicures. If fine shaping only is required, then just the fine side of the file is used during the filing of the nail.

The nail plate should ideally never be shaped (e.g. to an oval tip) until it has grown beyond the fingertip. This is so that it will not be necessary to file down into the corners of the free edge of the nail plate and weaken it. To develop nail strength, let the nails grow out straight at the sides for at least 1.5 mm ($\frac{1}{16}$ in.), then shape the tip into the desired shape. However, care must be taken not to leave a sharp 'corner' at the sides of the nails as this would catch on clothing and irritate the client.

Shape and length must be decided upon during consultation with the client, and selected according to her occupation and the shape of the fingers and hands. A basic oval shape is usually the best although some clients, especially those with long nails, prefer a more square effect; and a client who has to wear her nails short can make them look longer by having them filed to a narrower, almond shape (see pages 114–20).

During filing, a mental note must be made of any repairs which need to be carried out later.

Note that careless use of clippers and scissors can lead to the nail plate shattering, splitting or cracking. Use them only on nails which require a lot of length to be removed. Clip or cut into one side, then into the other, to accommodate the curvature of the nail. Attempting to clip or cut all the way across in one movement will result in a shattered nail. The length should be taken down nearly to the required length and then filed the rest of the way using an emery board. In this way if the nail does split, the shape is not ruined, and the free edge is sealed and bevelled correctly with the emery board to avoid future problems such as flaking.

Brittle nails can be soaked in hot soapy water to soften them before clipping or cutting. Most manicurists, however, never use clippers or scissors on natural nails, but quickly reduce excess length with coarse files before 'finishing off' the free edge with a fine emery file.

5 Buffing

If the nails are fine, fragile or splitting, then chamois leather buffing is carried out at this stage.

A small amount of paste polish is applied to the nail plate using a cuticle stick. It is then smudged across the surface of the nail with a fingertip. If there is too much polish the excess will be wasted and just serve to dirty the chamois leather buffer unnecessarily. Each of the client's fingers is held, in sequence, firmly between the thumb and first finger of the left hand (assuming, as before, that the manicurist is right-handed), whilst the right hand buffs the nail plate firmly from the matrix to the tip: this direction of movement stops paste polish from being pushed into the cuticles. If paste polish does get onto the surrounding tissues, it tends to dry them and can be difficult to remove without washing.

To prevent heat build-up, the buffer should be lifted from the nail surface after each stroke. A minimum of twenty firm actions per nail should be performed. At this stage in the manicure, buffing serves to increase the blood circulation to the nail bed and matrix. This improves the colour of the nail, making it pinker and more healthy-looking, and stimulates the nail growth. Buffing will also bind the nail layers together at the free edge, helping to eliminate any peeling of the nail plate and to give the nail a natural shine.

If nail buffing is intended simply to give the nail a smooth, polished look, rather than to prepare it for nail varnish application (as with a gentleman's manicure), it should be done at the end of the manicure. This type of buffing would involve the use of different types of buffer files followed by a drop of moisturising oil, rather than the paste polish and chamois leather method, which can leave a residue around the edge of the nail.

6 Application of cuticle cream

Cuticle cream is now applied to the nail plate with a cuticle stick (Figure 8.6) or directly from a tube. It is massaged into the nail plate,

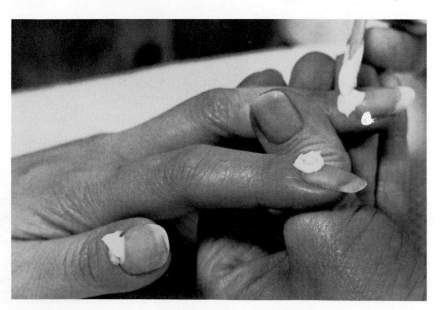

FIGURE 8.6 *Applying cuticle cream using a cuticle stick*

nail wall, cuticle, matrix, and down to the first joint of the finger, in a set sequence in order to achieve proper distribution of the cream and to give a professional approach to its application.

With the manicurist using the thumb, index and middle fingers of both hands, first the client's thumb and little finger are taken and massaged, followed by the index and ring finger, and finally the middle finger and thumb again (Figure 8.7). The thumb is massaged twice because of its large size. The cuticle cream penetrates and moisturises the nail plate and cuticle, and softens the skin and cuticle around the nail. In this it is aided by the warm, soapy water in the finger bowl.

7 Soaking

The fingers are placed in a manicure bowl containing warm, soapy water (Figure 8.8). Any liquid soap is suitable for this purpose and

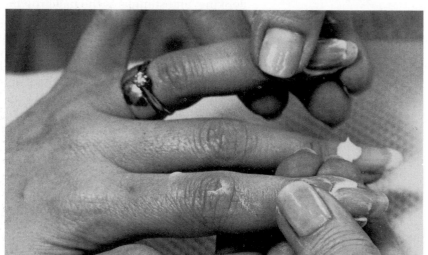

FIGURE 8.7 *Massaging in the cuticle cream*

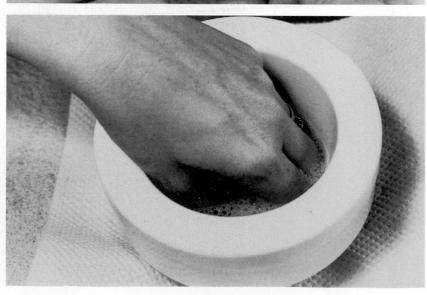

FIGURE 8.8 *The fingers in a manicure bowl containing warm soapy water*

softens the cuticle and nail wall. The water must not be too deep, to avoid accidents and spillage. A depth up to the first joint is sufficient. A non-spill bowl is the most suitable type to use.

8 Repeat for the other hand
Steps 4–6 are then repeated on the client's right hand.

9 Drying the hand
The left hand is removed from the manicure bowl and dried thoroughly (Figure 8.9). The water in the manicure bowl is changed and the client's right hand is placed in the clean, warm, soapy water. If a supply of clean water is not readily available then, because the hands have been previously checked for infections and cleansed with an antiseptic solution, it is acceptable to use the same bowl to soak the right hand. Do check to make sure that the water is still comfortably hot for the client.

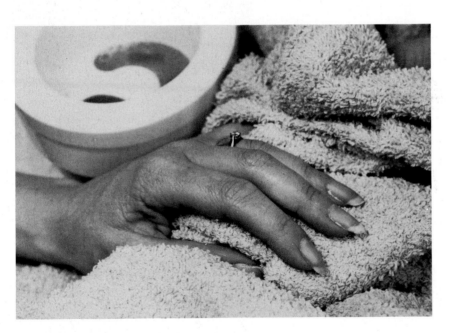

FIGURE 8.9 *The hand is removed from the bowl and thoroughly dried*

10 Cuticle work
Both the pointed and the rounded ends of the cuticle stick are now covered with a small, workable amount of cottonwool. There are three reasons for this:

1 to prevent the cuticle stick from scratching the nail plate during the cuticle work;
2 to cushion the cuticle from the cuticle stick, and thereby help to prevent any damage from occurring to the cuticle and nail wall;
3 for reasons of hygiene, as the cottonwool is used to collect any

dirt from around the nail and the dirty cottonwool is discarded after use on one hand and replaced with clean.

Cuticle remover is applied in four deft strokes to the area around the nail, as follows: one stroke under the free edge, one down the left nail wall, one down the right nail wall, and one across the cuticle. The remover is applied to all the nails of the left hand in succession (Figure 8.10).

Holding a small tissue in the left hand under each of the client's fingers in turn, the pointed end of the cuticle stick is placed in the centre under the free edge of the nail at a 45° angle and rolled first to the right of the nail and then from the centre to the left of the nail (Figure 8.11). These movements are repeated as often as necessary in

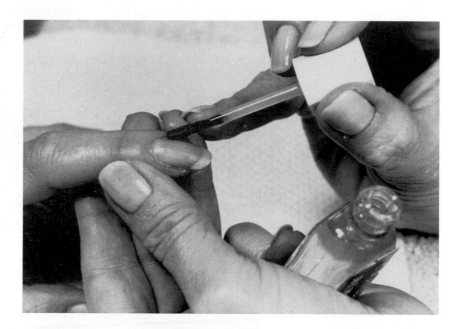

FIGURE 8.10 *Applying cuticle remover*

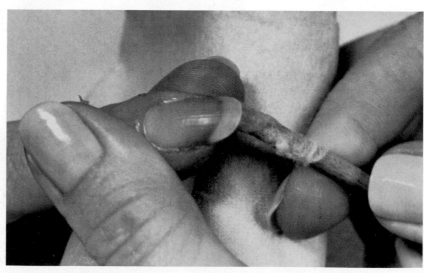

FIGURE 8.11 *Cleaning under the free edge: the cottonwool-covered cuticle stick is held at 45°*

order to remove any dirt lodging in this area. Care must be taken when doing this that the point does not press against the nail plate and nail bed junction: this area is richly supplied with nerve endings and any such pressure would be very painful to the client. The angle at which the orange stick is held is therefore crucial. Dirt removed from under each nail is transferred to the tissue. Finally, the tissue is used to remove the soiled cottonwool from the cuticle stick, and both cottonwool and tissue are discarded.

Next, using the rounded end of the cuticle stick and with the towel under each finger in turn, the cuticle stick is used with tiny circular movements and firm, but not hard, pressure, to ease and lift the cuticle back from the nail plate (Figure 8.12). The sides of the nail against the nail wall must also be included in this treatment. When

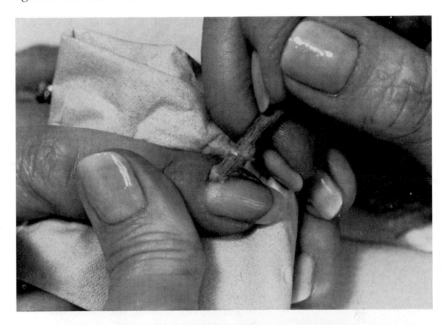

FIGURE 8.12 *Easing back the cuticle and lifting it from the nail plate, using firm pressure and tiny circular movements*

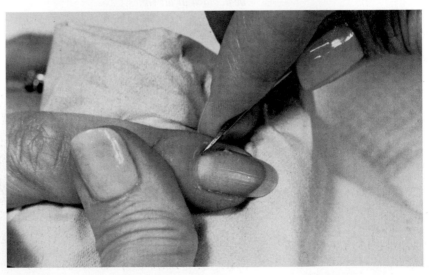

FIGURE 8.13 *Carefully easing back stubborn cuticle using a cuticle knife and light, tiny, circular movements. Plenty of cuticle remover must be used with the knife to prevent it scratching the nail plate*

completed, the cuticle should be well back and, if extensive, lifted into a frill. The nail plate too should be completely free of any adhering dead skin. Stubborn cuticle can be lifted using a knife (Figure 8.13). The cuticle remover should also be used to remove any stains from the surface of the nail, as far as possible. When all five nails are completed, the towel or a tissue should be used to remove the surplus cuticle remover from the nail and to effect a final pushing back of the cuticle.

At this stage, the cuticles are clipped if necessary. It is not good practice to clip the cuticles too much as this can in time lead to a thickening of the skin at the base of the nail. It is better to try to persuade the client to use a good hand cream regularly, a cuticle oil nightly, and push back the cuticles gently with a towel after every soaking in water. In this way, the cuticles can be encouraged to go back into a neat line without excessive future clipping.

Some clients, however, will have problem cuticles which will need clipping and this should be done carefully after they have been well loosened with the cuticle remover and cuticle stick (Figure 8.14). The cuticle should be trimmed just sufficiently to allow a tiny margin of cuticle to remain. More than this and the epidermis will be cut and will roll back, leaving an unsightly fringe of loose skin at the base of the nail.

Care must also be taken not to clip into the flesh line as this results in disproportionate and excessive bleeding due to the efficient blood circulation in this area. If the cuticle is accidentally clipped too deeply, a nasty cut can be caused which is often very painful and liable to infection because of its location. Antiseptic should be applied immediately if the skin is cut, and styptic powder or pressure used to stop the bleeding. A cotton pad must always be placed between any cut and the manicurist to prevent transmission of any blood-carried disease. (Note that if the manicurist has any cuts on her own hands, these must be protected by waterproof plasters, or rubber gloves or finger gloves, during the manicure. *Possible blood-to-blood contact must be avoided at all times.*)

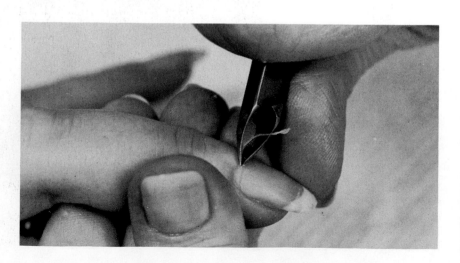

FIGURE 8.14 *Clipping away the cuticle (if necessary)*

A neat edge to the clipping is vital to the appearance of the nail and can be achieved by clipping the fringe of skin away in one complete strip, as opposed to nipping away at it in tiny sections. Any loose dead skin at the sides of the nail should also be clipped away, as should the dead skin portions of hangnails. When clipping is complete, wipe away any remnants of the cuticle remover using a tissue. Then remove any remaining frills of nail plate using the fine side of the emery board, held almost flat and underneath the nail plate.

Finally, place the left hand to rest on the sponge support.

11 Repeat for the other hand

Remove the right hand from the manicure bowl and dry thoroughly. Repeat sequence 10 on the right hand.

12 Cleaning the nails

At this stage, it is usual to scrub the nails with warm, soapy water and a soft nailbrush to remove any fragments of loose skin and remnants of cuticle remover. However, with the development of enclosed, non-spill manicure bowls, this process necessitates the use of another bowl of hot soapy water, or a basin where the client can wash her own hands. If neither of these is available, then a thorough wipe with a soft towel or tissue instead will suffice.

13 Application of hand cream and massage

Hand cream is applied to both hands in turn and gently massaged into the skin (Figure 8.15). The full hand and arm massage is carried out at this stage if required.

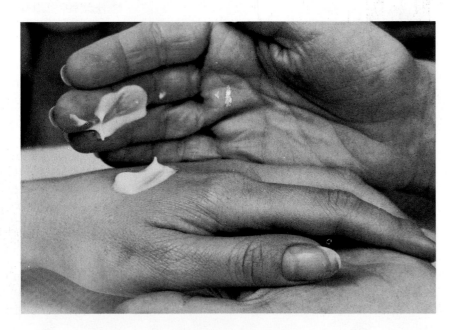

FIGURE 8.15 *Applying hand cream, which is then massaged in*

14 Checking that nails are 'squeaky-clean'

The nails are then wiped over firmly, in sequence, with a cottonwool pad soaked in non-oily and non-acetone nail varnish remover. Correctly done, sweeping the pad firmly to one and then the other side of the nail, this serves to remove all traces of oil and moisture from the surfaces of the nail and to prepare it for the application of nail varnish (Figure 8.16). When the surfaces of the nails are completely clean, they give out a squeaking noise at the end of this process – they are 'squeaky-clean'. This noise indicates that the job has been done correctly; if all the oils and moisture are *not* eliminated, then the nail varnish will bubble shortly after application. The cottonwool pad can be replaced to good effect at this stage by a viscose-fibre tissue or muslin-covered cottonwool pad. These latter two do not shed fibres as does plain cottonwool, so the follow-up application of varnish is made easier.

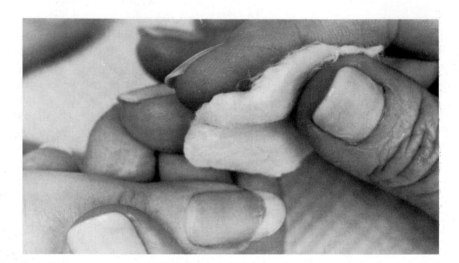

FIGURE 8.16 *Making the nail surface squeaky-clean using nail varnish remover*

15 Corrective treatments

Any repairs or corrective treatments required (e.g. nail wrapping) are carried out at this stage. Alternatively, single extensions or repairs can be done at the end of stage 3 (see 'Nail porosity', page 219).

16 Payment

The client's jewellery should now be replaced and payment taken for the services supplied. If she is in a hurry, then she can be helped on with her coat at this time. Carrying out these operations at this point helps to eliminate accidental smudging after the varnish has been applied.

17 Varnishing

Place a tissue on the manicure cushion and a cuticle stick into the nail varnish remover. These are used to clean up any varnish which may go onto the skin during the application. (To do this, take the cuticle stick out of the remover, touch to the tissue to release excess remover, wipe the affected skin with the damp cuticle stick, wipe the stick on the tissue, and replace it in the remover.

This cleaning up should take place as each mistake happens, nail by nail: do not leave cleaning up until the end of varnish application or the varnish will be difficult or impossible to remove, because it will have set.

The base coat is applied to the nail surface whilst following the correct digital sequence (Figure 8.17). This is followed by the nail varnish, and then by a top coat if necessary, again following the standard digital sequence. Varnish is applied with the minimum number of strokes and coats necessary to achieve a perfect finish. (See page 124 for discussion of the correct application of varnish.)

Nail varnish bottle tops must be wiped clean after use, to avoid air getting to the varnish in the bottle: this would cause evaporation of the solvent and thickening of the varnish. Wiping can be done using the soiled pad which was used to squeak the nails clean (Figure 8.20).

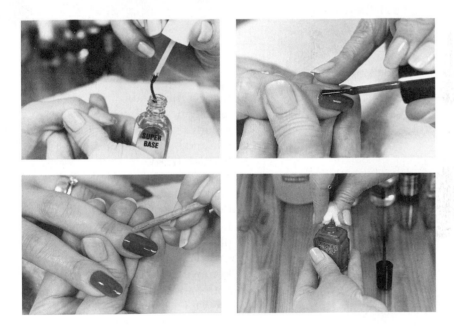

FIGURE 8.17 *Removing excess varnish from the brush before applying base coat to the nail surface; it is essential when working on the nails to maintain the correct sequence*

FIGURE 8.18 *The edge of the brush being used to achieve a straight edge when applying the nail varnish*

FIGURE 8.19 *Cleaning up after a mistake, using a cuticle stick dipped in remover; this must be done immediately*

FIGURE 8.20 *Wiping the bottle top before putting the varnish away*

18 Drying

A quick-drying spray or liquid may be applied to the nails at this stage to speed the drying of the nail varnish, but on no account must it be applied *between* applications of coats of varnish as this would give a greasy film to the surface of the nail and prevent correct adhesion of the varnish. The client should be asked to sit patiently until her nail varnish has dried, with drinks and magazines being available if required.

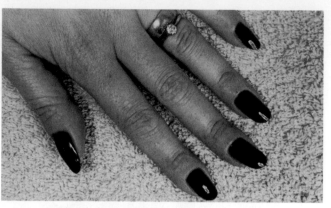

FIGURE 8.21 *The completed manicure*

The manicure sequence: a checklist

1   Inspect the hands.
2   Antiseptic – both hands.
3   Remove varnish – both hands.
4   File and bevel left hand.
5   Buff left hand.
6   Apply cuticle cream to left hand.
7   Soak left hand.
8   Repeat steps 4–6 on right hand.
9   Remove left hand from soak; dry; change water in the bowl; place right hand in soak.
10   Cuticle work on left hand; clip.
11   Remove right hand from soak; dry; cuticle work and clip.
12   Both hands: clean nails with warm soapy water and nailbrush; dry. *Or* wipe nails clean with a soft tissue.
13   Apply hand cream to both hands. Massage if required.
14   Wipe over nail plates with nail varnish remover until 'squeaky clean'.
15   Carry out any necessary repairs, reinforcements or extensions. Buff if varnish is not required.
16   Client replaces her jewellery; makes payment; puts on her coat if necessary.
17   Apply base coat.
18   Apply nail varnish and top coat if necessary. Wipe bottle tops before replacing the lids.
19   Apply quick-drying spray or liquid if required.

TIDYING THE MANICURE STATION

Immediately upon completion of the manicure, the following procedures should be carried out so that the station is left in readiness for the next client.

1 All the used materials – tissues, cottonwool, viscose tissues, emery boards and so on – should be disposed of into closed containers.
2 Used hand towels should be removed and put to be laundered.
3 The top of the manicure table should be wiped over. Isopropyl alcohol-impregnated disposable wipes are ideal for this purpose. If these are not available, a cloth rinsed in hot soapy water (and optionally containing a small amount of disinfectant) should be used.
4 The manicurist should wash and dry her hands.
5 Clean hand towels should be placed ready for the next client and the hand- and armrest covered with a clean piece of disposable tissue.
6 All used manicure implements should be scrubbed clean in hot soapy water, dried, and immersed in a suitable sterilising solution for the length of time recommended by the solution's manufacturer. After this time, the implements should be removed from the solution, rinsed, dried, and either used again immediately or placed into a dry sterilising cabinet to await their next use. If the manicurist has two sets of implements, this routine causes no problems.

    If implements have been in contact with blood, autoclave sterilisation may be necessary. However, recent advances in knowledge about hepatitis B virus (HBV) and human immunodeficiency virus (HIV) show them to be less resilient than was at first thought. This knowledge, coupled with advances in the effectiveness of chemical sterilisation liquids and techniques, renders the use of an autoclave unnecessary in such low-risk areas as manicuring, hairdressing and beauty therapy *as long as all the other daily sanitation and hygiene rules are closely adhered to as a matter of daily routine and cleanliness.* However, some local authorities may demand the use of an autoclave as a necessary requirement of running a manicure salon in their area. (Also, some examining boards may demand information about their use as part of their syllabus.)

Remember – a dirty salon is not a hygienic salon, nor will it attract or keep clients. Without clients, the manicurist does not have a job.

HOME CARE FOR NAILS AND HANDS

Hands and nails are such an important part of a person's appearance that they should be guarded and protected, to prevent skin from becoming roughened and stained and nails from becoming broken and flaky with dry, split and overgrown cuticles. They should not simply be presented occasionally to a manicurist for 'reconditioning' after being neglected in daily life.

The more the client looks after her hands and nails in between manicures, the less will need doing during the manicures (which reduces the expense for her), and the better her nails will look both after and between her manicures.

Here are some hints to pass on to clients for the home care of their hands and nails:

□ *Care of cuticles* To maintain cuticles in good condition, apply cuticle oil or cream to each nail nightly. This prevents the cuticles from overgrowing onto the surface of the nail, and thereby prevents hangnails, keeps a neat border to the nail between manicures, and almost eliminates the need to clip the cuticles during the manicure.

□ *Dry hands* If the hands are very dry, they should be massaged with plenty of treatment cream or warm oil (almond or olive, preferably with the addition of a capsule of vitamin E oil) last thing at night. A pair of plain cotton gloves can be worn to prevent soiling the bedclothes.

□ *Using the hands* Care should be taken when using the hands. Obvious danger areas are opening car and house doors, cutting vegetables with a knife, dialling old-style telephones, and using a typewriter. Ways should be found to minimise the damage to the free edges of the nails, such as dialling using a pencil instead of a fingertip.

□ *Gloves* Gloves should be worn while doing potentially damaging work. Rubber gloves give protection against hot water, soaps, detergents, bleaches, and the like; cotton or leather gloves give protection against work that may cause calluses or staining, such as gardening or cleaning silver or brasses. A liberal portion of hand cream applied before the gloves are put on will be of benefit to the hands.

□ *Barrier creams* When gloves are not being worn the use of barrier creams is effective in preventing stains.

□ *Preventing stains* Before doing really dirty jobs, the nails can be scraped across the surface of a bar of wet soap. This deposits soap under the nails; this can be washed out after the job has been done, thus preventing staining under the nail. This is a good thing to do when wearing rubber gloves for a really dirty job – it protects the nails if the fingertip of the glove splits halfway through the work!

□ *Drying the hands* Hands should be dried thoroughly after washing them and a good hand or hand and nail cream smoothed in immediately. This is made easier if pump dispensers of a good cream are kept by every basin in the house.

□ *Cold weather* Hands should be protected against cold weather by rubbing in hand cream and putting on a pair of gloves before going out into the cold.

☐ *Stains* Household stains can be removed immediately, before they have a chance to become embedded, using lemon juice. If the stain is too strong for this – as for fruit and berry juices, potato stains and dyes – then a chlorine bleach can be carefully used: a small amount can be applied using a cotton bud or cottonwool-covered cuticle stick, and then rinsed away with plenty of clean water once the stain has been removed.

☐ *Refreshing the varnish* If the client is freshening up her varnish at home, the drying time can be reduced by the use of an oil-based quick-drying spray (available from the salon), or by running the damp varnish underneath the cold water tap.

☐ *Preserving the varnish* The application of a clear top coat to the surface of the nail every day, or every other day, will serve to brighten up the varnish, prevent it from wearing away at the tips, and give added strength and protection to the nail plate and free edge.

9 NAIL SHAPE and LENGTH

SHAPE

There are many considerations to be taken into account when choosing a shape of nail which will suit the client, the first of which is her own preference regarding shape. However, time must be spent with a new client, educating her as to the nail shapes available and advising her as to which shape might be preferable for her occupation whilst taking into account the strength and natural shape of her nails.

It must always be remembered that it is the sides of the nail which give the nail plate its support. If these sides are filed away to give the nail a narrower appearance, then support is lost and the nail is weakened (Figures 9.1 and 9.2). This can easily be demonstrated to a client by bending her nail downwards. If the sides have been filed away then the nail will bend at a line of weakness level with where the filing has been started at the sides. Often there are cracks in this area which the client will require mending. She will also complain that when her nails break, they do so very low down when she has just grown her nails to a reasonable length (Figure 9.3). This is because the nail plate can no longer withstand the stresses incurred when a mechanical knock, magnified by the length of the nail, transmits pressure to the line of weakness. If the client is then shown the manicurist's own nail – which should be of the stronger straight-sided but rounded-tipped variety – and invited to bend this shape of nail, she will see that any pressures inflicted on this nail shape are evenly distributed over the whole surface and the nail does not bend at or possess a line of weakness in the same way as a pointed nail does (Figure 9.4). This demonstration alone should be sufficient to encourage a client to grow her nail into a stronger shape.

The second consideration for choosing a nail shape is the client's lifestyle. If she is keen on sports, bear in mind that long nails will prevent her from holding a racket efficiently, or break easily when subjected to the stresses of sailing and the like. However, if her sport is something in which the hands are not involved, such as jogging or aerobics, then long nails will present no problem. If she has young children, then long nails can cause difficulties: they may scratch the child, make it hard to fasten buttons, and so forth. Most mothers choose a shorter nail shape.

The third consideration is the client's occupation. A typist, check-out operator or pianist needs a strong nail shape in order to avoid breakage. Some clients from this group manage to keep their nails quite long as the constant tapping on the keys seems to stimulate the

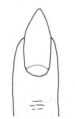

FIGURE 9.1 *A pointed nail*

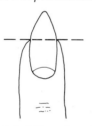

FIGURE 9.2 *A line of weakness is caused by filing away both sides of the nail: the nail will bend here whenever it hits a hard surface, and cracks will appear at the sides*

FIGURE 9.3 *The breakage of a pointed nail is low down, across the line of weakness*

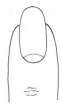

FIGURE 9.4 *A nail with straight sides and a rounded tip: here the sides give maximum support to the nail plate, so there is no line of weakness*

blood circulation and make the nails grow extremely strongly. However, the manicurist would not put long false nails onto a member of this group: the change from short to long would make the client unable to do her job properly, and the nails would not last as long as they should due to the knocks incurred. A shorter nail, straight-sided with a rounded tip, or a round nail, would be best for this client. If the client is in an occupation in which her hands are on show – such as employment as a jeweller, a sales assistant for lingerie, cosmetics or perfumes, an air hostess or an executive – then smart long nails are certainly desirable: they are an asset to her job.

The fourth consideration for a choice of nail shape is the shape of the client's hands and fingers. For example, short stubby fingers can be made to look longer and more slender if the nails are given a long oval shape; square nails on this type of hand would serve to emphasise the squat, square shape of the fingers and be most unflattering. A very long tapering finger would look spindly if the nail were to be long and tapering also: a shorter, more squared-off nail would add width to the fingers and give a more balanced effect.

A client with nails which curve downwards excessively, or nails which are very thick, would benefit from an oval or almond-shaped nail. This shape takes away a lot of the bulk of the nail, making it look more delicate. It also helps to give an illusion of straightness to the downward curve.

The fifth consideration, and this applies only if the client wishes to keep to her own natural nails and does not want false nails, is the structure and shape of the client's own nail plate (Figure 9.5). A flat nail (Figure 9.6) or a claw nail (Figure 9.7) will never be able to grow

FIGURE 9.5 *A normal nail: the gentle sideways and lengthways curves give structural strength to the nail plate*

FIGURE 9.6 *A flat nail: the flattened plate has little structural strength, and this nail will easily bend and break at the flesh line*

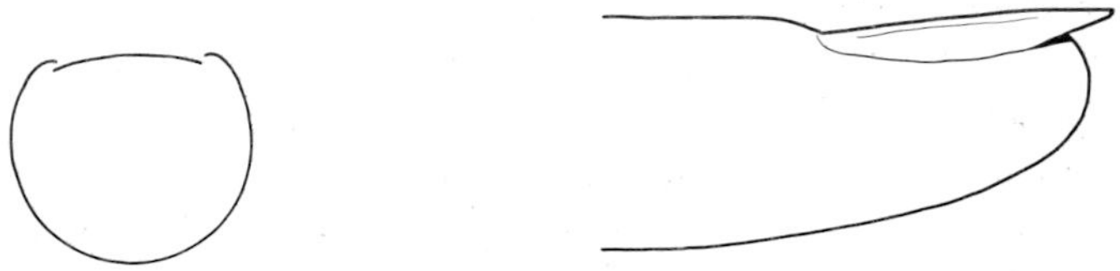

FIGURE 9.7 *A claw nail: although such nails are usually thick and strong, their hooked growth creates uneven pressures when they are knocked, which leads to breakage low down*

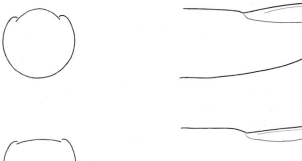

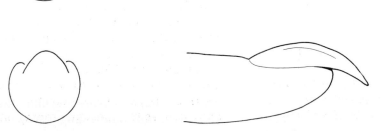

very long – the shape cannot withstand even normal pressures without bending over and cracking along the stress lines at the sides. Only clients with a normal nail or a nail slightly curved lengthwise will ever achieve the ideal of a length of half to the full length of the body of the nail again beyond the flesh line. Once this is understood, then the shape of the flat and claw-shaped nails can be modified to look attractive at a shorter, neat length.

Basic nail shapes

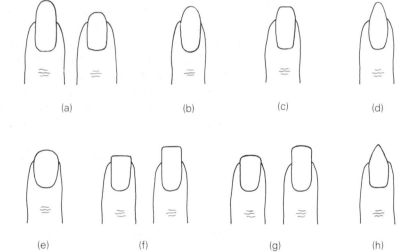

(a)   (b)   (c)   (d)

(e)   (f)   (g)   (h)

FIGURE 9.8 *Basic nail shapes: (a) straight-sided, with a slightly rounded tip; (b) oval; (c) square oval; (d) almond; (e) round; (f) square; (g) square with rounded corners; (h) pointed*

Straight-sided, with the nail slightly rounded at the tip

To create this shape, the sides are allowed to grow straight forward without filing, whilst the tip is gently rounded at the end (Figure 9.8a). This shape has maximum support from the sides, making it the strongest of the nail shapes. It also has an advantage over the other shapes in that if damage occurs to the side of a nail, the damage can be filed away to leave the nail slightly oval on either side, rather than having to file away the length of the nail in order to remove the damage. As the nail grows, the tip can be squared off a little at each filing and it will automatically regain its original shape. This shape is also one of the most attractive shapes and helps fingers to look straighter, longer and more slender.

Oval

The oval shape is created by filing the tip of the nail into an egg shape (pointed end) and filing away some of the sides of the nail

(Figure 9.8b). This weakens the nail to some extent, but is a flattering, feminine shape which a lot of ladies with short and mid-length nails like. It is ideally suited to nails which are thick or wide or which hook over, as it gives them a lighter, more delicate appearance.

Oval with a squared-off tip

This shape is created by filing away the sides slightly as if creating an oval nail, but the tip is squared off instead of being rounded (Figure 9.8c). It is useful to narrow a too-wide nail, and the squared-off tip adds to the strength by giving a more even weight distribution should the nail be banged against a hard surface.

Almond

The almond-shaped nail used to be thought of as the classical nail shape (Figure 9.8d). It is filed away at the sides and softly pointed at the tip so that the finished whole shape of the nail is similar to that of an almond kernel. This shape is not very strong and, if damage occurs to the side of the nail, the length of the nail has to be filed away to eliminate the damage. Because the nail is filed away at the side, the flesh of the finger shows on either side: this can make the fingers look fat. Although attractive and entirely suitable for short nails, this shape will not encourage the nail to grow to its maximum length which should be borne in mind if that is what is desired.

Round

This nail shape is ideal for a shorter nail. It is softly rounded on the tip after being encouraged to grow straight out for approximately 1.5 mm ($\frac{1}{16}$ in.) at the sides (Figure 9.8e). It is strong, neat and entirely suited to people who need to keep their nails short, such as health workers and most gentlemen.

Square

Square-shaped nails are created by allowing the sides to grow straight forward without any shaping, then filing the tip straight across at right angles to the rest of the nail plate without any curvature (Figure 9.8f). This shape of nail was in fashion in the early 1960s when the singer Cher helped to make it popular. However, it is really quite conspicuous and is usually only popular among clients with very long nails who wish to draw attention to them. Short square-shaped nails make hands look blunt and heavy. Long square-shaped nails make a good base for nail art designs.

Square with rounded corners

Square-shaped nails with rounded corners look somewhat prettier and softer than severely square nails, and do not catch on clothing as much as do the plain square-shaped nails (Figure 9.8g). This shape is flattering on very long nails and makes a good base for nail art designs. It is not suitable for short, wide-bodied nails or fan-shaped nails as it emphasises the shortness and makes the fingers look stubby. However, for people with narrow nails who need to keep their nails short (e.g. gentlemen), it provides an alternative choice of nail shape.

Pointed

Pointed nails are filed away at the sides and to a point at the tip (Figure 9.8h). Ladies who file their own nails at home often have this shape of nail: they mistakenly think that they have to file the sides every time they file the nail, and so a pointed shape develops. Then they find that they can never get any real length to the nails due to the weakness of this shape and this is usually the reason that they come for a professional manicure. The manicurist must tactfully point out to such clients that a pointed nail shape is the weakest as it has no strength or support at the sides. It has a tendency to break easily and very low down on the nail. It is also old-fashioned and unflattering to the hands. Ladies with this nail shape often think that it is very attractive but that is usually because they are unaware of alternative nail shapes and genuinely believe that this shape is the 'correct' shape for nails to be.

Problems

Curved fingers

Index and ring fingers are usually the problem here, the index finger often having a slant towards the little finger and the ring finger often bending towards the thumb. Extra care must be taken when shaping the nail. If the slant of the fingers is ignored and the nail tip shaped to follow the main body of the nail, then the curvature will be emphasised. The nail tip must be filed away more on one side than the other to give the finished appearance of a straight finger (Figure 9.9).

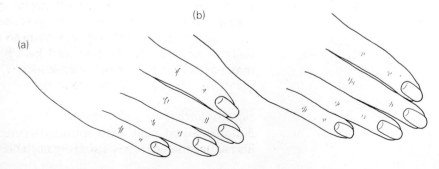

(a)   (b)

FIGURE 9.9 *Correct filing for a curved index finger: (a) the nail has been shaped normally; (b) more has been filed away on one side than the other to give the optical illusion of a straight finger*

Nail plate too narrow and small

To grow the nails long would draw attention to the smallness of the body of the nail. This nail type also has a tendency to curl under sideways, creating a point to the tip. Because of this, it is best not to let this type of nail grow too long and to file it into a shape which is square with rounded corners. This shape will give extra width, so the finished nail will look a reasonably normal shape once the curling has developed. It will also add bulk to the body of the nail, making it appear larger. If the nail plate is very curled, or very narrow, nail extensions can be used to straighten and widen the nail plate by a small amount.

Fan-shaped nails

A common and unfortunate nail shape is one where the body of the nail widens out as it gets nearer to the fingertip, thus giving a fan shape to the nail (Figure 9.10). Here, earlier instructions not to file away the sides of the nail must be disregarded as this is precisely what must be done. Filing away the sides as if trying to make an oval shape will give the desired straight-sided shape to the nail tip. This type of nail is often flat and therefore does not have the natural structural strength to grow very long. A short oval or round shape is probably the best shape to aim for.

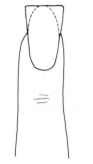

FIGURE 9.10 *Correct filing for a fan-shaped nail: file away the sides to leave a straight-sided or oval nail*

Duck-billed nails

These nails curve upwards when left to grow to any length (Figure 9.11). The solution here is never to let the nail grow past the point where it begins to curve upwards, and to choose an oval or almond shape as this will narrow the flat tip and lessen the appearance of any upswing. If longer nails are desired, then false nails must be used.

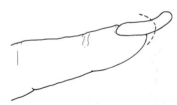

FIGURE 9.11 *Correct filing for a duck-billed nail: file away the length beyond which the nail grows upward, and use an oval or almond shape to minimise the flatness*

Claw nails

These nails curve downwards when left to grow to any length (Figure 9.12). This type of nail is often excessively curved sideways, too. It is best not to let this type of nail grow too long for two reasons: first, it will curl over and look unattractive; second, this nail shape is also at its weakest where it bends over the fingertip, where its curve is at its greatest. If the nail is banged, the pressure is greatest on this area which is thus most prone to cracking or breaking. If the nail is thick and wide, then it needs thinning at the sides to create a more delicate and attractive oval or almond shape. If the nail has excessive sideways curvature, then the sides must be left to grow straight forwards, adding width to the shape.

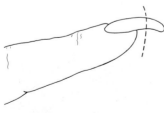

FIGURE 9.12 *Correct filing for a claw nail: file away the length as the nail begins to hook over*

Flat nails

These nails need to be filed away at the sides a little to eliminate bulk and create a flattering almond or oval shape. Their flatness means that they will be prone to bending backwards easily, so they will easily develop cracks at the side of the nail along lines of weakness. These will have to be filed out or repaired as they occur. It is best to select a reasonably short length for flat nails as they do break very easily.

LENGTH

For an elegant length which is still practical and manageable, it is desirable that the free edge of the nail be up to half as long again as the main body of the nail. This length is balanced and attractive, and most normal nails can support this length (or near to it) without too many problems. Beyond this length, extreme care has to be taken with the nails, but they can be grown if desired up to the length of the body of the nail again before all proportion with the hands is lost and simple jobs such as fastening jewellery or buttons become impossible. Nail length is really a matter of proportion with the hands, client choice, and the practicable length which the shape and strength of the nail will support. Each individual is different.

10 VARNISHING

PREPARING THE NAIL PLATE

It is in the client's own interests that she replaces her jewellery, pays her bill and puts her coat on before the nail varnish is applied. This will prevent undue smudging of the wet varnish.

Oils and moisture must be removed from the surface of the nails before nail varnish is applied or else the varnish may peel. If strong solvent residues (e.g. acetone) are left on the nail surface, these can also cause peeling and give rise to a dry, flaky nail condition.

The surface of the nail can be prepared for the varnish application in any of three ways:

1. The client can wash her hands in warm soapy water and dry them thoroughly.
2. The nail surface can be wiped 'squeaky clean' with a non-oily nail varnish remover or 70 per cent alcohol (methylated spirits), then wiped over again with pure water on a pad to remove the solvent.
3. One of the more modern, gentle, non-acetone and non-oily nail varnish removers may be found suitable for wiping over.

Although it has always been traditional to use cottonwool pads for the removal of nail varnish and the wiping over of the nail plate before nail varnish application, it will be found that small viscose-fibre tissues, or muslin-covered cottonwool pads (Nail Neats), will perform both functions more efficiently. When removing varnish, viscose fibre or Nail Neats soak up the dissolved varnish, preventing it from smearing onto the client's cuticle. Thus fewer pads, and consequently less remover, are needed to complete removal. Cotton-wool does not soak up the varnish but allows it to stay on the surface of the pad, necessitating the frequent turning and renewal of the pad if stale varnish is not to be transferred onto the surrounding skin. For wiping over the nail plate prior to nail varnish application, viscose-fibre tissues or Nail Neats are far superior as they do not shed fibres onto the surface of the nail and surrounding cuticle in the way that cottonwool does. Such stray fibres can make the following varnish application difficult. If cottonwool is used, the use of real cottonwool instead of synthetic varieties keeps shedding to a minimum, but it still occurs.

A disadvantage with the use of viscose-fibre tissues is that they cannot be held underneath the manicurist's fingers in the way that a cottonwool pad can, and so they are difficult to use without causing the smudging of the manicurist's own nail varnish. Another drawback to the use of Nail Neats and viscose-fibre tissues is that they cost far more than plain cottonwool. However, viscose-fibre tissue used in manicuring is similar to that which is manufactured as disposable kitchen wipes. A very cheap method of obtaining it, making it as cheap to use as cottonwool, is to buy the larger kitchen wipes and cut them up into 7–8 cm (3 in.) squares. These can be folded into four at the time of use to make them an ideal size and thickness.

PREPARING THE VARNISH

The nail varnish must be checked to ensure that it is of the correct consistency for use. The solvent ingredient of the varnish is chosen to have a quick evaporation rate so that the varnish will dry quickly when it is on the surface of the nails. However, this also means that the solvent will evaporate quickly all the time that the lid is off the varnish bottle and when the varnish is in use, causing the varnish to thicken in its consistency. Because of this, the application of varnishes must be rapid and on no account must bottles be left open to the air when not in use. This rapid evaporation of the solvent is the reason why it is important to always wipe the tops of nail varnish bottles clean before replacing the lid tightly, thus ensuring a good, airtight seal and no evaporation of solvent during storage. Manicurists in very hot climates find that keeping their nail varnishes in a refrigerator helps to reduce the evaporation of the solvents and maintain the consistency of their varnishes.

Varnish can be thinned using the same solvent or mixture of solvents as forms the base of the varnish. As different nail varnishes use different blends of solvents, it is important to use a thinner supplied by the same manufacturer as the varnish. A thinner based on a different solvent may not be compatible and could prevent the nail varnish from hardening or slow down its setting time. Nail varnish must *never* be thinned with nail varnish remover: removers contain oil, water and other impurities which would prevent the nail varnish from hardening.

It is advisable for the clients to choose their nail varnish colour prior to the treatment, so that the manicurist can check the consistency and add thinner if necessary, allowing time for the varnish to stand and the solvent to blend thoroughly with the other constituents before use. This is not always necessary (depending on the quality of the varnish being used) as the solvents used in modern high-grade varnishes disperse in the product very quickly. However, it is best always to ensure that the varnishes are the correct consistency *after* use and *before* returning them to the varnish store, so that they are always ready for use, as it frequently happens that the client changes her mind about the choice of colour immediately prior to the application. A colour wheel will help the client in making her selection – see Figure 8.1 (page 97).

APPLYING THE VARNISH

In anticipation of nail varnish application, a small tissue should be placed on the work area and a cuticle stick and the nail varnish remover placed readily to hand. These items are there to clean up immediately any varnish which may get onto the skin. Do not leave this clean-up process until the end of the application or a thorough and complete clean-up cannot be effected: do it straight away, nail by nail, whilst the varnish is still wet.

Cleaning up mistakes

The manicurist should have the rounded end of the cuticle stick standing in a container of nail varnish remover and, when a clean-up is necessary, take the stick from the remover, tap it onto the tissue to dislodge any excess liquid, and use it to wipe away any varnish on the skin (Figure 10.1). Only one wiping movement should be made at a time before the stick is wiped on the tissue, re-dipped in the remover, tapped on the tissue, and used again. In this way the stain is not spread but is removed efficiently. Care must be taken to pull the nail wall away from the nail whilst doing this, so that the varnish on the nail plate is not caught and smudged.

If the cuticle edge of the varnish is not as neat as it might be, it can be straightened by following the same method but using the pointed end of the cuticle stick to wipe a straight line to the edge.

It is important to tap away the excess remover before the cuticle stick is placed next to the nail: any excess remaining would flood the cuticle, where it could dry out the skin, affect the drying time of the varnish, and also disrupt the neatness of the edge of the varnish application.

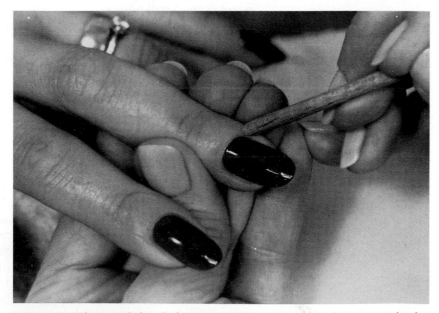

FIGURE 10.1 *The rounded end of a cuticle stick being used to clean up a mistake in the varnish application*

Application

The application of base coat, coloured varnish and top coat uses essentially the same technique, but obviously it must vary slightly to accommodate both the width of the nail plate and its shape around the cuticle. There are three basic shapes to be considered:

1   a normal-sized nail plate with an almond-shaped base margin;
2   a normal-sized nail plate with a square-shaped base margin;
3   a wide nail plate, such as a thumb or big toenail.

For all three shapes, the initial stages are the same.

The bottle of nail varnish must be shaken or rolled gently, or both, to distribute the pigment and solvent evenly without creating air bubbles in the varnish.

The bottle should be held, if the manicurist is right-handed, in the palm of the left hand, supported upright by the ring and little fingers (Figure 10.2). In this way the bottle is always held ready for use, and the thumb, index and middle fingers are left free to hold the finger of the nail which is being varnished.

To get the correct amount of varnish on the brush, the first time the brush is removed from the varnish this must be done slowly and with a circular movement, thereby pressing all sides of the shaft of the brush up against the inside of the neck of the bottle to remove all the varnish from the shaft. If this is not done, a drop of nail varnish is likely to gather on this shaft and roll down onto the nail plate during application, flooding the plate. When the end of the shaft is reached, the brush should be pressed up against the far side of the bottle and gently withdrawn (Figure 10.3). There will be sufficient varnish on the correct side of the brush for application to cover the surface of a normal-sized nail without re-dipping. When it is necessary to re-dip, dip the brush only, not the shaft, back into the varnish and repeat the last movement to withdraw it.

It is important to hold the client's fingers correctly between the index and middle fingers and the thumb of the left hand, with the fingers and thumb pulling the nail wall down away from the nail plate to be varnished and able to rotate the finger in any direction necessary to assist in the application of the varnish. The varnish brush must be held between the thumb, index and middle fingers of the right hand and the whole of the right hand must be stabilised by the little finger being placed on the tip of the middle finger of the left hand (Figure 10.4). Although this position feels awkward at first, after a short time it becomes easy and will result in a rapid application with no tremors or shaking affecting the final result.

Again to increase stability, the manicurist must lean part of her lower arms onto the table during the varnish application. There is no stability if she holds the client's hands up in the air, as is apparent when the manicurist has to varnish in a less than perfect situation, such as whilst the client is having her hair attended to. It is much more difficult to apply varnish in such circumstances.

The first touch of the varnish brush to the nail plate must be

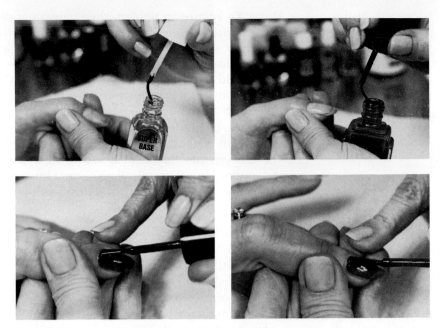

FIGURE 10.2 *Holding the bottle: it is supported between the palm of the hand and the little finger*

FIGURE 10.3 *Pressing the brush against the far side of the bottle to remove excess varnish*

FIGURE 10.4 *Holding the varnish brush; the hand applying the varnish is stabilised by the little finger to ensure a perfect application*

FIGURE 10.5 *Using the straight line of the brush head to give a straight edge to the nail varnish*

three-quarters of the way down the nail plate but nowhere near the cuticle. The brush will have a drop of varnish on its tip at this stage and if this was to come into contact with the cuticle, it would flood into the cuticle and be virtually impossible to remove completely.

This first placement of the brush, three-quarters of the way down the nail plate, puts the majority of the varnish in an area where it can be worked – underneath and to the back of the varnish brush. The brush is then gently pushed forward: the surface tension of the varnish will stop it from spreading, allowing the manicurist to create a straight line which she can place a hair's breadth away from the cuticle (Figure 10.5). As soon as this is done, the brush is pulled away from the cuticle in a long straight stroke to the tip of the nail plate. When holding the brush, do not hold it straight up with only the tip on the surface of the nail, but let the brush *angle downwards* so that the varnish is being spread by a good length of the brush: this will lead to a more even and smoother application. The excess varnish on the brush at this early stage of application will go to either side of the first stroke and can be worked in with following strokes.

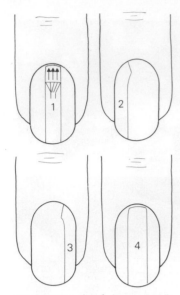

FIGURE 10.6 *Applying varnish to an almond-shaped nail base; the same technique is used in applying base coats*

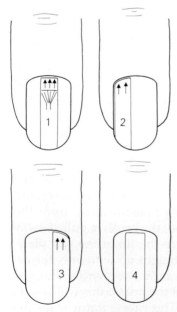

FIGURE 10.7 *Applying varnish to a square-shaped nail base*

To ensure an unblemished varnish application, it is important that this first stroke reaches all the way from the cuticle to the nail tip. If a short stroke – one not covering the full length – were made using a pearlised varnish, a brush mark would be left in the pearlising which would be impossible to eradicate. Although the placement and pushing of the varnish may seem difficult at first, this method is very quick and will give a perfect nail varnish application every time once it has been mastered.

This *first* movement applies to all the shapes of nail. *Subsequent* movements vary slightly according to the shape of nail being worked upon. However, all varnish must be applied using as few strokes as possible in order to achieve a smooth and even finish.

Almond-shaped nail base

Placing the tip of the brush towards the centre of the base of the nail, carefully sweep the brush to the left-hand side of the nail and let the varnish flow to create a neat edge to the varnish which follows the line of the cuticle wall but is a hair's breadth away (Figure 10.6). Do not angle the brush to the left but simply press down more to the left side of the nail. The sweep of the brush is then continued in a long straight stroke to the tip of the nail. This stroke is repeated on the right-hand side of the nail. The varnish application is completed by placing the brush next to the base of the nail plate at the centre and then making a long straight finishing stroke to the tip of the nail plate. This last stroke will bring together all the previous strokes and give an even finish to the varnish application.

(Note that base coats, because of their more fluid consistency and the fact that they are clear, are often applied this way regardless of the shape of the nail.)

Square-shaped nail base

Here the second stroke consists of placing the tip of the brush near the cuticle on the left, letting the varnish flow to the tip a little and pushing the varnish towards the cuticle to form a neat edge into the square of the nail (Figure 10.7). The stroke is completed by sweeping the brush in a long straight sweep to the tip of the nail plate. This movement is repeated on the right-hand side of the nail. The final stroke is down the centre, from the base to the tip, to give complete cover. Toenails are usually painted in this way as they are nearly always square-shaped.

Wide nail plates, such as the thumb and big toe

Because of the size of the nail the manicurist must expect to have to re-dip the brush into the varnish half-way through the application. Do not try to load enough varnish onto the brush to cover the whole nail at the first attempt: this will only lead to a thick and uneven application which will not dry properly.

The method here is the same as for square-shaped nails except that

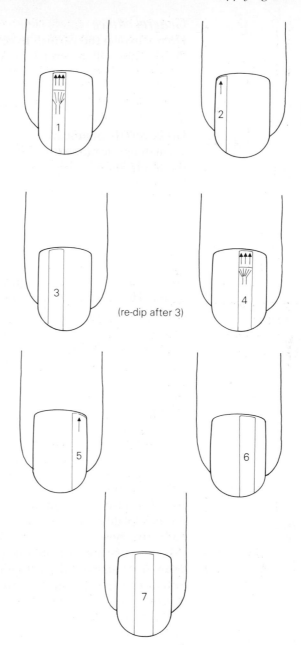

FIGURE 10.8 *Applying varnish to a wide nail base such as a thumbnail or big-toe nail*

up to seven strokes of the brush may be necessary to obtain an even finish. The first movement is started to the left of the centre of the nail plate. The second is from the base to the tip down the left-hand side. The third is from the base to the tip on the right of the second stroke. At this stage, the brush should be re-dipped to obtain more varnish. The next three strokes are a mirror image of the first three, on the right-hand side of the nail; and the final stroke is from the base to the tip straight down the centre of the nail plate.

General advice

Do not expect the varnish to cover evenly on the first coat. Whether it does or not will depend a great deal on the colour and consistency of the varnish being used, and if the varnish has poor covering power it is best, both for drying and lasting qualities, to apply very thin coats and increase the number of coats rather than the thickness of the application. Complete cover should be effected on the second coat. However, the manicurist should endeavour to get the margins of her varnish application correct on the first coat as this will then speed up the application of the second coat. If small mistakes are made in the first coat, they can often be covered up by the second coat. Large mistakes should be rectified by cleaning off the varnish and starting again.

Do not keep stroking the brush over the surface of the nail in an attempt to get the varnish application perfect. As the solvent evaporates from the varnish being worked, the varnish will become sticky and impossible to work with: the application will be made worse, not better. The manicurist should try to restrict herself to the advised four strokes on a normal nail and no more than seven on a larger nail. If the nail varnish application is uneven after this, it should be corrected by applying another thin coat after the previous coat is dry.

Base coats

It is important to use a base coat underneath any nail varnish application, including a clear application, because the formulation of base coats includes an adhesive resin which helps the base coat to adhere to the nail and the following varnish to adhere to the base coat. It is also important as a protective barrier to prevent staining of the nail plate by the coloured pigments contained in some coloured nail varnishes.

Base coats are available in plain or ridge-filler formulations. The latter are usually milky with a matt finish. When used on ridged and pitted nails, more of the product will settle into the dips and hollows of the nail than will coat the higher areas: the surface is thereby levelled, and the following varnish application looks more even. Ridge-filler base coats are often used on false nails and nail repairs.

It is vital that the base coat is thoroughly dry before the application of coloured varnish, or peeling or bubbling may occur and the varnish will not last as long as it should. Ridge-filler base coats take longer to dry than normal base coats and so the time of application is greater. Colour can be applied on top of colour before the previous coat is thoroughly dry, but base coats *must* be dry before proceeding.

Smudges

The client may smudge her nail varnish at the end of the treatment. If the varnish is not completely dry it will be found to be 'workable' using a dampened thumb pad. The varnish can be coaxed back into perfection, or nearly so, in this way. If a slight blemish remains, it can usually be smoothed away, with a coat of top coat if the varnish was a cream application, or with another coat of colour if it was a pearlised application. Almost all smudges can be returned to perfection in this way. If correction is unsuccessful, there is no alternative but to remove the varnish and start again. The client *must* leave the salon with her nails perfectly varnished.

One way in which a varnish application can be quickly ruined is for the satisfied client to sit back at the completion of the work and pat both hands firmly down on the work area. This causes dust to rise up from the work area and land on the wet varnish! It usually happens when the client has sat through a long treatment, such as the application of artificial nails. There is nothing that can be done to correct the situation except remove the varnish and start again. Prevention, however, is easy and simply means the manicurist getting into the habit of shaking clean her work area covering, or disposing of one covering and placing a clean one down before nail varnishing is commenced.

Nail-drying cosmetics

Various applications are available to speed up the drying time of nail varnish, including nail dry oils and sprays. These work partly by speeding up the drying, but also by putting an oily and slippery coating on the surface of the nail so that any slight scuffs slide off the surface of the nail, leaving no imprint on the varnish. The oily varieties also help to condition the cuticles.

Because of their oily content, it is important that these preparations are not used in between the coats of nail varnish: they would cause the varnish application to bubble and peel.

There are hot-air nail dryers now available, but note that forced rapid drying can result in a varnish application which chips easily. Care must be taken when selecting such equipment.

The number of coats needed

Clear varnish
1 Base coat.
2 Two coats of natural nail varnish followed by a glossy top coat *or* two coats of clear top coat.

Very pale pearlised varnishes
1   Base coat.
2   Three coats of the pale pearlised varnish.

Dark pearlised varnishes
1   Base coat.
2   Two coats of the dark pearlised varnish.

Cream varnishes
1   Base coat.
2   Two coats of cream varnish (three if the colour is *very* pale).
3   One coat of clear, glossy top coat.

The application of a top coat to damp pearlised varnishes can disrupt and spoil the pearlised finish. Pearlised varnishes are formulated so that they do not need a top coat. However, if it is desired to use a top coat so that the application will last longer, the manicurist must ensure that the pearlised varnish is dry before applying the top coat.

If the manicurist advises her client to apply a coat of clear top coat to the nails every other day at home, this will brighten the varnish and make the manicure last longer – a week on natural nails, and three weeks or more on artificial and very hard nails.

The reason that nail varnish lasts longer on artificial and hard nails than on a normal nail plate is that artificial nails do not bend when banged against objects, so the varnish is not subjected to stresses which may cause it to crack and chip. It will, however, wear away from the ends of artificial nails if top coat is not applied regularly as a preventive. Normal nails flex and bend when banged against anything and the varnish cannot bend with it completely and maintain its adhesion. It therefore lifts, cracks, and peels away.

A hard nail plate will hold onto its varnish longer than will a soft one, so the use of a hardener can in time help a client with the problem of cracking and peeling nail varnish. The use of plasticised, chip-proof top coats also helps to protect the varnish.

PROBLEMS DURING WEAR

Chipping

1   A flaky nail plate. If the client's nails are flaking, then as the flakes break away, so will the varnish. Nails in this condition need to have their edges buffed at each manicure to bevel and seal the flakes and help control the situation. Nail glue can be used on the tips before buffing if the condition is severe (see page 315).
2   No base coat, or an unsuitable one, was used.
3   The nail varnish was force-dried, using a fan or heater.
4   The varnish was applied too thinly.
5   The varnish used had been thinned down too much.

6 The surface of the nail was incorrectly prepared – oils or moisture or both were left on the nail plate prior to application of varnish *or* an unsuitable harsh or oily solvent was used to 'squeak clean' the nails and then left on the surface of the nail plate prior to application of the nail varnish.

Peeling

1 The surface of the nail was incorrectly prepared (as above).
2 The base coat was not thoroughly dry before the first coat of varnish was applied over the top.
3 An unsuitable base coat was used. Base coats should be of a thin, quick-drying consistency and contain adhesive resins to hold the varnish to the surface of the nail.
4 The varnish was applied too thickly.
5 The varnish used was too thick and needed to be thinned down.

Bubbling

1 The surface of the nail was incorrectly prepared (as above).
2 Nail dry cosmetics were applied between coats of nail varnish.

Very infrequently, problems with bubbling or peeling nail varnish on isolated individual clients are caused by:

1 The client being diabetic. Either the drugs or the condition can cause the nail surface to be 'slippery' so that varnish will not stay on the nail.
2 The client having an 'allergy' to the varnish, the only signs of this being that the varnish peels off in sheets shortly after application. Using a different brand of varnish can solve this problem.
3 The client having an 'allergy' (see 2) to the solvent left on the surface of the nail. This can be solved by wiping the nail with plain water or by washing and drying the hands before varnish application.

STYLES OF APPLICATION AND NAIL ART

'No varnish' varnish

Many ladies do not want to wear a coloured nail varnish, or cannot wear one because of their job (e.g. workers in the health and catering professions). Often these ladies are the most fastidious about their nails looking clean, though in fact a nail need not actually *be* dirty to *look* dirty. If a manicurist does a massage and then looks at her unvarnished nails, she will see that the oil makes her nails look discoloured underneath; this dirty appearance will not go until the nails have been scrubbed with soap and water a number of times. The nail plate can also be discoloured from peeling potatoes, smoking, or wearing coloured varnishes without a protective base coat.

The old-fashioned remedy to this problem was to resort to clear varnishes and wear nail white pencil underneath the nail tip to disguise any discoloration or dirt gathered there. However, the nail white pencil washes away when the hands are washed and needs to be continually reapplied if the nails are to look clean and healthy.

The modern techniques employ nail varnishes to re-create a natural, healthy look which can last from manicure to manicure without needing attention and also give the nails the protection of a nail varnish coating.

All that is needed are the usual base and top coat varnishes, plus a soft white varnish to create the tip and a translucent pale pink varnish for the body of the nail. These two colours are usually sold in pairs, especially for this purpose. It is vital to use the correct colours or the effect can look artificial.

Whichever of the following styles of nail varnish application is used, a cuticle stick should be placed in a container of nail varnish remover and a tissue placed on the work area so that corrections can be rectified, as explained earlier (page 123), immediately they occur and before the varnish dries on the skin. Mistakes must be expected during unusual varnish applications and must be corrected perfectly.

French style (French manicure – see front cover)
1 Prepare the nail plate and apply base coat as normal.
2 Using the white tip colour, create a tip to the nail by first touching the excess varnish to the centre of the tip of the nail, before sweeping the brush from the left, two-thirds of the way over the tip, then from the right, two-thirds of the way over the tip. Finish off if necessry with a sweep across the centre of the tip to create an even arc of off-white varnish. If one of the nails does not have much free edge (due to breakage), then the white tip can be used to create an illusion of length by showing the free edge to be a little wider than it actually is.
3 Apply a coat of the pale pink translucent varnish to the whole surface of the nail plate.
4 Apply top coat.

American style (American manicure)
1 Prepare the nail as normal, but also clean underneath the nail tip with solvent on a cottonwool-tipped cuticle stick. (Use the pointed end.)
2 To apply the white tip colour, the manicurist should hold the client's hands with the palms facing towards her so that she can see the undersides of the nail tips. The varnish must be taken from the bottle by pulling the brush towards the manicurist, thus leaving the varnish on the opposite side of the brush to the

normal one. The brush can then be used directly to paint in the underside of the free edge of the nail.

3 Apply base coat to the surface of the nails as normal.
4 Apply one or two coats of the translucent pink or clear to the surface of the nail to achieve the desired cover.
5 Apply top coat to finish.

There is little difference in appearance between the French and American ways of creating the 'no-varnish' varnish application: the choice of technique used is largely a matter of personal preference. The American way is not suitable for ladies with discoloured nail plates as the white has to show through the nail plate. However, if the nail plate is not discoloured, then the American method can be used, with a clear varnish or nail-hardening varnish application on the surface of the nail if desired, to give a really natural appearance. The French technique demands the use of a slightly coloured top varnish to stop the tip from appearing too white and to blend it in with the rest of the nail plate.

Half-moon

This is a method of nail varnish application which was popular in the 1940s and 50s and involves varnishing the nail plate but leaving the half-moon (lunula) free of varnish. It does have the optical effect of shortening the nail length.

1 Prepare the nail plate and apply base coat over the whole of the nail.
2 Using the 'flow' of the varnish around the base of the brush to create the clear line of the arch, apply the varnish in a similar way to painting almond-shaped nails. Leaving the lunula area unvarnished, take the first stroke around to the left side of the nail, the second stroke around to the right side of the nail, and the third stroke straight down the middle of the nail. Care must be taken to form a gentle arch of omission in the half-moon area. Note that it is easier to obtain a regular-shaped arch in this way than by trying to paint in an arch first and then filling in the nail plate. In the latter method it is virtually impossible to obtain an even arch: there will always be a tendency for it to be 'lop-sided'.
3 Apply a second coat of coloured varnish in the same way.
4 Apply a coat of top coat over the whole of the nail plate.

Shading

This is a simple, popular and effective introduction to nail art. Three (short nails) or four (long nails) blending shades of nail varnish are

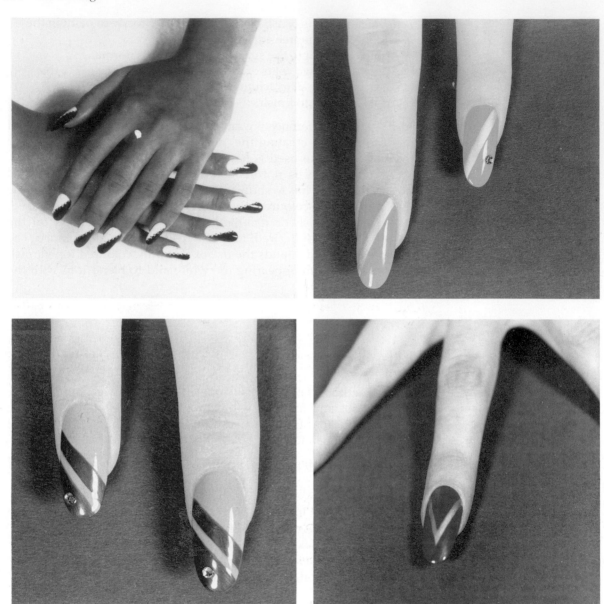

FIGURE 10.9 *Examples of nail art, all of which can be reproduced using the instructions below and suitable colours*

selected, such as pale pink, medium pink, deep pink, and a dark pinky red. It is inevitable that nail varnish will go onto the nail wall during this application, especially when the second colour is applied, so a thorough corrective technique is essential.

1 Prepare the nail plate as normal and apply base coat.
2 Apply two coats of the palest colour.
3 With the next colour, first dab the excess varnish into the centre of the nail and then use the brush to draw a line of varnish from

the outer base corner of the nail to the inner area where the nail tip leaves the flesh of its bed. Fill in the whole of the tip with the varnish. Make sure that the tip itself has only a thin covering of varnish but that the area next to the line, for about 0.5 cm ($\frac{1}{4}$ in.), is perfect in its coverage. This is to ensure a reasonable drying time – the subsequent build-up of coats on the tip increases the drying time.

4 The next colour is applied in the same way, only nearer to the tip of the nail. This coat has to be kept in balance so that if three colours are used each covers approximately a third of the area of the nail plate. If the nail is longer and four colours are used, the proportions have to be adjusted accordingly.

5 The whole application is then covered with a top coat, to merge the layers together and make it look as if the varnish was all applied as one. It is important that the top coat be applied on an angle too, or the colours may be drawn by the brush and streak over one another.

Increased time has to be allowed for the drying of this type of varnish application.

This basic technique can be used to create coloured diagonal effects and even 'V' shapes (Figure 10.9). Diamante or striping tape can be added to create more striking effects. They are added at the end, by sinking them into the final layer of varnish and sealing them in place with a layer of top coat. Striping tape must be cut just short of the edges of the nail plate to prevent it catching and lifting. Diamante can be picked up on the dampened sharp end of a cuticle stick to aid its placement.

SELECTING THE COLOUR

The choice of colour of nail varnish needs to be based on the client's preference, her skin tone, and the condition and size of her hands and nails.

Nails in poor condition, such as badly bitten or very short nails, should not have a varnish on them which will draw attention to them. Ideally, bright reds or gaudy colours should be avoided, something pale and subdued being preferable. When it is the hands which are in poor condition, however, as when the joints are deformed by arthritis, well-manicured nails and a bright varnish can draw attention *away* from the hands and onto the nails.

When trying on clothes, it rapidly becomes obvious that some colours flatter, adding a radiant healthy glow to the complexion and minimising any flaws, whilst other colours have the opposite effect of making the skin appear sallow, ruddy or grey. The nail varnish colour can have the same effect on the hands. The right shades will minimise lines and wrinkles and make the skin look healthy. The wrong colours will emphasise blemishes and make the skin look sallow, ruddy, blue or grey. So noticeable is this effect that the profession of 'colour coding' has arisen from its study. In its most primitive form, colour coding is based on the fact that all printed and manufactured colours are made up of varying combinations of three other colours – yellow, greenish-blue (cyan) and bluish-red (magenta): see Figure 10.10. Each of these colours – blue, red, and yellow – gives an underlying hue to the complete colour. In colour coding, all the colours are referred to as being blue-based (cool or synthetic) or yellow-based (warm or natural) – see Figure 10.11. Thus there can be a yellow-based red (clear, clean bright red or orange-red) and a blue-based red (fuchsia or raspberry red) with many shades of red in between these. Contrary to popular belief, any woman can wear a red nail varnish, as long as it is the right shade of red to match her skin tone. However, not every woman should wear purple for, as can be seen from the diagrams, it is a blue-based (cool) colour and therefore most suited to people with cool skin tones. Orange too cannot be worn by everyone as it is a yellow-based (warm) colour and therefore most suited to people who have a warm skin tone.

Colour coding is most frequently based around the four seasons, with Autumn and Spring types (warm) having a fair and freckled, or pinkish, cast to their skins; and Winter and Summer (cool) having a blue cast to their skins. Thus the Autumn and Spring types will best suit the warm, yellow-based colours, whilst Winter and Summer

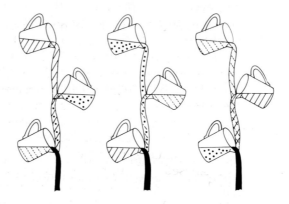
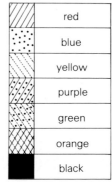

FIGURE 10.10 *The three basic colours when added together make black; red and blue together make purple, blue and yellow together make green, and red and yellow together make orange*

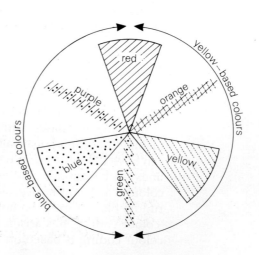

FIGURE 10.11 *A wheel showing colour mixing: red and blue make purple, blue and yellow make green, red and yellow make orange, and all the other colours are made with different proportions of the three basic pigments. Colours between red and green on the yellow side are known as yellow-based colours, and have an underlying yellow hue; those on the blue side are said to be blue-based*

types will suit the cool, blue-based colours. Spring and Summer types are just lighter, cleaner, brighter versions of the darker, mellower Winters and Autumns, and the colours they suit follow the same trend.

Of course, few things in life are this simple and the study of colour coding is much more involved, with clients often falling between categories and with many colours suiting more than one category. However, many clients have undergone colour analysis and may ask their manicurist's advice as to which colours will be best for their particular season. In addition to this, the manicurist needs to be able to assess the client's skin colouring and guide her to a suitable choice of colour. Colour coding gives suitable guidelines to help the manicurist to do this.

The skin colour should be assessed by looking at the wrist area or the palm of the hand: these areas are less likely to have been altered by exposure to sunlight and will consequently give a truer picture of the client's skin coloration. It is a good idea to place a white card or towel under the area being examined as it is easier to make a correct assessment if there are no distracting colour elements nearby.

Winter

The skin colouring for Winters is extremely varied. It can have a yellow cast (e.g. oriental skins), in which case the use of yellow-based colours will make the skin look sallow, whilst use of blue tones will whiten out the yellow tones in the skin and have a smoothing and softening effect. Winters can also have pale to dark olive skins, or pale to dark beige-based taupe skins, with or without rosy undertones. This group also includes pale to black skins. In all cases, use of a yellow-based colour will make the skin look sallow. This group also includes milk-white skins with dark hair, the 'Snow White' types. Blue-based and strong colours are needed, such as primary colours and vivid blue-based, cool colours, such as medium to dark pink-based plums, true red, bright burgundy, plum, taupe (beige-based grey), icy blue-based pink, icy violet, blue-based red, royal purple, bright fuchsia, magenta, shocking pink, deep hot pink. Avoid browns, golds or oranges.

Summer

The skin colouring for Summers has a definite blue undertone and usually an accompanying pink tinge. Some Summers have fair skin, others pink or rose-based beige. Sometimes they have white skins with blue veins showing through. Yellow-based colours will make the skin look dirty and emphasise any veins. Blue tones will whiten the skin, bringing out its delicacy and minimising the veins. A colour which is *too* blue will have a negative effect, draining the colour from the skin; that is why Summers' colours are lighter and brighter than Winters' colours, even though they are both blue-based. Choose soft pastels and cool colours with blue undertones, such as light to medium pinks and light-to-medium plums, soft fuchsia, raspberry, lavender, orchid, mauve, rose pinks, pastel and powder pinks, blue-based reds, burgundy, rose-based beige, rose-based brown, cocoa. Avoid oranges and golds.

Autumn

Autumn people are often strawberry blondes or redheads with freckles. They can have ruddy skin tones and the use of blue-based colours on these drains the skin of colour and emphasises any ruddiness. A yellow-based colour, however, will cool down the ruddiness and even out the skin tone. Autumn people always have golden undertones (sometimes even near orange) to their skins, which can vary from creamy peach and ivory to medium or deep copper. They need strong colours which are golden and yellow-based, such as orange, mocha, dark peach, dark apricot, russet, orange red, salmon, rust, terracotta, mustard, warm beige, gold, yellow gold, dark brown, bronze, coffee, caramel, mahogany. Avoid pink, burgundy or purple.

Spring

Spring people tend to have fair, pinkish, delicate blonde skin with pale freckles and golden undertones. They are a lighter, brighter version of the Autumns, and their skin can vary from a creamy ivory to peachy pink or pale biege. They often have rosy cheeks. Blue-based colours will drain the skin of colour, making it look unhealthy. Yellow-based colours, especially the yellowy pinks, will add warmth and a fresh healthy glow to the skin. The colours chosen should all be clear, delicate and bright, such as light peach, coral, coral pink, light orange, apricot, salmon and pastel pinks, orange-red, clear bright red, warm pinks, light beige, pale golden browns, medium violets, light gold. Avoid burgundy.

Sun-tanned skins

For a recent tan with golden beige skin tones, choose yellow-based colours such as corals, true reds, yellow-oranges. As the tan fades, avoid the yellow-based colours as these will then have a tendency to make the skin look sallow: change to colours with pink undertones, to bring back warmth.

Age

With age, the skin can become muddy-looking. The light, soft, muted pinky-browns normally chosen by this age group do nothing to lift the skin tones. The skin needs *more* colour, not less. A dusky pink (more pink than dusky) will add warmth and sparkle without being jazzy. It will brighten and clarify the skin tone. Particularly unkind are the dark browns and purples, which emphasise any lines and wrinkles.

Summer and winter

In the summer, it is more flattering to choose lighter, brighter members of the same colour families. In the winter, it is more flattering to choose darker, richer and deeper members of the same colour families.

Toenails

Fingernails and toenails look better if the nail varnish colours match. If this is not desired, then the choice should be to put the stronger, brighter colour on the toes, not the other way around. Dark, bright colours make the feet look cleaner, prettier and well cared for, much more so than do pale colours.

11 ADDITIONAL TREATMENTS

HOT OIL MANICURES

Hot oil manicures are recommended as a way of improving dry and flaky nail conditions, brittle nails and dry cuticles. The heat used in the treatment aids the penetration of oils and nutritive elements into the nail plate, cuticles and surrounding skin. Hot oil manicures can be as simple or as complicated as the manicurist wishes them to be. All are carried out during the course of a manicure at the stage when the soaking sequence would normally take place.

First the nail varnish is removed, then the nails are filed, and this is followed by the oil treatment instead of the usual cuticle soak. The oil treatment is followed by a massage, to work in the surplus oils; then the cuticle work is carried out and the manicure treatment completed by the application of varnish.

The most complicated of the hot oil treatments involves the use of a small infra-red lamp or a pair of electrically-heated mittens and a plastic bag, plus ten $2\frac{1}{2}$ cm (1 in.) bandages of approximately 20–30 cm (8–12 in.) length. The recommended oil mixture is two parts olive oil to one part almond oil. Each fingernail is wrapped in an oil-soaked bandage and the hand placed under the infra-red lamp *or* in a plastic bag and inside the electrically-heated mittens for fifteen minutes. After this time, the oil should have been absorbed. The bandages should be removed and the remnants of the oil massaged into the hands.

An easier method of carrying out a hot oil treatment involves the use of two parts olive oil to one part almond oil, or pure almond oil, which is heated, placed in a manicure bowl, and used for a soaking sequence of about ten minutes. The remnants of the oil are then massaged into the hands. If excess oil remains, it should be removed with soft disposable tissues.

Recent developments have included the manufacture of special nutritive creams designed to be used with electrically-heated bowls. The fingers are placed to soak in the warmed cream for a recommended time, usually about ten minutes, after which they are removed and the remnants of the cream massaged into the hands before the manicure is completed.

PARAFFIN WAXING

Paraffin waxing is a treatment which is used both on the hands and on the feet. It gives the following benefits:

1 it is a deep cleansing and toning treatment;
2 it stimulates the blood circulation, invigorating the tissues and improving their health;
3 it makes the skin soft and supple, making the cuticles easy to work and helping to eliminate hangnails and calluses;
4 it improves dry and chapped hands and feet;
5 it will temporarily plump out the wrinkles on hands, an effect that will last for several days;
6 it relieves pain in muscles and joints, such as the pain of arthritis, rheumatism, muscle spasms and inflamed joints: it is especially effective in relieving the pain of rheumatoid arthritis.

The wax

Many commercial waxes are blends of paraffin wax, which is obtained from the distillation of petroleum, and beeswax from beehives. Both waxes are solid at room temperature, but for the treatment of hands and feet they are warmed to 53 °C (127 °F) at which temperature they are liquid. (*Caution*: wax for use on the face is heated only to 43 °C (110–115 °F).)

Both waxes are highly inflammable, to the extent that their direct heating, even in a double boiler, is not recommended. They should be heated in purpose-built paraffin wax baths, in which the heating element is sealed away from the wax.

When the wax has been used for the body or the foot, or when essential oils have been added to the wax to increase the therapeutic value, the wax must be discarded after use. However, if the wax has been used solely on the hands, then it is permissible to recycle it by boiling it up with water in a pan. After it has been left to cool and settle, it will be found that any impurities have sunk to the bottom and can be scraped away, leaving the surface wax reusable.

The treatment

Before treatment commences, make sure that the surrounding areas are protected from splashes or spills by disposable tissues or plastic sheets. The wax is difficult to remove from fabrics and furnishings. If an accident does happen and wax spills onto fabric, the best way to remove it is to place the fabric between sheets of blotting or brown paper and go over the area with a hot iron. The wax will melt and be drawn out of the fabric and into the paper. This method cannot be used with all fabrics – prevention of accidents is better than cure!

Warm towels or insulated mittens should be ready for use, along with two plastic bags or clingfilm (saran wrap) to cover the hands or feet. The client's clothing should be adequately protected and her jewellery removed from the areas to be treated. The wax should be heated up and its temperature tested to ensure that it is not too hot.

1   The client should immerse the whole hand (with fingers spread apart) and lower arm, or the foot, into the wax bath (Figures 11.1 and 11.2).

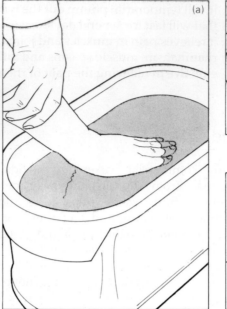
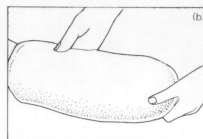
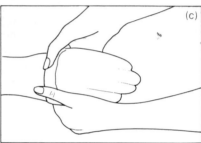

FIGURE 11.1 *A paraffin wax treatment for the hands: (a) the hand being dipped in the wax; (b) the hand wrapped in an insulated mitt; (c) the wax being peeled away*

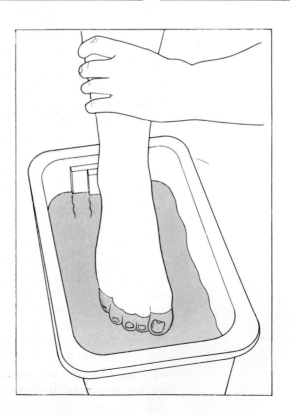

FIGURE 11.2 *A paraffin wax treatment for the feet*

2 Remove the limb from the wax bath, wait five to ten seconds for the wax to solidify, then immerse again.
3 Repeat until the limb has been dipped five to ten times.
4 Place the limb into a plastic bag or wrap in clingfilm (saran wrap). Then wrap the limb in warm towels. (An insulated mitten can be used instead of the towels.) Leave the limb in this way for 15–20 minutes or as long as the wax retains its heat.
5 Unwrap the limb and peel the wax off. The wax should be either discarded or recycled, as described on page 141.
6 The limb should now be massaged with a nutritive oil or cream, and the treatment followed by a manicure or pedicure.

NAIL BUFFING

Due to the advances made in buffing materials in recent years, nail buffing now falls into two distinct categories. The choice of method will depend on the original condition of the nail and on the desired end product.

Chamois leather buffing using paste polish

This method (see pages 100–1) is the original method of buffing and until recently the only one available. It is recommended as a way of improving the condition of fine, fragile, peeling and splitting nails with a poor colour of nail bed. It has two main effects on the nail plate.

First, the slight abrasive qualities of the paste polish used in conjunction with the buffer smooths the nail's surface into a shiny finish and helps to bind the nail layers together at the free edge of the nail plate. This helps to eliminate peeling of the nail layers. The action in this method is very gentle, and would not be sufficient to eradicate major problems such as psoriasis pitting or extensive ridging.

Secondly, the buffing action stimulates the blood circulation to the nail bed and matrix, improving the colour of the main body of the nail to a healthy pink shade. An improved blood circulation results in an improved and stronger nail condition as the new nail grows. It also stimulates the nail growth. For buffing to be effective in these ways it needs to be carried out daily over a long term (it takes about 4–6 months for a new nail to grow from base to tip – pages 278 and 331–2) without the abrasive paste polish used during the manicure sequence. Daily use of paste polish would wear away and weaken the nail plate.

Buffing using graduated buffer files

Recent advances in materials have led to the development of files whose sole purpose is to achieve a high gloss shine and a smooth surface to the nail plate. Their use has no effect on the blood circulation to the nail bed and matrix.

Buffing files are available in many forms. The misleadingly named 'three-sided' buffers are the ones most commonly used and sold to the client for her use at home. These are actually two-sided files: on one side are a fine-grade emery paper and an even finer grade, each taking up one half of a side of a strong foam file; on the other is a yet finer emery paper or a fabric. When used in sequence from the fine to the very fine grades, a high gloss shine can be built up on the surface of the nail plate. It is recommended that the coarsest grade of emery is used only at the first buffing. Subsequent buffings should utilise only the two finer sides, or even the one finest side, to maintain the shine. This is because a layer of nail is being rubbed away each time the coarse emery is used and frequent use would weaken the nail plate.

The different grades of emery and fabric are also available as individual files for professional use. Some systems use abrasive fabrics instead of emery papers; other systems supply squares of these fabrics and grades of emery which can be placed in special holders or clips. The choice is simply a matter of the manicurist's preference.

It is because the first emery is mildly abrasive that this type of buffing is so useful in correcting any rough nail plate conditions. Buffing files are invaluable for smoothing nail plates pitted by psoriasis or dermatitis, or ridged through an arthritic condition or other illness. They are used to buff a flaky nail condition smooth and to seal the edges of the nail tip. Buffing files will remove stains (e.g. cigarette stains) as they remove the top surface of the nail.

Buffing files are also used to smooth the nail plate and remove any fragments of nail glue still adhering to the nail's surface after false nails have been removed. They are used to buff out any irregularities and to put a high gloss finish on artificial nails. As artificial nails grow away from the cuticle with the nail plate, glues and buffer files are used to smooth and seal the join between the artificial and natural nail plate. Buffer files can even be used to buff scratches off the surface of gold nails.

Because they do not involve the use of messy paste polishes, and because they impart a high gloss to the surface of the nail, buffer files are often chosen for use in a manicure in which nail varnish is not required, such as a gentleman's manicure. Here the buffing would take place at the end of the manicure, in place of the application of nail varnish, and not after filing as would be the case if chamois leather buffing were being carried out.

The buffing technique used with buffer files – as opposed to the method used with chamois leather buffers and paste polish – is different in other ways too. With paste polish it is important that the buffing movement is from the matrix towards the tip of the nail, so that paste polish is not pushed into the cuticle area. This is not important with emery buffers. However, both techniques do demand that the buffer be lifted from the nail after each stroke, or every few strokes, to prevent heat build-up on the nail's surface.

GENTLEMAN'S MANICURE

A gentleman's manicure is carried out in basically the same way as a lady's manicure except that usually no nail varnish is applied.

Gentlemen usually require their nails to be filed short, neat, and with a round or square shape to the free edge (see page 117). Buffing is usually carried out to give a natural sheen to the nails; this can be done using either a chamois leather buffer and paste polish prior to soaking the nails, or with a three-sided buffer file at the end of the sequence. The condition of the nails will determine which of these options is chosen: if the gentleman is a heavy smoker, or if his nails are discoloured due to his occupation (e.g. with dyes or ink stains), then a three-sided buffer file can be used to eradicate these stains; if the nails are in relatively good condition, then chamois leather buffing will give a more natural sheen to the nails rather than a high gloss finish.

MANICURE MACHINES

Electric manicure machines normally fall into two categories: battery-operated machines, and machines working from mains electricity.

Battery-operated machines

These are usually quite small, the motor part designed to be desk-standing and connected to the working heads via a lightweight cable. (Very small, hand-held machines can be obtained in high-street retail shops.)

Usually four or five interchangeable cone- or disc-shaped working heads are supplied with these machines, these being designed to fulfil the requirements of basic filing, polishing, finishing, and hard skin (callus) removal:

1 a coarse, long-lasting sapphire disc, which is used for filing and shaping the nail;
2 one or two progressively finer discs or cones, to follow the sapphire disc: these are to bevel the nail edge and to give a finish on the surface of rough artificial or normal nails;
3 a fabric buffer (or mop), for use with paste polish to give a natural shine to the surface of normal or artificial nails;
4 a metal grating disc or cone for the removal of hard skin (callus) from the soles of the feet, and to flatten corns.

Most battery-operated manicure machines were originally made for the retail home market: they are seldom strong enough for salon use. Even the stronger models have a very limited usage in a salon. Hand filing of normal nails is more rapid, efficient and accurate than using a machine. Sculptured nail material is so hard that if a battery-operated machine is applied to the surface using any pressure, the machine will slow down and often stop. When buying such a machine, filing ability and rotation under pressure are the two main functions that should be checked before purchase.

Mains-operated machines

These machines (Figure 11.3), developed originally from dental drills, have been designed with the needs of the professional manicurist in mind. The motor is usually suspended from a stand, to keep the working area clear, to cushion the vibrations of the motor, and to allow air circulation to cool the motor. Flexible shafts lead from the machine to an on/off and speed foot-pedal control and to the working heads. The foot-pedal control leaves the hands free for working and enables the speed of the head to be varied between 5000 and 12 000 revolutions per minute.

FIGURE 11.3 *An electric manicure machine*

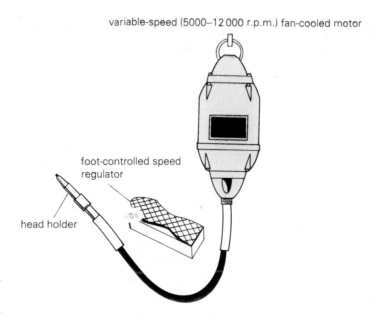

variable-speed (5000–12 000 r.p.m.) fan-cooled motor

foot-controlled speed regulator

head holder

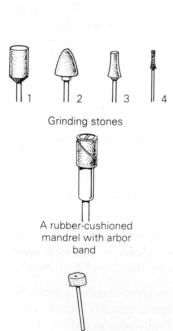

1　2　3　4

Grinding stones

A rubber-cushioned mandrel with arbor band

A 'mop' head for use with paste polish

FIGURE 11.4 *Head attachments for a manicure machine*

The working heads are attached to a heavy pen-like holder which initially may somewhat inhibit accuracy of movement. Practice is needed to master the use of the holder. A minimum of six heads are usually available with the machine; these are attached to the holder by a metal claw fastener which is opened and closed by means of a small rod or Allen key. The basic heads available are usually as follows:

1　*A rubber-cushioned mandrel with an arbor band* A mandrel is a drill head which is covered with rubber to provide some cushioning for the nail against the grit surface of the replaceable arbor band. The rubber cushion should be wetted before use in order to keep the arbor band on. Arbor bands are available in varying degrees of coarseness from coarse, through fine, to extra fine. Like emery

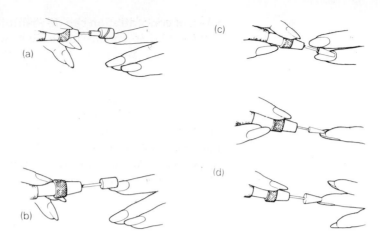

FIGURE 11.5 *Using head attachments: (a) The mandrel with an arbor band is used to file away excess acrylic material on the surface of the artificial nail. A coarse band should be used if a lot of filing needs to be done, and a fine band used to smooth the surface. (b) The fine grinding stone (no. 1) is used to obtain a smooth finish over the whole surface of acrylic nails. Stone no. 2, with its rounded edge, is used when working close to the cuticle. (c) The small cone-shaped stone (no. 4) is used for smoothing ridges of acrylic near the cuticle and for removing ridges of acrylic from underneath the nail tip. (d) The larger cone-shaped stone (no. 3) can also be used to file out the inside of built-up artificial nails*

boards, they have a limited lifespan and new ones should be used for each client. This attachment can be used to score the surface of the natural nail plate prior to the bonding of a false nail, or to progressively sand down the main surface of the applied artificial acrylic or gel nails if necessary.

Grinding stones These are made of fine sandstone and are available in a number of shapes, sizes and grades of fineness, selection of which depends on the area to be worked upon. Their purpose is to sand out or grind down irregularities on the surface of artificial acrylic or gel nails or at their junction with the natural nail plate. They are made to be used on areas for which the mandrel is too coarse in its size and effect, such as around the cuticles to smooth in a ridge, or underneath the free edge of an extension to remove any ridges which may have formed there. Grinding stones can also be used with care to remove the uneven surface of severely pitted or ridged natural nails, but caution should be exercised in this area. Chiropodists can use these attachments for reducing the thickness of toenails which have become distorted and thickened.

3 *'Mop' head attachments* These are made of synthetic fibres and are for use in conjunction with paste polishes to obtain a high gloss shine on both natural and artificial nail plates.

All the attachments are designed to be durable except the arbor bands, which need to be replaced for each client. Care must be taken to follow adequate sterilisation procedures for the detachable heads.

The advantages of manicure machines

Due to the powerful nature of the tool, working with an electric manicure machine can be quite difficult until skill is achieved. Extreme care must be taken not to rip the cuticle area. One moment's lapse of concentration can do painful and serious damage to this area.

An electric manicure machine is not needed to carry out a standard manicure or pedicure. Filing of the natural nail surface prior to artificial nail application is now discouraged totally or carried out with the finest abrasive materials available: a machine is definitely not required for this purpose. For very fine work, such as buffing nail tips level to the surface of the nail, it is important to be able to see at every stroke of the file whether the natural nail plate has been reached or is being filed into. The manicure machine can be too vigorous in its action to allow for this fine control unless the manicurist is very skilled with the machine.

The advances made in the manufacture and construction of manual files have led to more efficient and rapid finishing of the surfaces of artificial nails. The materials used for these nails have themselves been improved to the extent that only minor finishing is needed if the manicurist is skilled in her work. However, if the manicurist or nail technician does specialise in artificial nail application, then the fine sanding attachments and 'mops' of a manicure machine are useful for running over the edge and the entire surface of the nail extension product to leave it with a high gloss finish and indistinguishable from the natural nail plate. Used in this way they will also save the specialist nail technician valuable time.

Recent developments in the design of manicure machines for the professional nail technician have led to machine heads surrounded by a vacuum device which removes the dust from the filing of the false-nail product as it is created. This lessens the risk of dust inhalation, with its attendant health problems. Improvements are also being made in speed control and ease of handling, as well as in reduced noise emission.

12 MASSAGE: HANDS and ARMS

THE PRINCIPLES OF MASSAGE

Massage is the manipulation of the soft tissues of the body using the hands. It is one of the oldest forms of healing. In its simplest form, it is instinctive for a child or parent to rub – to massage – a part of the body that is hurting, as when the child has a stomach ache or pain after a fall, in order to make it better. On a more sophisticated level, there are records of highly developed forms of massage, such as shiatsu, being used in Chinese medicine as long as five thousand years ago.

The four main movements

The movements of massage are usually classed under four general headings: effleurage, petrissage, frictions, and tapotement.

Effleurage
This is the name given to a light or deeper stroking movement, applied with the palms of relaxed hands or with the palmar pads of the fingers. Pressure is exerted in the direction of the heart to aid both the venous and lymphatic flows, and the hands or fingers of the masseuse are returned to the starting point with no pressure whatsoever, but whilst still maintaining continuity via body contact.

Light, quick effleurage movements stimulate capillary blood flow and the tissues; they also stimulate the client. Deep, slow effleurage has a beneficial effect on the circulation of lymphatic fluids throughout the system and relaxes both the tissues and the client.

Petrissage
This is a more vigorous set of movements, designed to pick up, roll, wring, stretch and knead the muscular tissues of the body. They have both a mechanical and a reflex action on the circulation, allowing blood to flow more easily through the tissues. This can be seen and felt as redness (erythema) and a slight rise in the temperature of the tissues. The increased blood flow leads to an improvement in muscle and skin tone.

During petrissage, the muscle is lifted gently away from the bones, stretched, and then alternately squeezed and released. The veins and lymphatic vessels are thus alternatively emptied and filled.

Slow and rhythmic petrissage is soothing to the client. It speeds the absorption of fluid from the tissues by improving the lymphatic flow. It also softens any adhesions which may be present in the soft tissue.

Vigorous petrissage, however, has a pronounced stimulating effect on the tissues.

Frictions

These movements are made up of small circular motions of the thumb or finger pads, which are used to push muscles against bone, thereby breaking up any nodules or adhesions present in the tissues. The movements are directed at the underlying tissues and as such the circles made do not move *over* the surface of the skin but create their movement *beneath* the skin.

Tapotement

Sometimes known as *percussion*, this is a vigorous, highly stimulating and noisy set of 'hitting' movements, mainly comprising clapping with cupped hands, pummelling with the fists, and hacking with the sides of the hands and the fingers. It is used on the large muscle blocks and soft tissue areas of the body, such as the thighs and buttocks, and its purposes are to stimulate the circulation of the blood, to tone up the skin and to break up fatty tissue. As such, tapotement plays no part in the hand and arm, or foot and lower leg, massages.

There is a light tapping movement performed with the pads of the fingers which falls into this category. This movement is usually used as a stimulating and 'awakening' movement on the more delicate facial tissues; it has little effect when used on the areas involved in the manicurist's massage sequence.

Most of the benefits of massage can be attributed to its effects on the blood and lymphatic circulatory systems.

Where muscle tissue is pressed tightly up against bone in the body, blood has difficulty flowing through in sufficient quantities to ensure the optimum health of these tissues. The petrissage movements of massage lift the tissues away from the bones, allowing blood to flow easily through the capillaries of these stagnant areas. The blood flow acts to sweep away any poisonous wastes which may have collected in the tissues, including dissolved carbon dioxide, sarcolactic and lactic acids, and brings fresh nutrients and oxygen into the tissues.

Because the main pressures of massage are aimed at following the venous flow back to the heart, it is generally thought that one of the main purposes of massage is to stimulate the return of blood to the heart. This may be the case in clients with poor circulation, but the veins and arteries of a healthy person are quite capable – through a combination of muscular arterial walls, back pressure from the heart pump, and valves in the veins – of performing this function efficiently. These vessels lie deeply protected within the tissues and it is debatable as to just how much direct effect massage movements can have on them. Arteries and veins usually follow similar channels through the body, and a movement capable of exerting an effect on the venous return would have an equal effect in blocking the arterial flow to the area at the same time.

The circulatory system is aided by being stimulated at the capillary level, capillaries being the tiny vessels linking arteries and veins (see page 284). The greatest effect at the circulatory level, however, is on the functioning of the lymphatic system (see page 285). Lymph is a straw-coloured fluid containing white disease-fighting corpuscles, but no red, oxygen-carrying corpuscles. As well as forming part of the immune system, the lymphatic system is also responsible for aiding the removal of waste products and fluids from the body tissues. It does this by returning tissue fluids containing cellular waste products into the general circulation. These, as part of the lymph, move from the tissues into the small and large lymphatic ducts: these link up and finally empty the lymph into the bloodstream at the vena cava, just before it enters the heart. Waste products are processed and eliminated by the body through the organs of elimination: the lungs, the kidneys and the liver.

The pressure in the lymphatic vessels (ducts) is very low, much lower than in the main bloodstream, and the lymphatics ramify throughout all the soft tissues of the body, so they are very receptive to the pressures applied during massage movements. It is to assist with the vital lymphatic flow that each effleurage movement should follow the direction of lymphatic drainage back to the heart and aim to end, where practicable, with an increase of pressure at a group of lymph nodes.

The benefits of massage

1 Massage stimulates blood circulation: the blood sweeps away toxic waste in the tissues and brings in necessary oxygen and nutrients.
2 By increasing the circulation, the warmth and colour of the tissues is improved.
3 The improvement in muscle tone, caused by the effects of improved circulation, helps to firm the skin and the underlying muscles and tissues.
4 The appearance of the skin is improved. Surface debris, such as dry or loose skin cells, is removed. The skin is softened and made more pliable. The colour is improved.
5 Lymphatic drainage is improved, so the tissues benefit from the more efficient elimination of waste products and bacterial and malignant cells.

6 Massage relieves pain in tense and rheumatic muscle fibres. Nodules and muscle spasms are gently broken up and smoothed away.
7 Massage is soothing and relaxing to the client.
8 Regular massage prevents muscular wastage after injury.

Contra-indications

Massage should be avoided in the following circumstances:

1 Over very hairy areas, as massage can be irritating here, causing a rash and discomfort.
2 Over recent wounds or operation scars, as there is a danger of stretching scar tissue.
3 Over any bacterial inflammation, as massage could spread this.
4 Over any internal inflammation, such as an arthritic 'flare-up' with painful swollen finger joints. Massage can worsen such conditions and should be postponed until the inflammation has subsided.
5 If neuritis or neuralgia (inflammation or pain, or both, in the nerves) is present, as massage will irritate or aggravate the condition.
6 Over varicose veins, due to the danger of causing inflammation of the veins or perhaps even a thrombus (clot).

Massage mediums

So that the skin of the client is not uncomfortably stretched or pulled about, it is usual to use a lubricating massage medium. This medium can be a cream, an oil, or talcum powder.

In the manicure or pedicure situation creams are often chosen, primarily because they are the least messy. Oils can easily spill or drip, and the more nutritive plant oils such as almond oil, often used as carriers for aromatic essential oils, will soon cause staining of overalls and towels. Pure mineral oils do not cause this staining, nor do they go rancid with storage, as plant oils do when left exposed to the air. However, they contain no nutritive elements and are not absorbed into the skin, and therefore cannot be used as carrier mediums for essential (aromatic) oils. Talcs leave a white residue on the skin and towels which needs to be cleaned away at the end of the massage. Talc is also drying to the skin and if used regularly may clog the pores.

Creams are more controllable in their application and can be selected for nutritive and skin-conditioning properties as well as for their primary lubricant properties. A massage cream should be selected for its slow absorption rate so that a five- to ten-minute massage can be carried out without the need to apply more cream. Some creams can be used as carriers for essential oils.

Whichever medium is chosen, it is important to use enough of it to ensure client comfort during the sweeping effleurage movements, but not so much that the hands skate ineffectively over the skin during effleurage and friction movements or are unable to pick up the tissues during the petrissage movements.

HAND AND ARM MASSAGE

Before the start of the massage, the client must be made comfortable and her hands and arms supported on a soft but firm pad to prevent any muscle tension. Her clothing must be protected from the creams and oils to be used. Disposable paper tissues tucked around and under her cuffs and sleeve edges provide suitable protection.

During the massage, hand contact should be maintained at all times and the movements made to flow continuously into each other, the hands returning to starting points with a gentle contact only. Any pressures should be directed towards the heart.

The recommended frequencies of each movement are approximate because to give most benefit each movement should ideally be carried out until the tissues are relaxed and soft. However, time is often limited in the manicure sequence and so the number of movements have also to be limited.

Massage sequence

1 Using the relaxed palmar pads of the hands and fingers to mould to and apply an even pressure to the areas being massaged, effleurage from the wrist to the elbow (Figure 12.1). Hold the client's hand with the hand that is not massaging, in order to steady her arm. The movement is carried out three times up the outside and three times up the centre; change hands before continuing the movement three times up the inside without breaking the smooth and slow rhythmical flow. Repeat this whole sequence of movements twice more.

2 Using the palmar pads of the fingers to 'feel' firmly into the joint, carry out six circular movements around the elbow (Figure 12.2).

3 Using the fingers and thumbs in a large pinching movement, pick up the tissues and roll them thumb over fingers (petrissage) for approximately four movements up the outside from the wrist to the elbow (Figure 12.3). Repeat this twice more, supporting the arm in the same way as in 1. Then change hands and repeat the whole movement up the inside.

4 Apply effleurage to the back of the hand, using both hands and sweeping the thumbs alternately over the area, pulling down gently over the outside digits (Figure 12.4). As one hand is pulling, so the other hand is sweeping to give a synchronised relaxing movement. Repeat the movement approximately eight times with each hand.

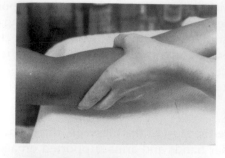
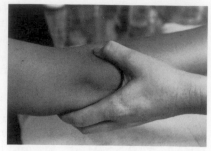

FIGURE 12.1 *Applying effleurage from the wrist to the elbow*

FIGURE 12.2 *Applying finger and thumb frictions into the elbow joint*

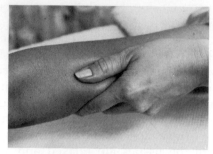
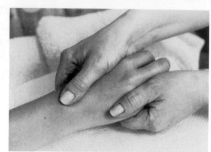

FIGURE 12.3 *Applying petrissage movements from the wrist to the elbow*

FIGURE 12.4 *Applying effleurage over the back of the hand*

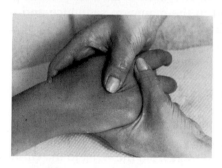
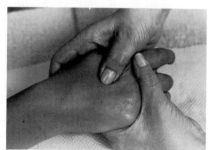

FIGURE 12.5 *Applying friction movements between the metacarpals, from the fingers to the wrist*

FIGURE 12.6 *Applying straight lymph drainage movements from the fingers to the wrist*

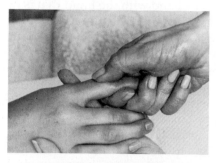
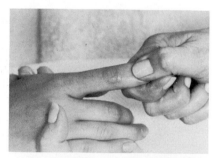

FIGURE 12.7 *Applying friction movements to a finger joint*

FIGURE 12.8 *Pulling and stretching a finger from the base to the tip*

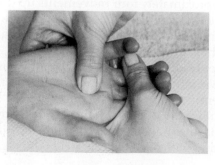
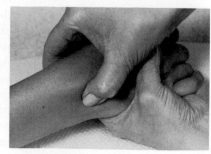

FIGURE 12.9 *Applying friction movements over the palm*

FIGURE 12.10 *Continuing the friction movements, now around the wrist*

5 Supporting the client's hand with one hand while working with the other, apply small friction movements (circles pressing the underlying tissue up against bone) in between the metacarpals, from the fingers to the wrist (Figure 12.5).

6 Using the thumbs in a straight-line pressing movement, slide them while applying constant pressure between the metacarpals, from the fingers to the wrist (Figure 12.6). (This movement, when used along the course of lymph vessels, is known as a lymph drainage movement.)

7 Apply friction movements to each finger in turn (Figure 12.7), concentrating the movements around the joints (three joints in each finger, two in each thumb). As each finger is finished, pull and stretch from its base to the tip, pausing to give most of the pull at the tip (Figure 12.8). (The joints of some clients may give a 'cracking' noise during this movement.) If the client's hands are too slippery to pull properly, wait until all the frictions have been completed and then grasp and pull each finger end in turn using a towel.

8 Turn the client's hand over and apply friction movements all over the palm, paying special attention to the metacarpal–phalangeal joints at the bases of the fingers and thumbs (Figure 12.9). Then apply friction movements into the joints of the wrist bones (Figure 12.10).

9 For this movement, the client's and the masseuse's fingers should be interlocked and the client's wrist rotated in as wide a circle as possible, three times one way, then three times the other way (Figure 12.11). Still maintaining the interlock, pull to apply a stretch to the wrist joints; then slide the interlock off whilst still applying traction (Figure 12.12).

10 Now hold the client's hand as if shaking the hand in greeting. This grip is used to move the hand (and therefore the wrist joints)

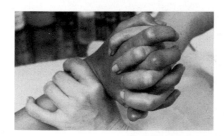
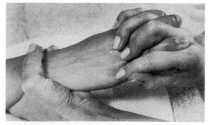
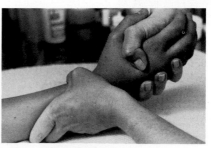

FIGURE 12.11 *Rotating the client's wrist, with the fingers interlocked*

FIGURE 12.12 *Sliding off the interlock and stretching the wrist*

FIGURE 12.13 *Shaking the hand up and down and from side to side*

up and down as far as it will go three times, and then from side to side as far as it will go three times (Figure 12.13).

11 The massage is completed by repeating a few effleurage movements to the hands as in 4. If time allows, movement 1 can also be repeated.

EXERCISING THE HANDS

To keep her hands flexible, the client should be encouraged to do the following exercises for a few minutes each day. They will also improve the blood circulation, which in turn will improve the colour

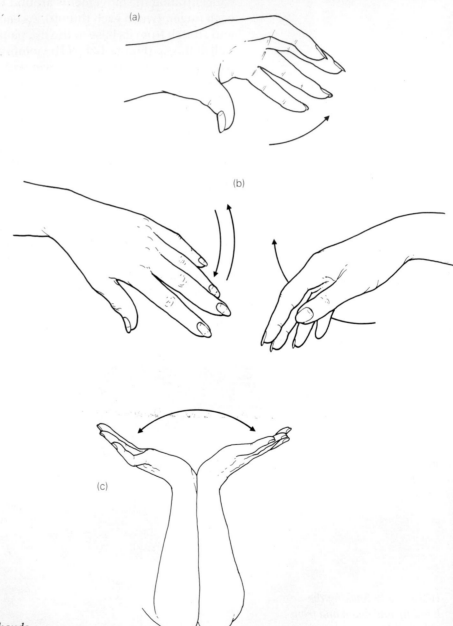

FIGURE 12.14 *Exercising the hands*

and tone of the skin and increase the growth and the strength of the nails.

1 The fist should be clenched as tightly as possible for 5 seconds, then sprung open and stretched wide, the stretching being held for 5 seconds before being released (Figure 12.14a). This movement should be repeated up to ten times.

2 The arms should be held out in front of the body, with the hands hanging limply. The hands are shaken up and down as hard as possible in a floppy movement, then relaxed (Figure 12.14b). This movement can be repeated up to ten times.

3 The arms are placed together from the elbows to the fingertips. The hands are then opened and stretched backwards as far as they will go from the wrists (Figure 12.14c). The stretch should be held for 5 seconds before relaxing. This exercise can be repeated up to ten times.

PART VI The pedicure

13 PRELIMINARIES

**PREPARING
THE PEDICURE
STATION**

The pedicure station should have everything that the pedicurist needs conveniently to hand (Figure 13.1), so that she has no need to break off the treatment procedure in order to go and get anything.

The pedicure station: a checklist

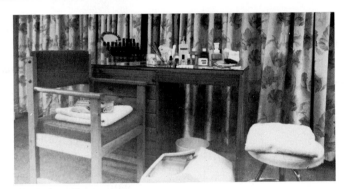

FIGURE 13.1 *A pedicure station*

1 A pedicurist's stool, low and without a back support.
2 A comfortable client's chair with armrests.
3 Magazines for the client to read.
4 Three large towels, one to cover the floor area or sponge pad, one to tuck around the client's knees, and one to use in carrying out the treatment.
5 A foot-bath, preferably one with a thermostatically-controlled heater (to maintain the water temperature) and a vibratory massage movement; a nearby power socket will be required if this type of bowl is to be used. If this is not available, then a simple plastic washing-up bowl will suffice.
6 A 10 cm (4 in.) deep foam pad on which to stand the foot-bath if it is of the vibratory type. The foam will absorb the vibrations and prevent the unit from being noisy.
7 A side table of sufficient size to accommodate a pedicure tray and leave a small space for working.
8 A waste disposal bin.

9   A dry sterilising cabinet nearby in which to keep sterile tools and buffers.

10   A pedicurist's sink and preparation area nearby, with hot and cold running water, antiseptic soap in a dispenser, a nailbrush in antiseptic solution, a paper towel dispenser and waste bin or a hot-air hand dryer, antiseptic and barrier creams for the pedicurist's hands, squeezy bottle dispensers of liquid soap, and antiseptic for use in the pedicure bowls.

11   A pedicure tray.

In the pedicure tray

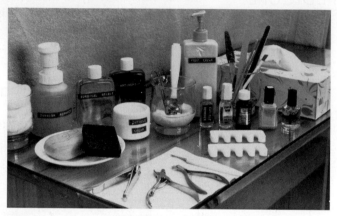

FIGURE 13.2 *The contents of the pedicure tray*

12   Cottonwool and small tissues in dispensers or jars.

13   Surgical spirits, antiseptic solution and non-oily nail varnish remover in either dish dispensers or bottles.

14   Foot cream, liquid, or a bar of, antiseptic soap, skin exfoliating cream and massage oil or cream, in pump dispensers, squeezy bottle dispensers, tubes or covered containers.

15   Cuticle cream and buffing cream (paste polish) in either tube dispensers or covered containers.

16   A jar containing two emery boards, two cuticle sticks, and a spatula to remove creams from their containers.

17   A jar containing a small amount of cottonwool at the base and sufficient surgical spirit or antiseptic solution with rust inhibitor to cover the blades of a cuticle knife, cuticle clippers (pliers), toenail pliers (if used), toenail clippers, a metal file, a corn plane, and a pair of nail scissors.

18   A chiropody sponge in a clean container, or a sterile hard skin rasp.

19   Toe separator pads.

20   Spare blades for the corn plane.

21   Small brush bottles containing cuticle remover, base coat, and top coat.

22   A small bottle of nail varnish thinner.

There should also be access to a good selection of nail varnish colours.

The pedicurist should carry a small magnifying glass with which to inspect anything unusual about the nails, such as a suspected fungal infection.

Due to the cutting and scratching potential of the equipment used during pedicuring, and the frequently dry and cracked nature of the skin and cuticles on the feet, the pedicurist should routinely wear fine rubber gloves (Figure 13.3) whilst working as a precaution against the transfer of blood-transmitted diseases.

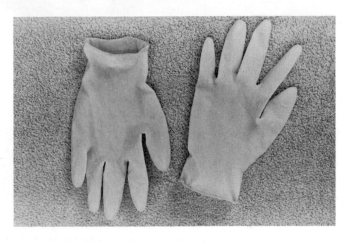

FIGURE 13.3 *Fine rubber surgical gloves, worn for protection*

Essentials for pedicuring: a checklist

Equipment
1 The client's chair.
2 The pedicurist's stool, side table and equipment tray.
3 Containers for cottonwool, implements and waste.
4 Three large towels.
5 A foot-bath.

Implements
6 Toenail clippers.
7 Emery boards (2).
8 Diamond Deb metal nail file.
9 Cuticle clippers and knife.
10 A corn plane with spare blades.
11 A chiropody sponge or callus file (hard skin rasp).
12 Toe separator pads.
13 Cuticle sticks (2).
14 A spatula.
15 A magnifying glass.
16 Fine rubber gloves.

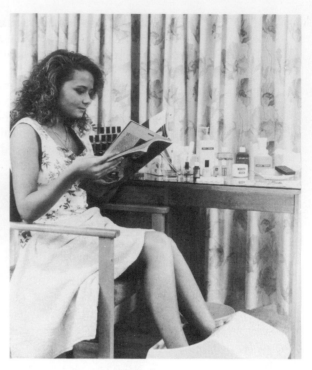

FIGURE 13.4 *The pedicure station in use*

Cosmetics

17 Foot exfoliating cream.
18 Foot cream.
19 Massage oil.
20 Cuticle cream.
21 Cuticle remover.
22 Antiseptic solution.
23 Surgical spirit.
24 Liquid, or a bar of, antiseptic soap.
25 A hot water supply, liquid soap and antiseptic.
26 Non-oily nail varnish remover.
27 Base coat, coloured nail varnishes, top coat and thinner.

Materials

28 Cottonwool.
29 Tissues.

Other

30 Magazines for the client.

CONTRA-INDICATIONS

Contra-indications to the pedicure treatment are the same as those given for the manicure treatment (page 93). Additional contagious conditions which must be avoided also include athlete's foot (tinea pedis) and verruca plantaris.

It is also inadvisable to carry out any cuticle clipping, hard skin paring or harsh rasping on diabetics or anyone else with poor peripheral circulation as their skin is both very slow to heal and prone to infection.

Corns are *not* a contra-indication, in fact if minor corns are treated in the same way as calluses, they often go away, or are at least kept under control.

14 The PEDICURE

The procedure outlined in this text is one of several ways to give a pedicure. Whatever procedure your instructor teaches you will be equally correct.

When the client books her pedicure appointment, she should be advised to bring a pair of open-toed sandals to wear home, if possible; if not, extra time must be allowed in the salon for her varnish to dry. Due to the coolness of the toes, nail varnish takes longer to dry on the feet than it does on the hands.

The desired colour of nail varnish should be selected *before* the treatment so that there is no need to disturb the client later. The pedicurist can check the consistency of the varnish and thin it if necessary, giving the pigments time to blend before use.

The pedicurist should wear rubber gloves, and the client should be aware that she has washed her hands before commencement of the treatment. During the pedicure all metal implements should be kept in an alcohol wet steriliser.

A cubicle should be available so that the client can remove and replace her tights or stockings in privacy. A dressing gown is sometimes needed for clients who arrive wearing tight-bottomed trousers which have to be removed.

PERFORMING THE PEDICURE

Before proceeding with the pedicure, ensure that the client is warm, is sitting comfortably and is relaxed, with magazines to read and a towel around her knees for modesty. The feet should be briefly inspected for contra-indications (Figure 14.1) before putting them to

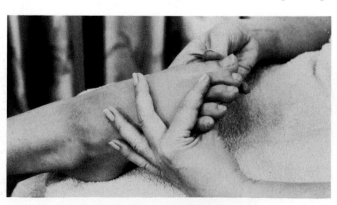

FIGURE 14.1 *The toenails and feet being inspected for contra-indications*

soak in the bowl for up to five minutes before the treatment commences.

The bowl should contain comfortably hot water to which has been added approximately 15 ml (1 tablespoonful) each of liquid soap and antiseptic.

The sequence of working

1 Inspection

The client's left foot is removed from the bowl, dried, and inspected thoroughly for any contra-indications to the treatment.

2 Varnish removal

Using a cottonwool pad saturated in nail varnish remover, and held between and beneath the first and second fingers to protect the pedicurist's own nail varnish, all old varnish is removed from the surface of the toenails with three or four firm, sweeping strokes. Darker coloured varnishes will require the pad to rest against them for a few seconds, to soften the varnish, before efficient removal can be effected.

During this removal, the nails are reinspected for any contra-indications or problems, such as fungal infections, which may have been hidden by varnish.

It is advisable to follow the same digital sequence of working on the toenails as has been learnt for the fingernails. Although the sequence is not as necessary on the toenails, it still forms the basis of a sound working routine, thus keeping mistakes and omissions to a minimum whilst helping to promote a professional image.

3 Clipping and filing

The nails are clipped almost to the required length using toenail clippers (Figure 14.2). Do not try to clip the whole width of large toenails in one movement or the nail may split or splinter. Clip one side of the nail straight to the centre, then the other side of the nail (Figure 14.3). Then, using an emery board or a 'Diamond Deb' to file,

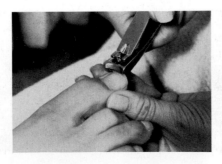
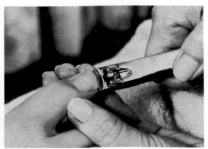

FIGURE 14.2 *Shortening the toenails by clipping them*

FIGURE 14.3 *The big-toe nail is clipped in two halves, to avoid splitting it*

file straight across the nail to square the tip and obtain the desired length. Any corners are then smoothed away, and the free edges of the nails bevelled in the same way as for fingernails (Figure 14.5). The completed nail should be squarely shaped with *slightly* rounded corners: it should extend no further than the end of the toe. (See the section on toenail shaping, page 173.)

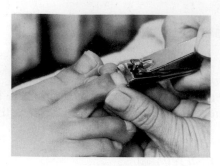
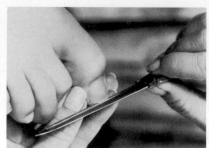

FIGURE 14.4 *A smaller nail being clipped straight across*

FIGURE 14.5 *A metal file being used to smooth the edge and corners*

4 The corn plane

Any very obvious thickened areas of hard skin (callus) can now be removed using a safety corn plane (Figure 14.6). Extra care must be taken during this procedure. If a slip is made, or the blade used over areas where there is no callus, the blade may cut the skin quite badly. Plenty of time must be taken to learn this technique under the supervision of an instructor. Never take away *all* the callus as this can leave the area sensitive for the client, especially if she is going to a hot climate and anticipates walking around barefoot: a thin veneer of callus must always be left to protect the feet. Constant touching of the area being treated, between sweeps of the blade, will soon give the pedicurist a 'feel' as to when enough callus has been removed. If at all doubtful, leave this stage out of the pedicure sequence until greater skill has been achieved.

The areas where callus is usually found include under the big toe, the ball of the foot (Figure 14.7), the heel margins, and the joints on the tops of the toes. Callus builds up as a protective layer to cushion bones in areas of fallen muscles and in areas where the foot rubs against footwear. Corns often appear in these places too, and small corns can be treated and removed in the same way as callus without problems. Larger corns require referral to a chiropodist.

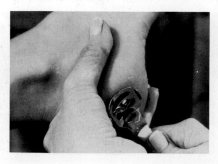
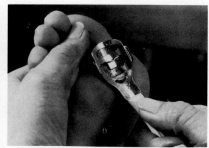

FIGURE 14.6 *Using a corn plane to pare excess dead skin from the heel*

FIGURE 14.7 *Paring skin from beneath the area of the metatarsal–phalangeal joints*

5 Cuticle cream

Cuticle cream is applied to the toenails and massaged into the nail plate, nail margins and down to the first joint of the toes, using the same method and sequence as used on the hands (Figures 14.8 and 14.9).

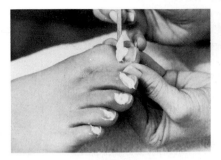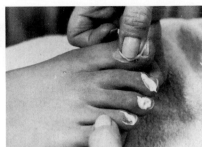

FIGURE 14.8 *Using a cuticle stick to apply cuticle cream*

FIGURE 14.9 *Massaging the cream into the nails*

6 First soaking

The left foot is returned to the soak.

7 Repeat with the other foot

Repeat steps 1–6 on the right foot.

Note If the client does not suffer with hard skin and callus, omit steps 4 and 9 and substitute the use of an exfoliating foot cream in step 8.

8 'Shampooing' (soap massage)

Take the left foot out of the bowl and cleanse it thoroughly using the liquid, or bar of, antiseptic soap. The incorporation of some relaxing effleurage and friction massage movements into this 'foot shampoo' will turn it into a most enjoyable experience for the client (Figure 14.10).

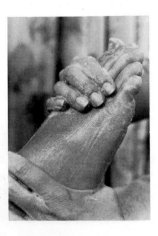

FIGURE 14.10 *The 'foot shampoo'*

9 *Chiropody sponge*

Whilst the foot is still lathered, remove the remaining hard skin using a chiropody sponge (Figures 14.11 and 14.12). The 'sponge' should be dipped into the water to moisten it, and soap applied to the side to be used. It is then rubbed firmly against the callus to remove the dead skin and leave the area smooth. Chiropody sponges must always be used wet and with lots of soap or they will scratch the skin. They should only be used on areas of callus. The use of a chiropody sponge only, without the prior use of a corn plane, is often sufficient on areas of light callus.

A hard skin rasp is a metal 'grater' shaped for use on the calluses of the feet. Rasps are not usually as efficient as a true chiropody sponge, but are used in the same way.

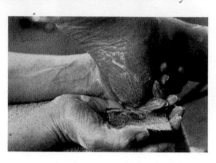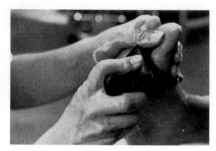

FIGURE 14.11 *Using a chiropody sponge to remove remaining hard skin from the heel . . .*

FIGURE 14.12 *. . . and from the ball of the foot*

10 *Second soaking*

Return the left foot to the soak.

11 *Repeat with the other foot*

Repeat steps 8–10 on the right foot.

12 *Drying the foot*

Take the left foot out of the soak and dry it thoroughly.

13 *Cuticle work*

Using cuticle remover and a small piece of tissue, in the same way as for a manicure (pages 103–7), clean under the toenails (wiping dirt on the tissue) and push back the cuticles with a cottonwool-covered cuticle stick (Figure 14.13). Loose and excess cuticle is now clipped away (Figure 14.14); then the excess debris and cuticle remover are wiped away with the tissue.

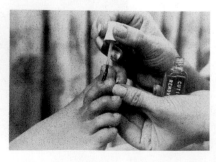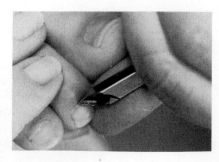

FIGURE 14.13 *The toenail cuticle is flooded with cuticle remover prior to pushing it back with a cuticle stick*

FIGURE 14.14 *Clipping away the pushed-back cuticle*

The easiest position for the pedicurist to work on the toes is with the client's knees bent, and her feet resting on the pedicurist's knees.

14 Foot cream

A non-greasy foot cream is now applied and massaged into the foot using soothing effleurage and friction movements. If a full foot and lower leg massage is not being carried out later, a quick, basic foot massage sequence can be incorporated here.

15 Keeping the foot warm

The left foot is now placed onto the base towel and wrapped in the towel to keep it warm.

16 Repeat for the other foot

The right foot is removed from the bowl and the bowl moved to one side, both for client comfort and to prevent any spillage. Steps 12–15 are repeated on the right foot.

17 Massage

If required, the full lower leg, ankle and foot massage is carried out at this stage. (See page 176 for technique.)

18 Position for varnishing

For ease of working, both of the client's feet are now placed on the pedicurist's knees. If the client finds this difficult, due to pregnancy, overweight or stiffness, then the left leg, followed by the right leg, must be treated in sequence throughout the following stages.

19 Toe separation

The toes are separated using clean (sterile) pre-formed sponge toe separators.

20 'Squeaky-clean' check

The toenails are wiped over to remove surface oils and moisture using a non-oily nail varnish remover on a cottonwool pad, or on a Nail Neat pad. The latter has the advantage of not shedding fibres onto the surface of the nail. Such stray fibres can make varnishing difficult.

A pedicurist needs to have a tissue, a cuticle stick and some nail varnish remover at hand with which to clean up any mistakes in nail varnish application as they occur. If mistakes are left until the end of the application the varnish will have hardened and a complete clean-up will be impossible.

21 Base coat

A base coat is applied, using the correct sequence.

22 Varnishing

Two or three coats of coloured nail varnish are applied, with the minimum number of strokes and coats necessary to achieve perfect coverage (see page 126). These are followed by a top coat if required.

The nail varnish bottle tops must be wiped clean before the lid is replaced, in order to maintain the consistency of the nail varnish. The soiled pad which was used to wipe over the nail surface prior to varnish application can be saved and used for this purpose.

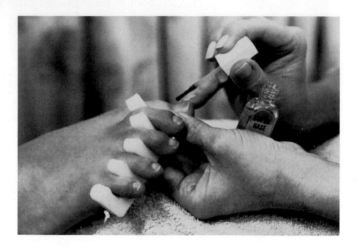

FIGURE 14.15 *Base coat, varnish and top coat are applied using the technique and the sequence of digits used for the fingers*

23 Drying

A drying time of 10–30 minutes, depending on the varnish used, must be allowed before the toe separators are removed and the client's shoes replaced. It is not advisable for the client to wear stockings, tights or closed-in shoes immediately after a pedicure. If these cannot be avoided, a quick-drying oil, solution or spray can be used to reduce the likelihood of smudging.

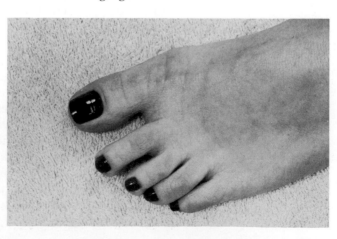

FIGURE 14.16 *The completed pedicure*

The pedicure sequence: a checklist

1 Brief inspection followed by soaking. Pre-select varnish colour.
2 Dry and inspect the left foot.
3 Remove nail varnish from the left foot.
4 Clip, file and shape the toenails of the left foot.
5 Remove obvious hard skin with the corn plane.
6 Apply cuticle cream and return the foot to soak.
7 Repeat steps 2–6 on the right foot.
8 Take the left foot out of the bowl and cleanse using a soap massage.
9 Remove the remaining hard skin using a chiropody sponge, rasp, or exfoliating foot cream.
10 Return the left foot to soak.
11 Repeat steps 8–10 on the right foot.
12 Take the left foot out of the soak and dry it thoroughly.
13 Apply cuticle remover to left foot, push back the cuticles and clip them. Wipe away any residue with a tissue.
14 Apply the foot cream and massage it in.
15 Place the left foot on the base towel and cover it to keep it warm.
16 Repeat steps 12–15 on the right foot.

A full foot and lower leg massage can be carried out here if required.

17 For both feet, separate the toes.
18 Wipe over the toenails with non-oily nail varnish remover.
19 Apply the base coat.
20 Apply coloured varnish and, if required, a top coat. Wipe the bottle top before the lid is replaced.

TIDYING THE PEDICURE STATION

Immediately upon completion of the pedicure, the work station should be tidied and cleaned in readiness for the next client, and all surfaces, materials and equipment cleaned, washed, sterilised or disposed of in accordance with the usual rules of hygiene in the salon (see page 36).

TOENAIL SHAPE AND LENGTH

The toenail shape should always be square with the corners gently rounded so that no sharp edges are left to dig into the flesh of the nail wall. The sides of the nail should never be filed away: such filing can be a cause of ingrowing toenails or unpleasant pressure soreness at the sides of the toes as the nail plate grows forwards. Socks, shoes

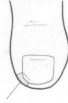

surgical adhesive fabric

FIGURE 14.17 *A cushioning piece of surgical adhesive fabric placed under the free edge of the nail to encourage the nail plate to grow straight out*

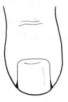

FIGURE 14.18 *The correct shape regained; the corrective treatment can now be discontinued*

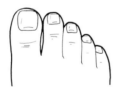

FIGURE 14.19 *The correct length and shape for toenails*

HOME CARE FOR NAILS AND FEET

and tights all press the flesh at the side of the toes, especially on the big toe, against the nail plate. If the nail plate is filed away, then the flesh is pressed over the area of missing nail. As new nail grows forwards, it pushes into this flesh, causing pain and often inflammation and infection if the flesh is cut into. If a client comes into the salon with nail walls which are infected due to this complaint, she must be referred to a chiropodist for help. If she is just experiencing discomfort due to incorrect prior filing, however, then the nail can be encouraged to grow straight out by placing a cushioning piece of surgical adhesive fabric under the corner of the offending nail area (Figure 14.17). The fabric can stay in place for a week or more before replacement and the free edge of the nail will grow forward over the top of it without cutting into the flesh or causing pain. After a few weeks, the correct shape of nail will be regained (Figure 14.18) and the pressure soreness will have gone; once this has happened, the use of the cushioning surgical fabric can be discontinued.

The correct length of nail to give the most pleasing and balanced appearance to the toes and feet is one which just reaches the end of the flesh line of the toes (Figure 14.19). Any longer than this and there is a danger of the nail plate being stubbed against furniture and being bent backwards, or of it pressing against the end of closed-in shoes. Both these mechanical traumas can cause pain, bruising, and lifting or even shedding of the toenail. This is why some clients, especially elderly people, gentlemen and sports people who wear close-fitting closed-in shoes all the time, may require their nails to be shorter than the ends of their toes. Other clients, however, such as ladies going on holiday who will be wearing open-toed sandals for much of the time, may require their nails to be left longer than the recommended length. The pedicurist must always be guided by client preference and ask the client at the start of the treatment which length she would prefer.

Often neglected because they are infrequently seen, toenails and feet need regular care in order to prevent the occurrence of physical problems as well as to maintain their cosmetic appearance. A regular monthly pedicure treatment should keep the feet and toenails in good condition, although excessive hard skin problems may necessitate more frequent treatments at two- or three-weekly intervals.

Between times, clients can look after their feet and toenails at home in the following ways:

1 To prevent infection and odour, feet should be washed daily and dried thoroughly. Talcum powder can be used to ensure dryness.
2 To prevent the formation of bunions or toe and nail deformation, shoes, socks, tights or stockings should not be too tight.
3 To prevent postural and arch problems, shoe-heel height should not be greater than 5 cm (2 in.). A 2.5 cm (1 in.) heel is best for the health of the feet.

4 If wearing shoes which are closed in over the toes, it is best not to let the nail length become too long: it could catch and press on the inside of the shoe. This can result in a lifting away of the nail from its bed or the breaking of the nail very low down on its bed. These problems are often seen on athletes. To avoid these problems, the toenail length should never be allowed to extend beyond the end of the toe, and should be shorter than this when closed-in footwear is worn.

5 If exercise sandals are worn, their use should be limited to 30 minutes each day. Over-exercise can cause the muscles to stretch and the arches to drop.

6 Hard skin can be kept under control at home by using purpose-made creams or pumice stones.

7 Socks should be changed daily and the same pair of shoes not worn on consecutive days, in order to keep the feet clean, dry and infection-free.

8 Exercises, such as those described on page 180, can be carried out two or three times each week to maintain the tone and suppleness of the foot.

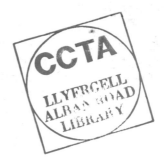

15 MASSAGE: FEET and LOWER LEGS

FOOT AND LEG MASSAGE

The notes given at the beginning of the hand and arm massage (page 149) also apply here, as do the instructions for carrying out the massage movements, which are given in the text. The client's clothing should be protected by a draped towel. This will already be in place for the pedicure sequence. The foot *not* being massaged should be kept warmly wrapped in a towel.

Massage movements on the foot should be carried out in a firm, no-nonsense manner. In this way tickling is entirely avoided. If tickling occurs, the technique of the masseuse is at fault.

Massage sequence

1 With the sole of the client's foot resting on the masseuse's knee so that the client's knee is bent, carry out effleurage from the rear of the ankle to the popliteal space (behind the knee), four times on the right side, then four times on the left (Figures 15.1 and 15.2). Repeat this movement. The hand not being used for massage can be used to support the foot.
2 Using both thumbs, apply friction up each side of the shin bone to the knee (Figure 15.3).
3 Using both hands – thumbs pointing up the shin bone, fingers slightly around to the back of the calf muscle – carry out effleurage four times up each side of the lower leg (Figure 15.4).
4 Repeat movements 2 and 3.
5 Now the client's leg is straightened by placing the back of her heel onto the masseuse's knee. Effleurage is applied to the foot by placing the fingers over the top of the metatarsal–phalangeal joints and the thumbs beneath the base of these joints and sweeping the hands downwards towards the heels (Figure 15.5). At the end of this movement the fingers should continue on to sweep around the ankle joints and down to the back of the heel (Figure 15.6). Each time this movement is repeated, the thumb pressures should be moved slightly so that the whole of the sole of the foot is covered. This movement is repeated approximately eight times.

6 Using the outer hand to hold the toes and hence the foot upright, the masseuse should place the heel of her other hand against the outer border of the base of the foot, with her fingers pointing at right angles and across the longitudinal arch of the foot. Effleurage movements are carried out by sliding the heel of this hand across the sole of the foot and upwards to the top of the foot (Figure 15.7). This movement should be repeated approximately eight times.

7 Frictions are now applied between the metatarsals on the upper surface of the foot, with pressures being directed towards the heart (Figure 15.8).

8 A sliding pressure lymph drainage movement, also between the metatarsals and directed towards the heart, now follows (Figure 15.9).

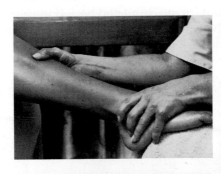
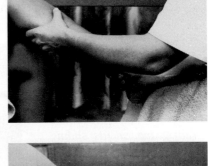
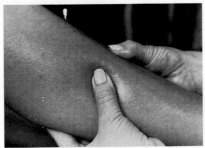
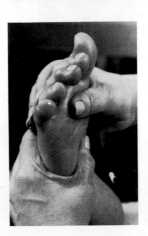
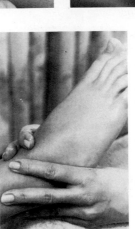
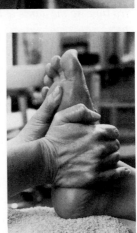

FIGURE 15.1 *Applying effleurage from the rear of the ankle to the popliteal space, on the right side . . .*

FIGURE 15.2 *. . . and on the left*

FIGURE 15.3 *Applying friction, using both thumbs, up both sides of the shin bone to the knee*

FIGURE 15.4 *Applying effleurage to each side of the lower leg*

FIGURE 15.5 *Applying effleurage to the top and base of the foot, from the metatarsal–phalangeal joints . . .*

FIGURE 15.6 *. . . to the heel, sweeping the fingers round the ankle joints*

FIGURE 15.7 *Sliding the heel of the hand across the longitudinal arch of the sole to the top of the foot*

9   Frictions are applied to the joints of the toes (Figure 15.10), and the toes are pulled to stretch the joints (Figure 15.11).

10   The masseuse should now position her hands as if she were about to start the foot effleurage movement described in 5. The fingers are used to bend the toes over the thumbs (Figure 15.12). This movement is repeated but moving the thumbs and fingers from side to side to stretch each metatarsal–phalangeal joint.

11   The masseuse should now grasp the foot with both hands, one on either side of the big toe and little toe. Moving one hand backwards and one hand forwards in unison, and reversing this movement about eight times, will give a shaking and loosening effect to the foot (Figure 15.13).

12   Frictions should now be applied over the whole of the sole of the foot (Figure 15.14), followed by two or three linking effleurage movements as in 4.

13   Thumb and finger frictions should be applied around the whole ankle joint, front and back (Figure 15.15).

14   Now the masseuse needs to hold and support the rear of the ankle joint with one hand while the other hand is used to hold the

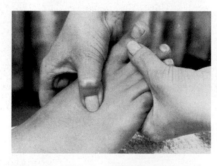
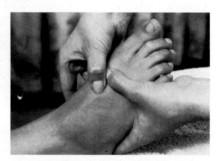

FIGURE 15.8 *Applying frictions between the metatarsal bones*

FIGURE 15.9 *Applying lymph drainage movements: sliding pressure is applied between the metatarsals, directed towards the leg*

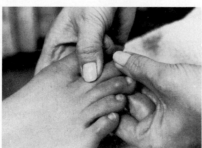
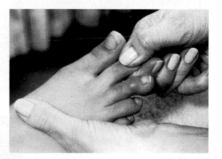

FIGURE 15.10 *Applying frictions to the joints of the toes*

FIGURE 15.11 *Stretching the joints by pulling the toes*

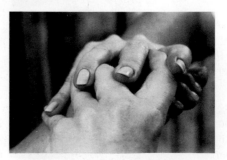

FIGURE 15.12 *Stretching the joints by bending the client's toes over the masseuse's thumbs*

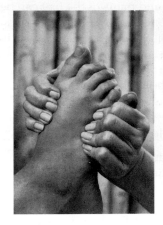
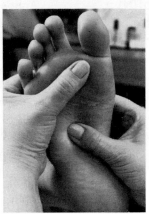

FIGURE 15.13 *Shaking the foot from side to side*

FIGURE 15.14 *Applying frictions over the whole sole of the foot*

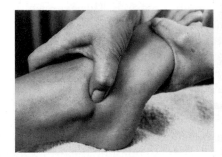
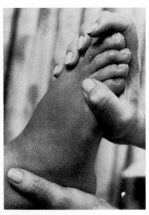

FIGURE 15.15 *Applying frictions around the whole ankle joint*

FIGURE 15.16 *Rotating the ankle joint*

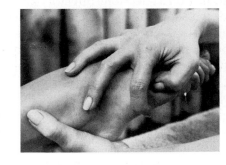
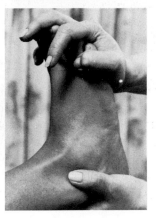

FIGURE 15.17 *Pulling the foot forward as far as it will go . . .*

FIGURE 15.18 *. . . and pushing it back as far as it will go*

foot firmly in the middle and rotate it three times one way and three times the other way, pushing it firmly so that the foot and hence the ankle are forced through as large a circle as possible (Figure 15.16). This will loosen the ankle joint.

15 Still holding the foot in this way, the foot is now pulled forward as far as it will go (Figure 15.17), then pushed back as far as it will go (Figure 15.18), again to loosen the ankle joint.

16 The massage is completed by repeating a few vertical and sideways effleurage movements (5 and 6).

EXERCISING THE FEET

Aches and pains of the feet can be avoided by exercising. Exercise will help tone up weakened muscles and counteract the cramping effects of high-heeled shoes. The exercises given below can be used to form the basis of an exercise routine to keep feet supple and strengthen the supporting structures around the arches of the feet, the toes, the ankle bones and calf muscles.

To help relieve foot problems caused by weak muscles, stretched ligaments and poor circulation, the client should be encouraged to do the following exercises for a few minutes each day.

1 Placing the weight on the outer borders of the feet (Figure 15.19a) relieves the strain on the muscles of the inner arch and makes the muscles of the outer arch work (contract). Walking forwards and backwards in this position for about a minute at a time helps to tone up the muscles of the outer arch.
2 Standing with the feet parallel and rising slowly up onto the toes and slowly down again (Figure 15.19b) exercises and strengthens both the leg and foot muscles, especially the gastrocnemius and the longitudinal arch. This exercise should be done five to ten times.
3 Extending the sole of the foot and pointing the toes so that they are in as straight a line as possible with the leg will tone the supporting muscles of the ankles, arches and toes (Figure 15.19c). It also has beneficial effects on the tarsal, metatarsal and phalangeal joints. The stretch should be held for 4–5 seconds before being released and the exercise done five times.
4 The beneficial effects of exercise 3 can be increased in this exercise. Again pointing the toes, rotate the foot slowly at the ankle as if trying to draw the largest circle possible with the big toe (Figure 15.19d). Carry out this movement five times in one direction, five times in the other.
5 Standing on a telephone directory and bending the toes down over the edge of the book will help to strengthen and tone the muscles at the front of the foot (Figure 15.19e). The completed movement should be held for 4–5 seconds before being released, and the exercise done five times. An alternative way to exercise these muscles is to try to pick up and hold a pencil with the toes. Hold for 5 seconds and repeat five times.

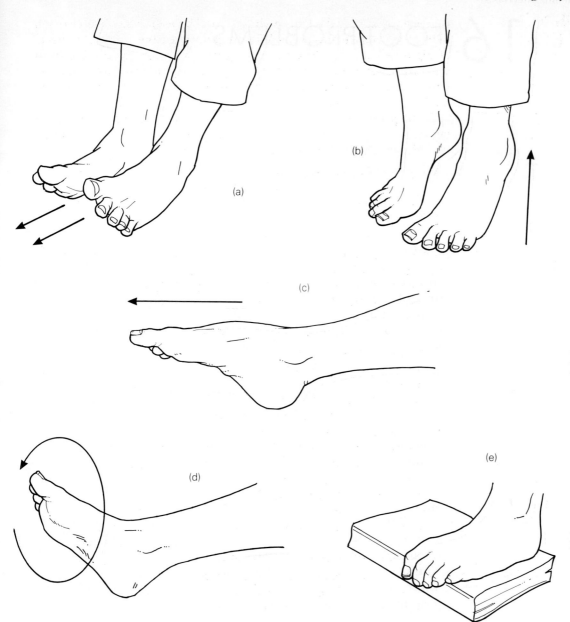

FIGURE 15.19 *Exercising the feet*

16 FOOT PROBLEMS

SOURCES OF PROBLEMS

The foot ranks as one of the world's greatest pieces of engineering. It contains 26 bones, 38 joints and 135 muscles and ligaments. The shape of these bones gives rise to arches which, together with the muscles, support the weight of the body whilst standing, and propel it forward in walking. It is flexible enough to adapt to uneven surfaces, yet it also forms a rigid bridge which does not collapse under the weight of the body.

In spite of its marvellous construction, the foot is often the most neglected area of the body. Not only is it expected to fulfil its duties uncomplainingly, it is often submitted to daily abuse according to the dictates of fashion.

Some people's feet spend most of their time encased in shoes with pointed toes and with stiletto, platform or high heels. They are further compressed by tights or tight socks. Flat, open sandals, flat plimsolls or exercise sandals, all meant for short-term wear, are worn indefinitely. Little wonder that chiropodists are faced with a deluge of unnecessary and often incurable foot problems!

The feet have a direct effect on the posture of the body. Any heel over 4–5 cm ($1\frac{1}{2}$–2 in.) high throws the weight of the body forward onto the metatarsal heads, causing pain and weakening of the front arch. This also gives rise to a 'protective' pad of hard skin forming over the ball of the foot; this leads to pain as it builds up and throws the foot still more out of balance. If a heel is over 5 cm (2 in.), the natural curvatures of the spine become distorted and the body's centre of gravity is altered in the effort to maintain an upright posture. This situation leads directly to the development of back problems and pain.

If a shoe is absolutely flat, as is a plimsoll, the arches can be stretched and may drop because the foot is constricted while being made to move over hard, unnatural, unyielding surfaces such as tarmac.

During human development, the foot evolved and adapted to walk on uneven, 'giving' surfaces, such as soil, without constriction in shoes. One of the best exercises for the feet, in fact, is to walk barefoot along sand or small stones.

It can be seen then how the vast majority of foot problems and many back problems trace directly back to unsuitable and ill-fitting footwear. The ideal shoe should have plenty of room in which the toes can flex and spread, the heel should be held firmly in place so that it does not slip, the arch should be slightly supported, and the heel should be around 2½ cm (1 in.) high.

The nails and skin of the feet can suffer from the same problems as the nails and skin of the hands (pages 301–31), including tinea unguium (ringworm) infection, or a brittle and flaky condition. However, feet also have problems which are unique to them, some of which are described below.

SOME COMMON PROBLEMS

Strain and wear and tear on the feet occur as a direct result of long standing, cramped and unsuitable footwear, overweight and bad posture. All these factors produce direct effects and side-effects as follows.

Arthritis

This can be an illness (e.g. rheumatoid arthritis) or due to wear and tear caused by incorrect weight-bearing. In both instances, the synovial membranes and capsules of the joints become inflamed and swollen, with fluid retained and associated pain.

Although massage must not be carried out during an arthritic flare-up when inflammation is present, massage afterwards will help to eliminate fluid and keep the joints mobile. Medical attention is needed and will probably already be being given.

Athlete's foot (tinea pedis)

Sometimes known as ringworm of the foot, athlete's foot is a fungal infection which receives its name from the fact that athletes are often associated with the perfect conditions for the infection to spread: warmth and damp, such as are found in sweaty clothing, socks, towels, matting or boards on the floors of bathrooms, swimming pool surrounds, showers, changing rooms and other communal facilities. The condition is acquired by walking with bare feet on infected floors.

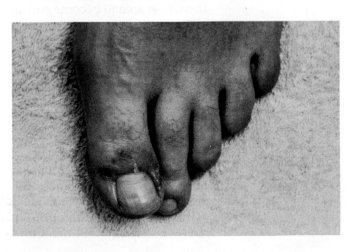

FIGURE 16.1 *A fungal infection of the skin around the big-toe nail*

It is aggravated by hot weather, when sweating will give the fungus an ideal environment in which to multiply.

There are two varieties of athlete's foot. In the first, described as 'vesicular', the area is covered with small blisters. This form begins on the soles of the feet. In the second, 'intertriginous', the skin between the toes becomes white and 'sodden', splitting and peeling away to leave raw, red areas. Both types can be accompanied by an itchy rash. If neglected, toenails, usually one or two, can become affected. They are very resistant to treatment, needing medical care and tablets. It is important to have the condition diagnosed by a doctor because a similar appearance may be produced by another infecting organism or by excessive sweating.

After correct medical diagnosis, athlete's foot, as long as the toenails have not become involved, can be treated successfully at home with pharmacy-bought liquids and powders; it should clear up in a few weeks. During treatment, socks (preferably not made of synthetic fibres, as these encourage sweating) should be changed daily, and shoes, socks, slippers and sandals dusted with athlete's foot powders to prevent cross- and reinfection.

A person with athlete's foot should not walk barefoot and should ensure that there is no chance of other people using the same socks, shoes, clothing or towels.

A pedicure should not be given to a person suffering from athlete's foot because of the risk of transmission to other clients. If an infected person is treated inadvertently, everything their feet have come in contact with should be disinfected.

(Compare onychomycosis, page 320.)

Bunions (hallux valgus)

Bunions occur when the big toe deviates towards the other toes. The joint (metatarsal–phalangeal) becomes prominent and enlarged and the body produces a cushion of fluid to act as a shock absorber. With time, this fluid solidifies and continued friction and pressure cause the whole area to become painful and inflamed.

The main causes of bunions are shoes which are too short or pointed, and socks, stockings or tights that are too short or not wide enough across the toes. The pressure rubs and thickens the skin, and the big toe is pushed under the second one to give rise to the joint problem. Another cause of bunions is a weakness in the arches of the feet, which again leads to the big toe sliding under the second toe and the metatarsal–phalangeal joint being opened and irritated.

Bunions can be helped in their early stages by massage and exercise. The massage helps to keep the joint mobile, break up and mobilise solidifying fluid, or remove existing fluid swelling. Massage and exercise will both help to strengthen the muscles of the foot arches. However, these must be seen as an accessory to proper treatment by a chiropodist or remedial practitioner, and not a substitute for other treatment.

Bursitis

This is a condition caused by footwear that is too tight rubbing the little protective pad of tissue between the Achilles tendon and the heel. This causes inflammation, swelling (due to fluid retained in order to cushion the area), and soreness. The footwear should be changed and a doctor consulted.

Callus (hard skin)

One of the most common of all foot problems, callus (hard skin) is nearly always the result of friction and pressure by the shoe on the skin of the foot (Figure 16.2). The skin is 'sandwiched' between the bone and the shoe and the continuous irritation causes the cornified layers to build up until they form a hard, thick, dead protective layer. Some people produce lots of callus upon irritation, other people hardly any; whilst some people seem to produce it all the time for no obvious or known reason. Overweight people tend to have more callus than normal-weight people, probably because their extra weight causes more pressure on the feet.

Callus does not have a central part (nucleus). The foot grows it as a protection over bony prominences, such as the ball of the foot if a dropped transverse arch causes the bones to sag, or the edges of the heels, especially when backless sandals are worn frequently. Callus can give a burning sensation in the feet due to the pressure of the hard skin on the nerves.

An experienced pedicurist can remove callus during a normal pedicure using a corn plane and a chiropody sponge (see page 168). Regular pedicures – once every 2–4 weeks depending on the severity of the problem – and a change in the type of footwear worn can help either to eliminate the problem or to keep it under control.

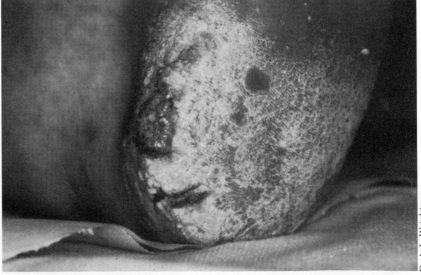

FIGURE 16.2 *A callused heel*

Dr A. L. Wright

Chilblains

These are associated with cold, damp weather, and also with poor circulation. The symptoms are redness, tingling and itching, accompanied by inflammation and swelling. They are aggravated by shoe pressure.

Chilblains are a medical problem and need to be treated by a doctor. However, the condition can be helped at home in the following ways. Chilblain ointment should be used early, *before* the skin breaks. Regular foot exercises and hot and cold contrast bathing – alternate bathing of the feet in basins of warm and cold water (30 seconds in each for a total of 5 minutes), finishing with cold water, then drying the feet thoroughly – will help to stimulate the circulation and keep the problem at bay.

Corns

Corns (Figure 16.3) can be said to be a special type of callus. They are caused by the same factors as callus – friction and pressure – but with a corn the build-up of hard skin is cone-shaped with the pointed part, called the nucleus, facing inwards. When the nucleus presses onto a nerve it causes pain.

There are several types of corn, the most common being the hard corn which is frequently found on the tops or tips of the toes, although it can also be seen interspersed in the callus on the base of the foot. Soft corns are found between the toes, where perspiration collects. These too are caused by pressure, are also painful, but remain soft due to the moisture.

If small corns are treated in the same way as callus during the pedicure, they will often disappear (but only if the pressure source, incorrect footwear, is removed). However, large or painful corns must be referred to a chiropodist.

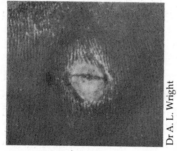

FIGURE 16.3 *A corn*

Dr A. L. Wright

Excessive perspiration

This is often accompanied by foot odour. It is caused by a functional disorder of the sweat glands known as hyperhidrosis. It can be relieved by the use of special foot powders containing anti-perspirants (to stop perspiration) and deodorants (to disguise any odour). Daily washing, thorough drying and the daily use of dry anti-perspirant sprays is also recommended, as is the frequent changing of socks and shoes, and wearing shoes made of leather instead of synthetic materials. Leather allows the foot to 'breathe', whereas plastic-based synthetics encourage perspiration.

Hammer toes

This is a condition where one or more toes become permanently flexed and humped. It is caused by ill-fitting footwear, and a chiropodist should be consulted if necessary.

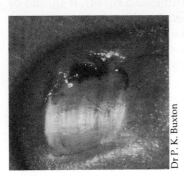

FIGURE 16.4 *An ingrowing toenail (onychocryptosis)*

Dr P. K. Buxton

Ingrowing toenails (onychocryptosis)

A true ingrowing toenail occurs when the edge of the nail and the nail wall are pushed so tightly up against each other that the nail cuts into the nail wall (Figure 16.4). This is a very painful condition and is often accompanied by inflammation, bacterial infection and the formation of pus. If this is the case, the pedicurist must not touch the affected toe but must refer the client to a chiropodist.

Ingrowing toenails can be due to a congenital defect (a deformity present from birth) or to the wearing of too-tight footwear or socks. They can also be caused by clipping the corners and sides of the nail away, so that the flesh is pushed into the area no longer covered by the nail; as the nail grows forward it cuts into the flesh instead of having its usual wide and natural bed to follow. This is the reason why toenails must be shaped squarely with simply the sharp edge of the corners smoothed away when they are being reduced in length.

Ingrowing toenails caused by a congenital defect are usually rectified by surgery to cut away a portion of the nail matrix, thus reducing the width of the nail. Established problems caused by incorrect shaping or footwear also sometimes require minor surgery. However minor discomfort can be eased and corrected by tucking a piece of sticking-plaster or fabric under the nail as it grows forward (see page 174). This will stop the nail from cutting into the flesh, and will also encourage the nail to resume its rightful path along its bed.

Meta-tarsalgia

This is a condition caused by ill-fitting or unsuitable footwear. The heads of the metatarsals are forced to take the body weight directly, eventually leading to a dropped front arch. Extreme pain and aching occurs under the front part of the foot due to the stretching of the ligaments, and the joints can become inflamed. A change in style of footwear is essential and a doctor or chiropodist should be consulted.

Nail lifting away (onychomadesis)

Most commonly seen on the big toe, the nail lifting away from its bed can be due to something heavy being dropped onto the toe nail (a doctor should be consulted; usually this will already have been done). If this is not the cause, then it is usually due to the nail pressing too tightly against the roof of the shoe. It is a problem frequently seen in athletes, where friction and pressure against footwear subjects the nail to a trauma sufficient to lift it from its bed. This situation is usually not painful, and often the first indication of it is the sight of the old nail ending towards the base, with a new nail following immediately behind, as if the growth of one nail has been terminated and the growth of the following nail has started immediately. This is in fact exactly what does happen, due to the trauma. It can be avoided by wearing footwear with a roomy toe area and by keeping the big-toe nail clipped short.

To treat the condition, the lifted nail should be clipped as short as possible so that it does not catch on anything and rip off. It should be allowed to move forwards, being pushed by the new nail growing forward from the nail matrix. As the nail gets looser and looser, a plaster should be worn to stop it from catching, and finally the nail will come away of its own accord, usually leaving a perfect new nail growing up underneath. Forcing the old nail to come off by pulling can damage the new nail coming from the matrix, sometimes permanently.

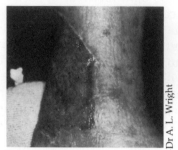

FIGURE 16.5 *A swollen ankle (with a leg ulcer)*

Swollen feet and ankles

These are often due to poor circulation, aggravated by lengthy standing. If the swelling is not relieved or eased, it remains and thickens, looking unsightly and causing joint problems later (Figure 16.5). It can be relieved by regular massage, exercises, and resting with the feet positioned higher than the head. All these help to stimulate the circulation and lymphatic drainage so that the fluid can be removed. However, swollen feet and ankles are usually an indication of general fluid retention in the body. As this is a medical or a dietary problem, a doctor's advice should be sought.

Thickened toenail plates (onychauxis or hypertrophy)

Elderly people often have extremely thickened and yellow big-toe nails, often resembling horns and very difficult to cut. They are frequently a side-effect of old age, or the result of pressure on the nail, trauma, psoriasis, fungal infection or the ingestion of certain drugs.

A client with thickened nails which prove too difficult to cut and file in a normal pedicure should be referred to a chiropodist: chiropodists are trained to thin the nail using electric nail files. A pedicurist must *never* attempt to thin the nail herself as it is easy to file through to the nail bed and cause damage if the filing is not done correctly.

Tired aching feet

Feet will ache if they are subjected to long periods of standing, or because of foot problems such as arthritis, bunions, calluses, corns, fallen arches or swollen feet.

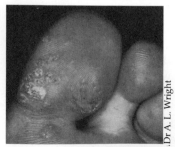

FIGURE 16.6 *Verrucae (foot warts)*

Verrucae (verucca plantaris)

These are foot warts which can multiply rapidly or grow bigger if not treated immediately (Figure 16.6). They are caused by a viral infection, and tend to be common in young children who run about barefoot in gyms or around swimming pools. Verrucae look like corns but are usually moist and often have a black speck in the centre of them. They occur mostly on the soles of the feet, but can also be found on other parts (e.g. between or on top of the toes).

Home treatment is not recommended: a doctor or chiropodist must be consulted. Verrucae must not be treated in the salon, neither must a pedicure be given to a client with them: as they are caused by a virus, standard disinfection procedures are not sufficient to guard against their transmission. Sterilisation procedures are needed. If contact is made with them inadvertently, all items which cannot be sterilised must be destroyed. Towels must be boil-washed in water to which a small amount of bleach has been added.

Weak feet and fallen arches

These develop when the supporting muscles become strained and the ligaments lose their tone (tightness). Because the foot structure lacks strength, the arches weaken and fall (drop). Flat feet are an example: here the ligaments of the joints stretch and give, the muscles lose their tone, and the bony arches 'drop' and flatten out. The bones start to come uncomfortably in contact with the ground, causing aching feet and postural problems. The body tries to cushion the bones by forming layers of hard skin (callus).

This problem often results from overstrain due to pregnancy, overweight or excessive standing. It is also seen in sedentary people who do not offset their inactivity by exercising their feet, or in people who over-exercise their foot muscles to collapsing point by the continuous wearing of exercise sandals (designed only for short-term wear).

Massage and the right corrective exercises can both help to strengthen weakened arches. However, if the condition is painful or causing problems, then a chiropodist should be seen. She can give treatments such as faradic foot-baths, in which the muscles of the foot are stimulated to contract at regular intervals during the treatment, thereby strengthening the muscles of the arches. She can also design a corrective home exercise programme and fit arch supports into the client's shoes to help alleviate discomfort.

PART VII Advanced nail techniques

17 The BASIC PRINCIPLES

It is no longer sufficient for a manicurist simply to be able to carry out a manicure and a pedicure treatment. Modern technology has put within her reach a vast array of products and techniques which may be used to carry out permanent or semi-permanent repairs and extensions to broken, damaged, bitten or short nails. It is the duty of a manicurist to be competent to provide these for her client, immediately and on request. Such a manicurist is now more accurately known as a 'nail technician' – one who uses current advances in modern technology to provide the best possible nail service for her client.

Note
It is logical to study the different techniques of nail *extension* before studying methods of *repairing* nails, because the most efficient and durable repairs are carried out using modified nail extension materials and techniques.

NAIL EXTENSION TECHNIQUES: AN INTRODUCTION

Nail extensions fall within two main categories: temporary and permanent.

Temporary extensions

These are pre-formed complete nail covers which are designed to last from one to fourteen days, depending on the type of adhesive used.

'Permanent' extensions

These are built up and extended from the client's natural nail (Figure 17.1). They were originally designed for permanent and continuous wear, partly because of the difficulty of their removal! Improvements in products mean that many of the 'permanent' nails can now be removed at any time with no damage to the natural nail beneath. In order to wear these nails for any length of time, they need salon

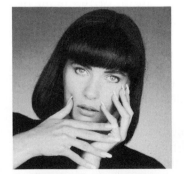

FIGURE 17.1 *A set of nail extensions*

maintenance treatments every two weeks to deal with problems associated with the area of natural nail growth at their base. These nails fall into three main categories:

1 *Sculptured nails* using *acrylic* or allied products, in which a powder and a liquid are brought together to form a quick-setting paste which is used to create the nail extension. (These are sometimes known as sculptured nails.)
2 *Gels*, which are brushed over an extension tip or nail form and then set with a light source or a catalyst spray.
3 *Fibreglass* or allied products, a combination of webbing, resin and a catalyst, applied as a strengthener and support over an extension tip.

CONSULTATION

Before a client books, there must be an extensive, two-way consultation procedure. The potential client must understand thoroughly just what she is embarking upon. She must be made aware of the types of nail available and the differences between them; how long they will last and whether they need to be worn with nail varnish or not; the expense of the initial treatment and any other expenses involved, such as special nail adhesives for emergency repairs and special nail varnish removers; the cost of removing the nails or of products to remove them at home, and the cost and frequency of any maintenance treatments which may be needed.

Honest advice must be given here – for example, a bride requiring nails for a two-week period for her wedding and honeymoon, before returning to a profession as nurse, cook or shorthand typist, would be best advised to have either cheaper, temporary extensions which would last her two weeks only and would have to be worn with nail varnish at all times, or more expensive, but lighter and more natural-looking fibreglass or other easily dissolvable extensions, which could be worn with or without nail varnish. Both these types can be easily and quickly removed, either at home or in the salon, before she has to return to her work. Her own nails would not be damaged; further, if she has the false ones removed in the salon and followed by a manicure, she will be made aware of the manicure service and will probably return for this again.

Always be honest and perceptive with clients. Never look upon a client as just another source of income: each person is an individual whose nail care programme needs tailoring to fit her, her income and her lifestyle. Time spent on initial consultations will ultimately benefit the nail technician by producing satisfied clients and helping to minimise potential future problems.

Conversely, is the nail technician willing to accept responsibility for the nails of this potential customer? This might sound strange, but a client who consistently increases the length of time between nail-fill treatments not only makes booking difficult in a busy schedule, but confronts the manicurist with sometimes quite horrific problems –

lifted extensions, glue all over her varnish and built up under the nail product, brittle product due to over-use of cheap store-bought glues, and worst of all natural nail plates thinned, damaged and possibly infected with bacteria due to the continual self-inflicted lifting and gluing. Does a busy and conscientious nail technician really need such problems? If the client is obliged on this occasion, and her nails sorted out by time-consuming treatment, she may simply repeat the incident and eventually criticise both the nails and the manicurist for ruining her natural nails. She may even sue the salon – and she would be quite within her rights to do so. The nail technician, as a professional person, is legally liable for the condition of her client's nails, and by not stopping her damaging behaviour and discouraging her from wearing the nails, she is condoning the situation.

To avoid incidents like this, the manicurist *must* stress at the initial consultation the necessary aftercare. Two-weekly fills must be insisted upon, with *additional* weekly manicures (checks) and shorter nail lengths for clients with badly bitten nails or those who are in heavy manual work. *The nail technician would be both foolish and unprofessional if she neglected to inform future clients of essential aftercare procedures, or if she accepted any client who was not prepared to follow the recommendations given to her.*

Contra-indications

Contra-indications include those for a manicure (page 93); there are also some additional ones, for temporary extensions (page 202) and for permanent extensions (page 221).

ADMINIS-TRATION

Record-keeping

Record-keeping (Figure 17.2) is essential for many reasons:

1 To satisfy the requirements of the salon's insurance policy.
2 To record the client's name, address and telephone number. This makes it possible to contact her if necessary, for example to cancel her treatment if the manicurist should be ill, to remind her of her appointment, to enquire as to why she has not kept an appointment and reschedule it if necessary, to send her details of any salon promotions or promotional gifts (e.g. a birthday or Christmas card or voucher), or even to inform her should the salon be moving or changing its telephone number. Be very careful to record whether the client wishes to be known as 'Mrs', 'Miss' or 'Ms': ladies are usually very sensitive on this point and can take offence easily.
3 To record what previous services have been carried out on the nails in any salon, their effectiveness, and whether any allergies were encountered. This gives a guide as to what treatments to choose in the future.

Surname _____	Forename _____	Marital status _____

Address _____   Birth date _____

_____   Tel. (home) _____

_____   Tel. (work) _____

Prior history or comments _____

_____

Referrals   1) _____

2) _____

3) _____

Date	Service and product	Shape	Varnish	Cost	Comments

Prior history or comments *Badly bitten nails with a pad of flesh protruding at end of nail plate. Rec. 2-3 sets ex. nails then f/g. nails to gain length, then regular manicures + use of nail hardeners.*

Date	Service and product	Shape	Varnish	Cost	Comments
3/7/92	Express (full) nails	Short Oval	Pale lilac	14.50	Only leave 10 days. Nail plate short
15/7/92	Rem. nails + new set	"	Sugar pink	17.50	Only leave 10 days.
24/7/92	Rem. nails + full set f/g. ext.	Medium square	French	40.00	Free edge now 1/16" so o.k. for fibre glass extensions.
7/8/92	1st fill and shorten	"	Beige dream	12.00	No problems.
21/8/92	2nd fill and shorten	"	True red	18.00	No problems.
4/9/92	1st fill and shorten	"	"	12.00	Free edge growing nicely. Perhaps return to own nails next.
18/9/92	Rem. f/g ext. + man. + buff	Rounded square	Sugar pink	15.00	Nail hardener £6-95 Cuticle oil £6-95
25/9/92	Man.	"		8.00	Nails O.K. and quite hard.
2/10/92	Man.	"	Clover	8.00	Nail varnish £4.95.
9/10/92	Man.	"	True red	8.00	Nails very hard and strong.
16/10/92	Man.	"	"	8.00	Could go to 2-weekly mans.
					if desired but no longer.

FIGURE 17.2 *An example of a record card*

4 To record the condition of the client's nail plate and cuticles prior to treatment. Were the nails in good condition, or was an attempt being made to rectify an existing problem? Was a service postponed or another substituted because of a problem, such as badly bitten nails, fungal infection, a lifting nail plate, or pitting or ridging of the nail plate?

5 To record the client's occupation. This may influence the wear and tear the nails will be subjected to, and how suitable they would be for her. For instance, the mother of a young baby would be advised not to have her nails long as she might scratch her child; a retail sales assistant in a jewellery shop would find that wearing long nails would actually enhance her sales of rings.

6 To record the date the nails were applied and the date of any nail fill-ins. This allows the manicurist to check that her client is booking her fills regularly, and to follow up on any 'offenders'.

7 To record the type of nail applied, and the products and procedures used.

8 To record any reactions to the products, or any allergies encountered.

9 To record the shape of the nails worn by the client.

10 To record the cost of the services and products which the client has bought. This shows the nail technician how much the client has invested in her nails and indicates her spending power.

11 To record the colour of the nail varnish used, and any products purchased, so that if the client wishes the same colour or product in the future, the manicurist knows exactly what she means.

12 To record any referrals made by the client, such as recommending the salon to a friend. It is good business to thank and even to reward a client for any successful referrals.

13 Occasionally, 'trivial' information can be recorded, to assist the nail technician in remembering conversational details about her client. Examples are the names and ages of her children or of special pets. Remembering points like this makes the client feel special and welcome in the salon.

Advance booking

Each nail technician will develop her own system of booking, unique to her and her type of trade or clientele. However, a major point which needs to be borne in mind is that people wearing nail extensions need regular two- or three-weekly fill-in treatments. Because of this, pre-scheduled, standing appointments for fill-ins should be booked whilst the client is having her initial treatment. These bookings can be scheduled three months or more in advance so that the client can be assured of the time and day which is most suitable to her. She will not be very impressed if the salon has a casual 'book-when-you-please' attitude and in consequence she cannot get her fills when she wants them because the manicurist is booked up!

In such circumstances, she will look elsewhere to obtain satisfaction. Conversely, the manicurist will not be pleased if she has booked one hour to do a fill-in and the client arrives with her nails in need of extra attention because she has 'been meaning to make an appointment for the past five weeks'! At the very least, the client should book her next appointment as she leaves the salon. If she is not willing to do this, she will not make a good client.

Advanced bookings can lead to clients not turning up for appointments and time is money for the nail technician. This can be discouraged in several ways:

- ☐ *Always* give out appointment cards with the salon's number on, at the time of booking. Do not trust the client's belief that she 'will remember'. With regular, pre-scheduled bookings, put three or six months of bookings on one specially designed appointment card.
- ☐ Take substantial deposits (up to 50 per cent) with initial bookings from clients not previously known to the salon. If they book over the phone, tell them that it is a provisional booking until a certain date, before which they must post or bring a deposit to the salon. A genuine client will comply with these requests.
- ☐ Telephone clients the evening before their appointment, to confirm their booking. This is essential when long periods of the manicurist's time are booked out with one client.
- ☐ If a client does not come for her appointment, this might be for a genuine reason, such as a car crash on the way, or it might be because she is scatterbrained and simply does not care. Time is money for the nail technician and she must judge accordingly. Three 'no-shows' with no genuine reason in one year is enough; the manicurist must thereafter call a halt and could pretend to be booked up every time that particular client calls, in order to encourage her to go elsewhere. A good manicurist will have a waiting list of potential clients eager to fill such slots.
- ☐ A persistent latecomer is easier to deal with. First try the usual requests, but some people seem destined to go through life being late for everything! In such instances, schedule the appointment in the book but write a time 15 minutes earlier on the client's appointment card. In the event that she one day arrives 'on time', profuse apologies about running late will usually pacify her.

A nail technician will get to know her clients – the ones who *do* need reminding or who come late, and the ones who come every time, on time. If she builds up her regular clientele and keeps a good advanced booking system, she will rapidly become booked up. (The maximum capacity for one manicurist is about sixty regular false-nail clients.) The fact that she is booked up will enhance her reputation and clients will not want to miss their appointment because of the difficulty of getting another 'slot'.

If a client does have to cancel at the last minute and an alternative space is not available, keep her name and number in a special column in the appointment book reserved for clients waiting for a cancellation. As a cancellation occurs, such clients can be telephoned in sequence until one is found to fill the space.

PREPARING THE NAIL PLATE

In order to achieve a natural-looking nail extension which adheres firmly round the base, it is essential to give prior attention to the cuticle area. Overgrown cuticles not only spoil the appearance of the finished nails but cause lifting around the base of the extension if the extension material overlaps onto any cuticle particles. The cuticles need to be pushed back from the nail plate to leave a clean surface for the nail to adhere to, and clipped where necessary to give a neat and tidy appearance to the base of the finished nail.

In practice, a nail technician with a number of years' experience can achieve this by the application of cuticle remover to the area, followed by pushing back the overgrown cuticle with a rubber hoof stick or a cuticle knife (or both), followed by careful clipping to achieve a smooth line. This quick method, ideal for single emergency extensions, can be advocated only when carried out by a good manicurist who will *never* cause a wound by clipping.

In theory, and essential in practice for recently trained manicurists, cuticles must never be clipped immediately prior to the application of extensions. This is because the chemicals and glues used in the treatment could cause an allergic reaction to a cut and sensitive area. In cases like this, the client should visit the salon three or four days before the extensions are to be applied: the nails can be pre-manicured and if any damage does occur to the cuticle area, there is time for it to settle down and heal before any chemicals are used on the area.

After the cuticles have been attended to, the manicurist should quickly neaten the free edge of the natural nail with an emery board, so that it will accommodate a tip or nail form easily. A free edge of 1.5 mm ($\frac{1}{16}$ in.) is ideal, though not essential, for most extension techniques.

Finally, the client should be sent to scrub her hands and nails with a good-quality antiseptic soap, drying them on a disposable towel or with a hot-air dryer. This is to guard against any possible infections being trapped under the false nail cover, and also to degrease the surface of the natural nail to encourage better adhesion. Care must be taken to ensure that the surface of the nail is completely dry before any nail application is made.

From here on, each product available will have different primers, pre-primers and recommended application techniques: it is vital that the instructions enclosed with the product in use be read and followed carefully. Below are *generalised* instructions for the selection, application and care of the major groups of nail extension.

TEMPORARY EXTENSIONS

Temporary extensions fall into two broad categories: those most suited for the client's use at home, and those most suited for application and removal in the salon. Both these categories utilise a pre-formed plastic nail which can be of neutral colouring and ready to accept a nail varnish of the client's choosing, or pre-coloured in a uniform colour or a fancy nail art design.

There are many widths, lengths and shapes available and one should be selected which is the nearest possible to the final desired fit, both around the cuticle area and in the width. Minor adjustments can be made around the base with assorted files, taking care to bevel the plastic to achieve a smooth and tapering finish. The correct length is not important with salon fitting as this can easily be obtained by cutting and filing once the nail has been firmly fixed in position. With nails for home use, however, the correct length must be obtained *before* fitting as the adhesive is not strong enough to allow shaping when the nail has been fixed in position.

TEMPORARY EXTENSIONS FOR HOME USE

Temporary extensions are ideal in the following circumstances:

1 For covering, and thus protecting, a torn or split nail until it can be mended permanently.
2 For extending a single nail, or a full set of nails, for a short time (24 hours or longer), depending on the occupation of the client and the care she takes with her hands. A very careful client who does not wash up or otherwise put her nails at risk should manage to keep them for up to a week before they need removing and the adhesive renewing.
3 For retailing to clients for home use.

The older type of temporary extensions utilised adhesives which remained soft and rubbery when set, allowing the extension to be gently pulled off when no longer needed. Any surplus glue could easily be rubbed away without causing any damage. The current method of adhesion utilises double-sided sticky pads, one side of which sticks to the natural nail, the other to the false nail. The false nail can be removed by gently pulling it away from the sticky pad and rubbing the pad away from the surface of the nail plate using a fingertip. Whichever type of adhesive is used, the false nails should not be worn longer than a week before giving the nail plate an overnight 'breathing' period.

The advantages of the sticky pad method of adhesion are that no damage is done to the natural nail plate and that the false nails are able to be reused as they are not damaged during removal.

Fitting home nail extensions

Materials
- □ Soap (preferably antiseptic) and warm water.
- □ A nailbrush.
- □ False nails, pre-formed and shaped to fit the natural nails.
- □ Adhesive nail tabs.
- □ Small, sharp scissors.

Technique
1 After pre-manicuring the natural nails, wash the hands and scrub the natural nails thoroughly with soap and water. This will remove any surface oils from the nail plate and allow the adhesive to stick firmly. Dry them thoroughly on a clean towel.
2 Select an adhesive pad of the right size to cover the surface of the nail or trim a larger-sized pad to fit. Remove the paper backing from one side of the pad and press the sticky side evenly and firmly onto the surface of the natural nail.
3 Remove the protective paper from the top of the sticky pad, position the false nail over the top, and press it firmly into place.
4 For as long as possible, avoid placing the hands into water.

TEMPORARY EXTENSIONS FOR SALON USE

It is recommended that a full, pre-formed nail cover which is attached to the natural nail plate by the fast (five-second) nail glues is only suitable for supervised salon use and not home use for the following reasons:

1 A lack of hygiene (failing to use antiseptic soaps) before home application, coupled with the possibility of creating air bubbles during application, can easily lead to bacterial infections.
2 A tendency to keep the nails on for too long, or to wait until they fall off or become loose and are pulled off, followed by immediate re-gluing, may cause problems (see page 202).

Such nails are ideal for fitting in the salon, however, for:

1 Short-term wear (up to 2 weeks).
2 Very badly bitten nails, such that the client is ashamed of the appearance of her nails but really wants to grow her own. This

type of temporary extension will last her up to ten days, covering her embarrassment and breaking the nail-biting habit, whilst her own nails grow protected underneath. It may take two or three sets of false nails before sufficient length is obtained for regular manicures (plus the use of nail hardeners) or for the application of a more permanent type of false nail.

3 As an interim protective extension whilst badly bitten nails (those with a bulbous fleshy protrusion beyond their tip) grow to a length which will accommodate permanent nails more easily. If permanent nails are applied immediately in cases where this bulbous flesh is present, the bulb of flesh will exert undue pressure on the false nail bond each time the client touches anything, thus reducing its effectiveness. This, coupled with the fact that the permanent nail extension is bonded only to a tiny area, means that the extension will not survive well. This is also why a temporary extension, even with care, will only last 7–10 days on these nails instead of the 14 trouble-free days which can be expected on normal nails.

Temporary extensions are *unsuitable* in these circumstances:

1 For single nail extensions when nail varnish is not going to be worn, or if pale coloured varnishes are desired. The whiteness of the false nail would be obvious.

2 For applying as a full set if no varnish or French varnish is required (i.e. a natural look), or if pale nail varnish colours are requested. The whiteness would show through and looks false.

3 For clients who will not follow the removal instructions properly. When these nails are pulled off instead of being dissolved away in acetone, it is not the glue bond which breaks away, but the first nail layer. This leaves the natural nail thin, weak, damaged – with areas of nail torn away in places, to different depths – and flaky. This effect can be remedied somewhat by buffing, with or without the prior use of nail glues (depending on the severity of the damage), followed by the use of a good protective, varnish-type nail hardener. In effect, however, this damage has to grow out, a process which can take up to six months. ('Bad' clients often pull the nails off and re-glue them for the sake of 'economy'.)

4 For a very lengthwise curved, 'parrot's beak' shape of natural nail: a large gap would be left at the tip and would show from the back of the nails.

This type of nail is available in different lengths and shapes, curved or straight lengthwise with different-shaped bases. Experience has shown the straight varieties to be the strongest and most durable, although the curved varieties are the most natural-looking. Length varies from country to country, with the Americans wearing their nails *long* and producing 'European' shorter-length nails for the English market which *still* have to be trimmed down for almost all clients!

Pre-coloured nails are available: these shorten the application time as there is no need to varnish them.

Adhesives vary and are a matter of choice. They are all variations of the 'super-glue' genre and care must be taken with their use. Removal of the nails with acetone will not remove these glues, which must be removed by careful buffing away using suitable buffing files. Solvents are now available for some glues.

Fitting temporary nail extensions

Materials (in addition to the usual manicure station)

- A selection of sizes of false nails (0–9).
- Small, sharp scissors with which to trim the false nails (e.g. needlework scissors).
- Files: one 100 grit (very coarse for rough shaping); one 240–260 grit (coarse for final shaping and shaping the base to fit).
- A double-sided small file with foam between the emeries, which might be 240–260 grit and 600 grit (for shaping the base to fit and for bevelling both the base and the completed tip). These files are often shaped, as hearts, squares or circles.
- A three-sided buffer file, 600 grit and finer. (This is needed only if glue gets onto the nail plate to re-smooth the surface – essential when learning.)
- Quick-setting nail glue.
- Methylated spirits (70 per cent alcohol).
- A cuticle stick.
- Cottonwool (to roll around the tip of the cuticle stick, making an applicator swab for the methylated spirits).
- Tissue roll (one sheet is needed to soak up any excess glue which may be mistakenly applied).
- Ridge-filler base coat.

Technique

Prior preparation: the nails should have been pre-manicured and scrubbed with an antiseptic soap.

1 *Inspection* Ask the client to place both hands palm down on the manicure towel. Examine the nails minutely for contra-indications and for any areas which will need special care later (e.g. a single badly bitten nail).

2 *Degreasing* Dip the cottonwool-tipped cuticle stick into the methylated spirits and use it to wipe firmly and thoroughly over the surface of the nails. This removes any oils and moisture from the surface of the nail, allowing proper adhesion, and it also helps to kill any potential infection on the nail surface.

3 *Sizing-up* Now the correct sizes of nails must be selected to cover and extend the natural nail. The width of the selected nail is crucial: it must be neither too narrow, such that the natural nail shows at the side, nor too wide, such that the nail looks spoon-shaped or obviously clumsy and false. Application of too-wide nails is the most common fault; not only do they look unsightly, but the overlap onto the nail wall creates a space for moisture and dirt to collect, thus shortening the life of the nails by encouraging lifting. The second most common fault is failure to shape the base of the false nail to the natural line of the cuticle. In most cases, some shaping is needed here, followed by bevelling to give both a comfortable fit (no sharp edges) and a tapered (as opposed to a thick) finish. The two-sided sponge files are ideal for this work.

Nails are also available curved or flat from side to side, so a good fit with no stress on the nail plate or the false nail can be achieved, thus making the false nails last longer.

As each nail is sized up, place it in a linear sequence to the right of the work-space, with the tip nearest the edge of the manicurist's side of the table, to make the set easy to pick up later.

4 *Removing the shine* Using a fine buffer file (certainly no more than 600 grit), gently take the shine off the surface of the natural nail plate. This is to allow the glue to bond better to the surface, which will be slightly scuffed instead of completely smooth. It is also to remove surface grease. At one time, this scuffing process was unnecessarily vigorous and damaging to the nail plate; improvements in the adhesion properties of the materials used are leading towards this stage being eliminated completely.

5 *Degreasing* Repeat step 2.

6 *Sticking* Make sure that the glue, tissues and nails are ready to hand. It is quickest if one starts the sticking procedure from the client's right little finger and works straight across all ten nails.

Make sure that the methylated spirit has completely evaporated away from the surface of the starting nail. If it has not, the fumes will cause the glue to start to set immediately and make the application of the false nail impossible. If this happens, quickly wipe the glue away with the tissue, apply some more glue and continue.

Taking one nail at a time, place a line of nail glue down the centre of the nail, starting about 2.5 mm ($\frac{1}{8}$ in.) away from the cuticle. If the glue flows down the sides of the plate onto the finger, then too much glue has been used. Use sufficient so that the surface tension of the glue holds it in place in a long drop.

Immediately put the glue container down and pick up the relevant false nail, initially holding it at an angle to the nail plate. Place the base of the false nail onto the nail plate, level with the base of the glue drop. 'Pick up' the glue with the base of the false nail and take it to the base of the nail plate, without flooding the

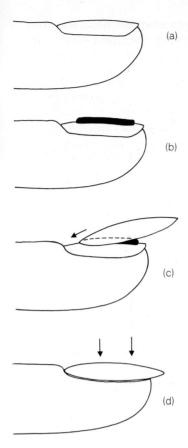

FIGURE 18.1 *Fitting temporary false nail extensions: (a) The prepared nail, with the cuticle pushed back, the surface degreased and the shine removed. (b) The line of glue, held in place by surface tension. (c) The angled false nail, picking up the glue and sliding it towards the base. (d) The false nail being lowered onto the nail plate, with the glue evenly distributed beneath it; surface pressure completes the bonding*

cuticles, by sliding the false nail down the nail plate and up against the cuticle, meanwhile lowering the rest of the false nail onto the nail plate. In this way the glue is distributed evenly underneath the false nail and air bubbles are avoided. Do not push the false nail into the cuticle or it will cause irritation, but also do not leave a gap or it will not look right. A natural, snug fit is correct.

Press down firmly on the top surface of the nail (when learning, be prepared to clean up excess glue with the tissue), wait about ten seconds, and fitting is complete. Repeat for the next nine nails in sequence.

At the end of fitting, check around the edges and under the tips of the nails to make sure that contact is total and that there are no air gaps. If these gaps are present, fill with glue, wiping away the excess. Gaps can easily be seen through the false nail.

If an air bubble has been created under the false nail, then the nail must be removed and another one applied or there is risk of lack of adhesion and, more seriously, of bacterial infection. At this stage, if some acetone is placed onto a cottonwool ball and rubbed firmly up and down the false nail plate, the false nail will easily be removed.

7 *Cutting* Selecting a first (index) finger, discuss with the client as to what length she would like the extensions. It must be explained that for optimum strength, the extension should be no longer than half as long again as the natural nail plate. Anything longer than this will decrease the length of time that the false nails will adhere to the natural nails. A client with naturally short nails is not used to handling long nails and will probably repeatedly catch and bang them. This will cause the nail layers to begin to flake away and the false nail to start to 'lift' and come off. Not only this, but repeated knocks can start to lift the *natural* nail from its bed, causing damage in this area as well as the possibility of bacterial or fungal infection.

After discussion, cut the extension straight across, slightly longer than you think – a bit more can always be filed away, but it is impossible to stick any back on! Then cut the sides roughly to shape. Show the client and continue cutting this nail until the right length has been agreed. Now the other nails can be cut, with one cut straight across and one cut to take each corner away – a total of three quick cuts per nail.

8 *Filing to shape* Selecting the 100 grit file, file all the nails to the correct shape and length. Fine shaping can be done using the 240–260 grit file, and the frills can be removed using the two-sided sponge sandwich file. Use each file on all ten nails before moving on to the next file so that time is not wasted through constantly putting down and picking up files. If there is any glue on the surface of the nails, this must be removed using the three-sided buffer.

9 *Cleaning up* Shake away the dust and bits from the hand towel on the station, tidy up, and wipe all the dust off the client's hands in readiness for varnishing.

10 *Varnishing* A ridge-filler base coat should be used, as some plastic nails show 'stress lines' after application and these can only be seen after the varnish is applied. They show more with pearlised varnishes than with cream varnishes, but use of a ridge-filling base coat smooths them over. The usual number of coats of varnish should be applied and the nails finished with a top coat.

If the client is advised to apply a coat of top coat to the nails every second or third day, the varnish will last her as long as the nails do: false nails are not flexible and so will not bend and break away from the varnish as soft natural nails do (a major cause of flaking and peeling). The only thing which will cause the deterioration of the varnish is its wearing away in use. A regularly applied top coat will stop this.

REMOVING TEMPORARY EXTENSIONS

Materials
- □ Pottery or glass dishes, 8–10 cm (3–4 in.) in diameter and 5–7 cm (2–3 in.) deep (2).
- □ Sufficient acetone to fill these dishes, approx. 2–3 cm (1 in.) deep. (Refer to the warning on page 59.)
- □ 15 ml (1 tablespoon) of oil (vegetable or mineral, e.g. baby oil) for each dish.
- □ A tissue sheet to protect the manicure station.
- □ Cottonwool or Nail Neats.
- □ Small scissors.
- □ A three-sided buffer file.

Technique
1 Remove the nail varnish.
2 Roughly cut away the excess length of the nail extension, taking care not to cut the natural nail underneath.
3 Place the fingers in the dishes containing the acetone and the oil. The oil coats the fingers and prevents the acetone from drying out the skin.
4 It helps greatly if the client will agitate her finger ends in the bowl, rubbing them against each other and against the bottom of the bowl.
5 Take one hand out of the acetone and, holding the fingers over the bowl to catch the drips, firmly wipe the melting surface of each false nail in turn with a piece of cottonwool or a Nail Neat which has been dipped into the acetone. Return the fingers to the acetone.
6 Keep repeating 5 with alternate hands until all the false nail has dissolved or melted away. There will still be some glue residue on

the nail surface which will not dissolve in the acetone.

7 Ask the client to wash her hands, to remove the acetone and oil.
8 Proceed to manicure the nails as normal, during the course of which the remnants of the glue on the surface of the nail can be removed and the natural nail brought to a high gloss with the careful use of buffer files.

It is recommended that one use a varnish-type nail hardener after wearing these nails, to rectify any weakness or softness which may occur.

19 'PERMANENT' EXTENSIONS: an INTRODUCTION

SPECIAL EQUIPMENT, IMPLEMENTS, COSMETICS AND MATERIALS

The following items are needed in addition to the usual manicure tools and supplies.

Equipment

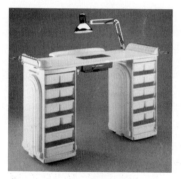

FIGURE 19.1 *A well-lit and ventilated manicure desk*

A well-lit and ventilated work desk

Ventilation is essential as the dust and fumes created during nail extension treatments are harmful in the long term if precautions are not taken to avoid excessive inhalation. Most nail extension cosmetics carry warnings to the effect that they must only be used in a well-ventilated area.

A comfortable work stool with adjustable height and a backrest

Throughout the working day, the stool determines the posture and hence the comfort of the manicurist. Incorrect posture can result in injuries, including backache or even tenosynivitis (repetitive strain injury of the hands and wrists).

A comfortable client's chair

A must when clients are attending for frequent 1–2-hour treatments.

A dryer

The natural nail plate must be thoroughly dry before any type of extension or repair is applied: a dryer will ensure that this is so. A hairdryer will suffice if a commercial dryer is not available.

Protective spectacles

These are needed both by the client and by the manicurist. They must be worn during the clipping-back procedure to guard the eyes from flying particles. They can be bought with wrap-around lenses which will fit over the top of most eyeglasses.

A light-source lamp

This is used in setting the gels if gel light nail extensions are to be carried out.

Terry towels

The deep pile of terry towels on the manicure area collects filings and nail dust. When filing, the manicurist should continually re-fold one of these towels on her work station to trap product dust. When filing is completed, the towel should be moved away and laundered, a clean one being placed on the work area. This minimises allergic reactions and eczemas which can occur on the manicurist's arms, hands and wrists as a result of exposure to product dusts. This practice also reduces the possibility of dust spoiling the nail varnish application.

Implements

Tip nippers

Short-bladed, sturdy, sprung-handled clippers, ideal for cutting and shaping nail tips.

Acrylic nippers

Strong clippers with fine tips, specifically designed to cut hard acrylic. Like all clippers, they should be oiled and sharpened regularly. Acrylic nippers are available with double springs which eliminate metal-on-metal rubbing and virtually eliminate the breaking of springs.

Fabric scissors

These are often shaped like a stork, giving rise to their common name, 'stork scissors' (Figure 19.2). They are a very fine scissor especially selected for cutting the finest of nail-wrapping materials. These scissors should be used for nothing but cutting fine fabrics or else the blades will be spoilt.

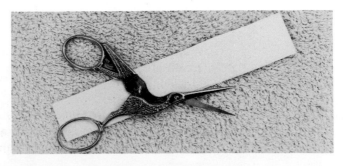

FIGURE 19.2 *Fine 'stork' scissors and fibreglass webbing*

Small product containers (e.g. Dappen dishes)

Small dishes (Figure 19.3) are needed to hold small quantities of the polymers (powders) and monomers (liquids) used when applying acrylic nails. They need to be small to minimise evaporation, which causes fumes and loss of the product whilst working. The powders and liquids must never be returned to their original containers or contamination (resulting in activation and spoiling of the bulk liquids and powders) will occur: small dishes mean small amounts will be dispensed and only small amounts will have to be thrown away at the end of the treatment.

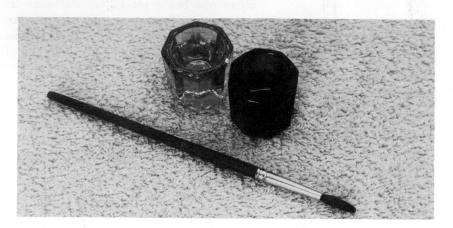

FIGURE 19.3 *Dappen dishes and a sable brush*

Some nail technicians prefer to keep their monomer liquid in stainless-steel pump dispensers. These dispensers include a mushroom-shaped plug in the centre of the holding dish. This plug prevents liquid which has combined with acrylic product from draining back into the pump mechanism and clogging the dispenser. A standard dispenser, for use with nail varnish removers, antiseptics and the like, does not contain this plug and is therefore unsuitable.

The correct dispenser, designed to eliminate evaporation, fumes and waste, is excellent as long as the manicurist does not overpump, flooding the contaminated product back into the dispenser via the air holes in the rim of the dish, and does not use the lid of the dispenser to wipe excess acrylic off the brush. The latter can cause activated liquid and powder to run down the wire hinge of the lid, get inside the pump mechanism, and glue the moving parts together.

Nail scrubbing brushes

These are essential; used with antiseptic soaps the client (and the manicurist) can clean her hands and nails thoroughly prior to the nail treatment.

Product applicator brushes (for acrylics and gels)

The brushes for gel application are made of semi-stiff special nylon filaments which give a smooth and even application of the gel. They should be cleaned regularly with brush cleaners and allowed to dry before reuse.

The brushes for the application of acrylic products are completely different. Sable brushes are preferred, both for performance and durability. They may have a rounded or a pointed tip, the choice being a matter of personal preference. Size varies too, for example a size 6 brush is quite full and will hold a lot of acrylic. Therefore it is often the choice for application of full sets of complete nails. A size 4 brush is smaller and good for doing nail fills, or for the manicurist who prefers to work with smaller quantities of acrylic on her brush. Sable brushes should be cleaned after every use, reshaped, and allowed to air-dry with the bristles pointing upwards.

Pottery or glass finger bowls

These are for use when dissolving products to remove them from the natural nail surface. Acetone or some similar solvent is used in the removal process: such solvents will dissolve most plastic containers but not pottery or glass.

Nail forms

These are adjustable platforms which are applied to fingertips under the free edge of the nail plate (Figure 19.4). The acrylic or gel is then applied to the nail plate and extended over the platform to create an extension of the natural nail plate. A nail form must be able to hold a C-curve under the weight of the acrylic. It must fit the natural nail plate without leaving gaps at the side. It must be adhesive enough to hold in place on the finger throughout the treatment, yet able to be removed easily when the nail material has set.

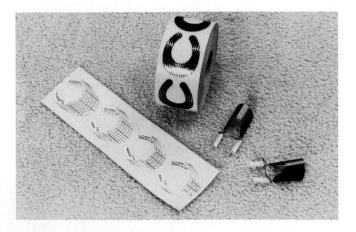

FIGURE 19.4 *Paper-backed foil nail forms of standard shapes with cut-away sides, and (right) Teflon-coated reusable nail forms*

There are various types of nail form, available with and without printed guidelines:

1 *Sticky-backed foil* These are very manoeuvrable, but thin. Manicurists often use two together for added support.

2 *Sticky-backed foil with paper backing* The support is better here, but care must be taken when fitting that corners (folds in the form) are not created. This is the most popular disposable nail form and is available in standard and 'cut-away' shapes. The 'cut-away' shape allows straighter sides to be formed to the extension, thus eliminating sidewall stress points and minimising breakage and cracking. It is also easier to shape a square-shaped nail on this type of form as the nail created is given a more even depth of product.

3 *Reusable nail forms* Made of non-stick Teflon, these forms have little handles and a gentle but firm metal clip to attach the form to the finger. One size fits all nails (the foil forms need to be available in various sizes) and the clip ensures a snug, immovable fit with a really good C-curve. The clip releases easily to remove the form from the completed nail, and the Teflon ensures that the form is easily wiped clean ready for immediate reuse.

A large face powder brush or manicure brush

This is used in brushing any dust off the surface of the nails.

Cosmetics

Nail tips

These are nail shapes made out of plastic or nylon (Figure 19.5). They are used, with glues, to extend a short nail (this type of extension, in which the tip starts halfway up the natural nail, is often strengthened with a gel, acrylic or wrap overlay) or to completely cover and extend a natural nail. Nail tips can be long, short, straight or curved lengthways, and very curved or flatter from side to side. The choice of shapes, coupled with approximately ten size choices, means that most natural nails can be fitted with a tip, although some customisation is usually necessary.

From the point of view of technique, however, they can have a concave and short overlap (sometimes called a well), or a convex and

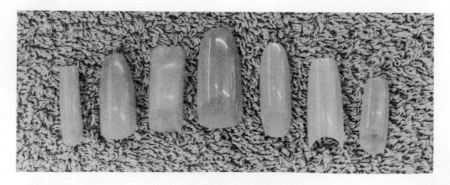

FIGURE 19.5 *Nail tips and full nails in assorted shapes and sizes*

short or long overlap. The concave with short overlap are ideal when used with transparent gels and fibreglass overlays to reduce the amount of 'blending in' that the tip needs. In fact, with skill a French manicure effect is easily created in this way. Some manicurists use this type of tip on badly bitten nails where there is not much nail surface onto which to glue the tip.

The deeper overlaps, or wells, are used to give greater overall stability and extra reinforcement at the sides of the nail (good when a client is hard on her hands). The mid portion of this kind of tip has to be filed away before the overlay is applied or it may show, depending on the transparency of the tip. This type is the one chosen by nail technicians doing the full-cover temporary nail extension (sometimes called the 'express nail extension' because of its speed of application).

Tips can be made of nylon. These will bend in any direction without cracking or breaking. Fibres can often be seen in the nail. They are good tips, but many products will not stick to them. Nylon tips are often sold with gel systems, which will adhere to them.

ABS Plastic is the usual material used for nail tips. The tips are formed by injection moulding and the 'trees' (supports) formed at the same time are ground up when the tips have been removed and the grindings (regrind) are added back to the initial plastic to be made into more tips. As the process continues there is a build-up of regrind in the manufacturing material, which can be detected by the colour of the completed tip. A white tip has no regrind in it; a yellow tip has a lot of regrind in it. A tip with too much regrind in it will be brittle and crack easily due to the frequent heating and cooling the regrind has undergone. A tip with no regrind in at all does not stick to the natural nail or to product easily. The best nail tip is an in-between one with some regrind in it.

Antiseptic soap

Any soap used with hot water has antibacterial properties. However, liquid soaps with added antibacterial chemicals such as Hexachlorophane are available in hygienic pump dispensers especially for pre-treatment use by staff and clients in the manicure salon.

Acrylic products (primers, polymers, and monomers)

Primers are products used to prepare the surface of the nail so that the acrylic material will stick to it. For many years they were made of methacrylic acid, and more recently from the less damaging acrylic ester monomers. Their effect is chemically to burn off the bacteria and grease from the surface of the nail and to etch the surface so that the acrylic can form a bond. This highly caustic action is the reason that primer must not come into contact with the surrounding skin. *Many primers damage the nail surface and over-use of such primers will cause excessive damage to the nail plate and underlying tissues.* Fortunately, primers like this will be replaced as technology progresses. Already products are available which help adhesion by balancing the pH of the nail surface to that of the acrylic without causing any damage to the nail surface. This, combined with the antiseptic, drying and degreasing properties, is the proper function of a nail primer.

Pre-primers are separate products included in some product lines for the additional dehydration and sanitation of the nail surface. They are applied before primers and are only necessary if the product range in use includes one. Sanitisers, containing alcohols and anti-bacterial agents, are also sometimes used as pre-primers. (These are sometimes called Thermolise solutions.)

Sculptured nail powders, for example polymethyl methacrylate, are polymers and acrylic esters. (A *polymer* is a long molecule: a chain of many identical short chemical units. A *monomer* is a single such unit. And an *oligomer* is a short chain, comprising just a few units.)

Sculptured nail liquids, such as ethyl methacrylate, are monomers – small individual chemical units whose molecules can join together to form a polymer.

The mixture of the polymer and monomer results in a chemical reaction which alters the chemical make-up of the two. The combination of the chemicals results in a cross-linking which makes the finished product hard. In effect, the polymer and monomers combine to form a different polymer: further polymerisation takes place. The polymer (powder) contains a catalyst, usually benzyl peroxide, which acts to initiate the chemical reaction. The monomer (liquid) also contains a promoter such as N,N-dimethyl-p-toluidine.

Methyl methacrylate used to be the monomer used. Its use was stopped in 1975 because it caused extreme allergic reactions in some clients; it created a lot of heat during polymerisation, which sometimes caused burns to the nail bed and cuticle area; and it formed a *very* strong bond which made the acrylic virtually impossible to remove. Today, ethyl or isobutyl methacrylate is the monomer of choice. These do not produce as much heat as they set (polymerise), and they are easier to remove using suitable solvents.

Methacrylic vapours can irritate the eyes, nose and throat or produce headaches and drowsiness. (Once the acrylic is dry, there is no further problem.) It is therefore necessary to work in a well-ventilated area. It is also essential to avoid inhaling the dust from filing acrylic. Some form of ventilation, extraction fans, or vacuum-extraction manicure machines are ideal solutions to this problem.

Note that the absence of odour does *not* mean that no dangerous chemicals are present – carbon monoxide, for instance, is odourless yet poisonous. The new generation of odour-free acrylics still need to be used in well-ventilated areas.

Sculptured nail liquids, primers and brush cleaners often comprise the same chemicals combined in slightly different proportions.

Gel products

Light-setting gels, which set in visible light and ultraviolet light, can be viewed as second-generation acrylic products (although they are made of different ingredients). The gels contain a monomer and an oligomer resin together with a photo-initiator. The latter, when illuminated, triggers the formation of a polymer network from the monomer and oligomer. This hardens the gel. Gels are often based on acrylester resins, a high-grade plastic rather than the usual acrylic.

A typical gel might contain methacrylic or acrylic ester monomers, polyurethane and a curing agent. Gels usually contain cellulose. This is noted for turning yellow in ultraviolet light (which is why some pale nail varnishes turn yellow in the sunshine). Consequently, gels also have to contain anti-yellowing agents. Gels are available in different colours, to create nail art designs or French manicure finishes.

Spray-setting gels are similar in concept to the light-setting gels, except that the photo-initiator is replaced by a chemical initiator which is triggered by the use of a spray chemical (for example, N-methyl-palotoluene) once the gel is in place. Spray-setting gels are usually cyanoacrylate-based. The spray-on activators are usually carried in freon or trichloroethane.

Some gels are set with a brush-on activator solution. This type of activator is usually esteracetate-based and has the added advantage that it can also be used to set cyanoacrylate glues.

Wrap products

☐ *Fabrics* These include paper, silk, fibreglass and linen, and may be self-adhesive or otherwise.

☐ *Adhesives* These are usually cyanoacrylate glues, obtainable in different viscosities (thicknesses).

☐ *Adhesive-setting sprays* (catalysts) Like the sprays used to set the gels, these are often setting agents such as N-methyl-palotoluene contained in a carrier fluid, usually freon or trichloroethane.

Fibreglass products

☐ *Fibreglass fabric* The support system which is to be embedded in the resin to give the finished product flexibility and prevent its cracking or shattering.

☐ *Fibreglass resin* This contains a monomer (e.g. ethyl cyanoacrylate) and a polymer (e.g. stabilised epoxide polyester resins), plus other additives. These resins will dry and stick without the use of the catalyst spray, but in such a case the product will be porous and break down quickly in wear.

☐ *Fibreglass setting spray* (a catalyst) A setting agent in a spray fluid, usually similar in composition to those used with wrapping adhesives. A setting spray is needed to make the product non-porous and stable. (These sprays will also set cyanoacrylate glues.)

Product removers

These are sold by manufacturers to dissolve their products away from the surface of the natural nail when they are no longer required. Different products require different solvents.

Baby oil

If acetone is used to remove wraps or extensions, the addition of one tablespoon of baby oil to each dish of acetone before soaking is helpful as the oil coats the fingers and prevents the skin and nails from drying out, yet does not hinder the removal process.

Cuticle oil

This should be worked into the cuticle and surrounding skin at the completion of the nail service to combat any dryness resulting from the filing and to make the finished job look better.

Non-acetone nail varnish remover

Acetone is damaging to most nail extensions and covers and so any nail varnish removers must be strictly acetone-free.

Brush cleaner

This is essential for softening hardened acrylic on the bristles of the applicator brush, making it easy to remove and lengthening the life of the brush. It is also useful in cleaning the small product receptacles.

Nail glue

This is used in applying nail tips and levelling the ledge between the nail tip base and the natural nail before buffing in. Many nail technicians use it for resealing edges and repairing cracks in acrylic during fills. This should not be necessary and is not ideal: the glue lifts more easily than acrylic.

Materials

Files

Good, well-maintained files are preferable to, and just as quick as, an electric manicure machine. Files are graded in coarseness according to the size and therefore quantity of the grit on their surface (Figure 19.6). Comparatively 'large' pieces of grit take up more room and give a very rough and abrasive surface to the file. An example of this is a coarse 100-grit file, used for very rough shaping on artificial nail material only.

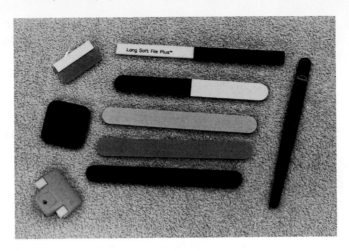

FIGURE 19.6 *Assorted buffers and files for use with nail extensions*

Much smaller pieces of grit take up less room on the file so there are more of them in a given area, producing a finer file. An example of this is a medium 240–260 grit file, used for the initial buffing of a false nail product over its surface and around the edge where it blends into the natural nail.

Even smaller pieces will make a finer still 600 grit file, used to continue the buffing over and around the false nail product. A 600 grit file would be the one to choose for gently scuffing the surface of the natural nail if this was required prior to any application. A 600 grit file is also good for bevelling the bases and tips of false nails to smooth them and eliminate 'frills'.

It is very important to have smooth edges to these files so that the client's cuticles are not inadvertently cut with a sharp side. Files can be bought with the edges smoothed away or protected in plastic; otherwise, draw one edge of a new file up against another before use to file away the sharp edges.

Buffer files

Usually sponge-inlaid files covered with three grades of emery, 600 grit and below; used in succession these create a smooth glossy finish to the artificial nail. Sometimes these buffers are used wet to achieve a high gloss finish, and sometimes the buffer is not made of emery but of gently abrasive fabrics.

Nail tidy pads (Nail Neats)

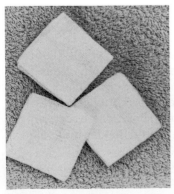

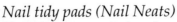

FIGURE 19.7 *Nail Neats*

These are cottonwool pads which are encased in gauze (Figure 19.7). Because of the gauze covering, they have a gentle, non-scratching abrasive action and are therefore ideal for the removal of any nail wrap and extension product after it has been soaked in remover. They are also the ideal pad to use for the removal of nail varnish or for wiping over the nail prior to varnish application, especially when gel systems are in use: few cotton fibres escape, which minimises the risk of their getting into the gel or new varnish application. Similar products for the same purpose, but made of synthetic fabrics, are now becoming available.

Disposable towels

In order to prevent infections occurring underneath the nail covers or extensions, it is essential to dry the hands and nails with clean disposable towels after the use of antiseptic soaps. It is as important for the nail technician as it is for the client to use these products prior to a treatment.

Small paper towels

These are used for wiping the brushes during acrylic nail applications, so that the acrylic does not build up on the bristles.

GENERAL POINTS

Allergies

Before the client arrives, always check her record card for any previous allergic reactions or problems. If she is a new client, she must be given a full consultation before booking or treatment in order to avoid future problems.

A regular client must have her nails examined carefully at each appointment to check for any sensitivity or allergic reaction which may occur with prolonged use of adhesives and other products. Signs to look for are: separation of the hyponychium; sensitivity and slight discomfort when pressure is applied to the nail bed; and separation of the nail plate from the nail bed – this may look like an extended free edge. If any of these signs is seen, the product should be removed and its use discontinued. If the nail plate has separated from the nail bed, the client must be referred to her doctor.

Record cards must be brought up to date at the end of each treatment so that a full past history is always available.

Patch tests

If there is the slightest risk of an allergic reaction (e.g. if the client has exhibited an allergy to gel nails but wishes to try another, chemically-unrelated product, for example fibreglass, or if the client has a history of general allergies), the manicurist must do a patch test with the nail liquid or gel and allow 24 hours for a reaction. For a patch test, simply apply the product to a plaster and place it on the inside of her elbow. Redness would indicate an adverse reaction.

Alternatively, she could fit one nail on the client and then wait for 48 hours to check that there is no adverse reaction to the product before fitting a full set.

Nail porosity

The natural nail plate is porous. It will absorb oils and moisture, swelling minutely in the process. Shrinking back then occurs as the nail dries out again. Hence, use of any oils or soaking methods prior to fitting extensions will cause lifting of the product. To maximise adhesion, the nails must be oil-free and dried thoroughly with the aid of a dryer before any technique is started.

If a client is requesting repairs or a single extension as part of a manicure, carry these out at the start of the manicure prior to any soaking or nail plate application.

Lifting

The nail plate is very flexible, especially at the base near to the cuticle. Pressure will cause it to bend. The false nail product however is inflexible, or at least much less flexible. Applying too much direct pressure to the surface of the false nail in areas where it is thin will cause the nail plate to flex and break its adhesion from the false nail product, thus causing lifting. Three prime examples of this are the use of too much pressure during surface filing, especially around the cuticle and nail wall areas; the use of too much pressure when pushing the cuticles back prior to nail fill-in treatments; and the too-vigorous use of acrylic nippers to cut away loose product prior to filling-in. If the nipper heads are too big or pressed down on the nail plate too hard, the nail plate will flex and more lifting will be caused. The nippers should be placed against the *product*, not the nail plate, and any loose material broken away with a rolling motion towards the manicurist.

Filing

When filing the surface of the false nail, keep the file moving around the area; do not file for too long in one spot. This will avoid friction burning and flat spots.

Also, do not over-file the surface of false nail products as this can break down the structure of the false nail, especially with a product that is built up in layers. There is little point in putting on product only to remove it with excessive filing! If low spots show up during filing, fill up the hollows with more product, do not file down the rest of the nail to the hollow.

When filing around the edges of the false nail product, keep the file flat to the nail. If the file is held at an angle it will file into and damage the natural nail at the base.

Products

Do not intermix product ranges. It is impossible to predict what chemical reactions will take place.

Always read and follow the instructions given by the manufacturer of the product in use. The guidelines given here are general and basic only. Each manufacturer will recommend important variations on technique of application – for instance, a primer may have to be left wet on the nail surface before application of product, instead of being allowed to dry out as described in the following techniques.

Problems during wear

It is essential for the client to have fill-in treatments at two- or three-weekly intervals. This is to prevent any lifting or to rectify any lifting which has already occurred. It is also important in maintaining the stability and support mechanism of the nail.

If the nail is left unattended, the false nail 'grows' forwards, leaving a progressively longer neglected regrowth area (Figure 19.8). After 4–7 weeks (depending on the rate of growth) the nail is tip-heavy with product and does not have enough support lower down to maintain its stability. If the nail is banged against a hard surface, the false nail product will remain rigid but the nail plate underneath will flex because it is not adequately supported. This may cause bruising of the nail bed or partial lifting of the product, which can also lead to cracking across the nail plate at the demarcation line between the affixed and lifted product. This cracking often penetrates right through to the nail bed in badly neglected nails and if it is not dealt with straight away, infection will almost certainly ensue.

If cracking does occur, great care and caution must be exercised. Firstly, soak off the product from the surface of the nail. This will really sting as the solvent (e.g. acetone) will be going into an open wound. Next, examine the area. If the damage has literally only just happened, then proceed further. If the damage happened the previous day or even a number of hours ago, the chances are that the crack or cut will already be infected. To seal over the top of this would be most unwise: the infection would be sealed in. Apply antiseptic cream and a plaster and instruct the client to keep a careful watch on the area. If it gets hot, red or sore, she should contact her doctor for antibiotics.

After a few days, when the area has healed and there is no sign of infection, or if the crack or cut is completely clean, then it is essential to repair the crack or it will keep catching on things, become sore, and re-open. The least of the problems is that it will also be unsightly. After cleansing and thorough sanitising, hold the crack firmly together and apply fibreglass resin and spray. Continue to repair the crack in the usual way by strengthening the whole of the nail with fibreglass. (Fibreglass is recommended as being the product least likely to cause an allergic reaction on the open wound. Many of the fibreglass resins currently on sale have medical applications, as well as functions within the nail industry, so they are the safest products to use for this type of repair.) After reinforcement to repair the damage, do not leave the nail length too long as the nail bed will be bruised and sore and further mechanical damage must be avoided.

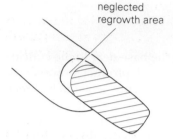

neglected regrowth area

FIGURE 19.8 *This nail is too long, and has insufficient support for the false nail lower down: pressure on the tip may bruise the nail bed or cause partial lifting, leading to cracking across the nail plate, even completely through to the nail bed below*

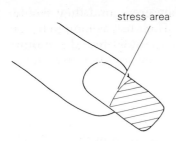

stress area

FIGURE 19.9 *A very old repair or extension which has been allowed to become tip-heavy: the natural nail will not support it and will crack and break in the area shown – the false nail material should have been removed well before this stage*

Repairs

When a nail is repaired using a false nail product, it is not usual to take the product all the way down to the base of the nail, but rather to 'feather it in' about two-thirds of the way down. In this way the repair can grow out as the nail grows. However, if the product has been applied too thickly, or if the free edge is very long, an old repair can get tip-heavy (Figure 19.9). In this case, the natural nail will not support the tip and will finally crack and break along the line where the product ends on the surface of the nail. This results in a complete extension then being necessary and defeats the object of the repair in the first place – that the client keep her own nails.

To avoid this happening, a careful watch should be kept on repairs each time the client attends for her manicure. As soon as nail growth allows for the original crack to be filed out, the false nail product should be removed from the nail surface.

Preparation

It is not a good thing to have to file the surface of the natural nail prior to false nail application. Over-filing can cause mechanical damage, remove the keratin from the surface of the nail, and make the nail plate more susceptible to bacterial growth. Products are available which eliminate this need for prior filing. If it must be done, it should be kept to a minimum so that only the shine is removed, and carried out with base-to-tip movements with a fine-grade file, certainly no coarser than 600 grit.

Moisturising

Due to the extensive filing necessary when finishing off false nails, the cuticle and nail wall areas can become dried out. To counteract this, it is necessary to apply a conditioning oil at the end of the treatment. Care should be taken here that too much oil is not applied or the client may transfer this oil to her clothing, causing a stain. To avoid this, either apply the oil prior to the varnish, so that it will be wiped off the nail surface and only left on the surrounding skin; or choose a spray product which delivers a very fine mist which absorbs quickly. The advantage of spraying at the end is that the spray also dries the nail varnish application.

CONTRA-INDICATIONS

Contra-indications obviously include all those which would also contra-indicate a manicure (see page 93). Additional contra-indications are as follows.

Curvature

An extreme curvature to the natural nail, either upwards or downwards, would contra-indicate the fitting of a full set of nail extensions.

They would not keep a good shape as they grew, and they would tend to break due to the stresses involved. Their use as temporary or single extensions would not always be contra-indicated, depending on the extent of the curvature, and in fact they could be used for a special occasion to camouflage an unsightly curve.

Nail separation

If there is any separation of the natural nail plate from the nail bed, nail extensions must be avoided. The increased length would only result in more mechanical damage to the nail and more lifting from the nail bed. There is also the possibility that the lifting is due to a fungal infection.

Nail thickness

A thin nail plate would not be able to support a nail extension properly and the accidental loss of an extension would further weaken the natural nail plate. If extensions are really wanted, then they must be short and fills must be scheduled more frequently to cope with lifting due to the flexible nature of the weak nail plate.

Damaged cuticles

To fit nail extensions where the cuticles are inflamed or broken, or where there is infection around the nails, is to invite an allergic reaction. Once such a reaction has occurred, it is highly likely to recur every time that product is used on that person as she will have become sensitised to the product. It is much better to heal the problem, then fit the nails.

Diabetes

Diabetics have flesh that heals poorly, and an increased susceptibility to infection. Because of this, they do not make good candidates for permanent nail extensions. If a file slipped and cut them, it could result in a bad infection.

Cold hands

People with poor blood circulation often suffer from cold hands – a problem which can cause lifting of the product due to the ineffective initial adhesion.

Drugs

Certain drugs (e.g. anti-malarial compounds) alter the surface of the nails making them more 'slippery': products literally will not stick to the nail surface. Some drugs (e.g. tetracyclines) make people photosensitive and can cause unusual reactions if systems are used on them.

Nail length

On nails where the free edge is so badly bitten down as to show a fleshy protrusion in front of the nail plate (see page 202), 1.5 mm ($\frac{1}{16}$ in.) is the optimum length of the free edge for fitting nail extensions correctly.

ALLERGIC REACTIONS

Very early indications of an allergic reaction to a product would be a slight red swelling in the cuticle area and possibly an aching in the nail bed. At a later stage, the client might report her finger pads and cuticle areas becoming tender, hot, red, and sensitive to the touch. They might also become itchy and sometimes swollen, especially around the nail. This is most likely to happen immediately after a nail application or fill, and could last from a few hours to a few days before stopping (until the next fill, when it would occur again, more violently). After this reaction, the nail wall and cuticle would probably become dry and peel. More severe cases do not stop after a few days, but can develop into sores around the cuticle wall, followed by pus and scab formation.

In all instances of allergy, the product must be removed immediately and its use totally discontinued. Once the client has become sensitised to a product, it is usual that she will always react to that product thereafter. This does not mean that she can never have extensions or repairs again, only that another product of a completely different chemical composition will have to be used. However, a patch test for allergic reaction must be carried out before anything else is used.

Allergic reactions are usually to the liquid component of a product, which is why it is important not to allow primers to touch the client's skin and for the nail technician to take care that she does not get the liquids onto her own hands. This is also the reason that the majority of allergies now occur with gel nails and slow-setting products. For example, a manicurist can often find it difficult to work with gels without getting them and the sticky residues onto her own hands. Constant contact with the wet product in this way can rapidly lead to an allergic reaction.

For the client, if the product is not completely cured (it may have been applied too thickly or not put under the lamp for long enough) then she will be in contact with the unset product for quite a time. In fact, some manufacturers advise against the client putting her hands into water for 24 hours after application, as the gel continues to cure throughout that time! It is this lengthy contact with unset product that is most likely to give rise to allergic reactions. From this it can be seen that great care must be taken when handling these chemicals if allergy is to be avoided.

A manicurist's allergy usually takes the form of an eczematous rash on the hands. It can be itchy and red, or broken and weeping, according to the severity. Cortisone creams can control it, but the manicurist is best advised to change her products and take greater care to avoid contact with the new products in future. Use of a non-greasy barrier cream after every hand wash is also helpful.

INFECTIONS

Proper maintenance and careful fill-ins usually prohibit the growth of bacteria under false nails. (Primers and some products contain aseptic agents.) However, if a nail has been lifted for a few days, or has lifted and the client has glued it back without sterilising it, perhaps leaving an air bubble as well, ideal conditions are created for the growth of bacteria such as *Pseudomonas* species. Bacteria are found in soil, and are all around us in the air. They proliferate in warm, damp conditions and darkness; the moist space under a varnished false nail is ideal. Bacterial infection could also occur under false nails if the manicurist does not remove all the loose product before a fill, or if she puts false nail product onto a damp nail, thereby creating damp spaces as she works (see pages 322–3).

Infection is usually first noticed when the manicurist removes the client's nail varnish at the start of a treatment, when it appears as a small or large greenish-black area underneath the false nail. When the loose nail is clipped away, it can be seen that the infection has stained the nail plate a greeny-black colour.

A professional decision must be made here. If the client has many such areas on her nails, due to neglect, then the extensions must be removed. (If the problem were allowed to develop further, the infection might invade the nail bed, possibly leading to separation of the nail from the bed and even ultimately nail loss.) After removal of the extensions, the client should be instructed to soak her nails in one of the solutions mentioned below for five minutes every day for a week before returning to the salon for a check – just to be sure. However, if the client is usually very careful with her nails and this infection is a small one, the manicurist can treat it and continue with her fill-in treatment.

Treatment consists of clipping back the nail extension material to expose all of the discoloured area, then soaking the nail plate in *either* three parts chlorine bleach to one part water, *or* neat 70 per cent alcohol, surgical spirits or methylated spirits, for 10 minutes. Any of these solutions will kill the bacteria; the bleach may also fade the discoloration. (The colour will grow out otherwise with the nail plate, and can be disguised with dark varnishes.) After this, the nail can be scrubbed with an antiseptic soap to remove any trace of the chemicals before proceeding with a fill. A careful watch must be kept as to the future size of the discoloured patch to ensure that all the bacterial infection has been killed.

The manicurist must be especially careful to sterilise all her towels, equipment and working areas after dealing with such an infection, and where appropriate materials (e.g. emery boards and cuticle sticks) must be disposed of. (See also page 38.)

Pseudomonas is a particularly resilient and troublesome species of bacteria, found almost everywhere, even in hospitals. It is common in water, and grows on bars of soap. It is characterized by a greenish-black discoloration.

AFTERCARE

When a client comes into the salon with short nails, and goes out with long nails, certain adjustments have to be made to the way she uses her hands. The first time she opens a door, she will bang her nails against the wood. If her telephone is an old-style dial type, she will be trying to dial with her nails instead of a pencil. All these everyday hazards add up to broken and lifting extensions. It is therefore important not to put over-long extensions on a new client and to schedule an early fill appointment for the first time.

The client will become used to using her hands in a different way to minimise such incidents, but some guidelines need to be given to her:

☐ The false and natural nails will become damaged if excessive pressure or jarring is constantly applied to the tips. If she is in an occupation where this is likely to happen, she would be advised to keep her nails reasonably short.

☐ Gardening without gloves is to be avoided. The soil particles work their way under the edges of the product, causing lifting and infections.

☐ Sun-tan oils and sand also wreak havoc with extensions, again working their way under the product and causing severe lifting.

☐ Rubber gloves must be worn to protect the nails from washing-up liquid and all harsh household cleaning agents.

☐ Non-acetone products must be used to remove the nail varnish as acetone can be damaging. It is best not to change the varnish more than once a week. Explain to the client that if she uses a clear top coat every other day, her varnish will stay in excellent condition and will not need replacing. Varnish does not chip or peel off false nails, but will wear away if not protected with a top coat.

☐ It is best not to use glue on lifted areas as the glue can turn the product brittle or encourage bacterial growth. Over-use of glues can also cause allergies and damage the nail surface. The client needs to return to the salon for a fill if lifting is occurring.

If she cannot get to the salon, however, instruct her to clean underneath and around the lifted nail with 70 per cent alcohol or methylated spirits. (An old toothbrush or similar will help to clean underneath the lift.) This will sterilise the area and take away oils and moisture so that the adhesive will stick better. Then the area must be dried completely before re-sticking with a good-quality, compatible adhesive supplied by the salon.

LIFTING

Lifting may occur in various circumstances:

- The product has been applied too near to, or even overlapping, the cuticle. It should be kept 1.5 mm ($\frac{1}{16}$ in.) away for best results.
- The product has been applied too thickly near the cuticle and the nail wall.
- Too much pressure has been used during the finishing-off filing, the filing around the edges prior to fill-ins, or the cuticle work prior to fill-ins. All these will break the product away from the flexible nail plate.
- The client has let too long a time elapse between fill-ins.
- The nail extension is too long for the body of the nail to support. For optimum strength and support, a new extension should be no longer than half as long again as the natural nail plate.
- The client has a systemic disturbance, such as poor circulation or the taking of certain kinds of drugs.
- The client is abusing the extensions.

Other problems can occur. A nail technician specialising in nail extensions needs to be sensible in her work and aware of problems which may occur through a flaw in her technique. Hairline cracks, for example, could be due to her applying the product too thinly. She needs to build up a high degree of skill, being aware of the general technical guidelines in the following sections. Never work with a new product on a client until practice has brought proficiency.

REMOVAL

Numerous products for the softening, dissolving and removing of false nail materials are available. Be sure to choose a removal product which is made or recommended by the same manufacturer as the material to be removed.

These removers are strong solvents: they must therefore be used only in non-reactive containers such as glass or pottery bowls. If they are sold to clients for home use, this warning must be stressed to them. They must be instructed not to put solvents in contact with plastics. It is not unknown for clients to tip the used remover down a plastic sink, melting the bowl in the process. The solvent should be poured down a toilet or directly into an outside drain, and flushed away.

The procedure for removal is as follows.

Materials
- Paper towels.
- Nail clippers.
- Two pottery or glass bowls 8–10 cm (3–4 in.) across and 5–8 cm (2–3 in.) deep.
- The relevant false nail solvent.
- Nail Neat pads.

Technique

1 Protect the work station with paper towels and remove any nail varnish from the surface of the nails.

2 Remove any excess length to the nail, using nail clippers. Take care not to damage the underlying nail. If this stage causes problems at all, leave the length in place. (Some products can be thick and brittle and will snap and tear the nail underneath if clipped. Others will clip as easily as natural nails.)

3 Pour the remover into the two small bowls. Use only as much remover as is required to cover the nails when the fingers are placed in the bowls.

4 Soak all the nails, at the same time, for the recommended length of time. It often helps if the client agitates her fingernails against the base of the bowl and her other fingers during this soaking time.

   At the end of this time, different products will have behaved in different ways, some dissolving completely, others just softening and needing to be prised away. The following are two potential alternative ways of removal.

5 *Either* Removing one hand from the solution, wipe the surface of the nails with a Nail Neat soaked in the solution. Return the hand to the solution and repeat this stage on the other hand. Continue soaking and wiping in this way until all the product has been removed.

   Or Keeping the nails under the solution, prise the softened material away from the nail surface using a cottonwool-covered cuticle stick. When most of the material has been removed, rub with a soaked Nail Neat to remove the residue.

6 Remove the fingers from the solvent and dry them on a paper towel. At this stage it may be a good idea for the client to wash her hands to remove any oil or solvent residue.

7 Using a fine buffer, buff the surface of the natural nails to remove any residue, and return the nails to a gloss finish.

20 'PERMANENT' EXTENSIONS: TECHNIQUES

ACRYLIC (SCULPTURED) NAILS

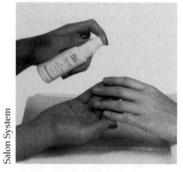

FIGURE 20.1 *After pre-manicuring and buffing to remove the surface shine, sanitiser is applied to disinfect the nail surface*

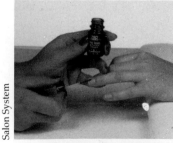

FIGURE 20.2 *A thin coat of primer being applied to each nail plate and allowed to dry naturally*

'Acrylic' is a general term: acrylic products differ in their chemical make-up and each manufacturer's instructions for use must be read through thoroughly before using the product.

Acrylic (sculptured) nails must always be applied at room temperature (70–80 °F, 21–27 °C). If the room temperature is too cold, the product may set ('cure') too slowly or even crystallise. If too warm, the product can cure too rapidly to stick properly or work with.

Acrylic nails have the advantage of being very strong, natural-looking and durable, and product development has made the method simple and reasonably quick once skills have been developed. A disadvantage is the thinning of the natural nail plate with constant wear. Although undesirable, this damage is not permanent and will grow out as the natural nail plate grows.

Bacterial growth underneath the acrylic can present a problem if thorough sanitisation techniques are not practised throughout all aspects of the process, or if the client does not attend for regular infills to avoid problems with lifting of the acrylic. Allergies too can occur, either in the nail technician or the client, but no more than with any other product.

Materials
In addition to the usual manicure station:

- ☐ Dappen dishes (2 or 3).
- ☐ A sable applicator brush.
- ☐ A cuticle stick.
- ☐ Sanitising solution.
- ☐ Primer.
- ☐ Acrylic powder – all clear, or some clear and some white.
- ☐ Acrylic liquid.
- ☐ Nail forms.
- ☐ Files and buffers.
- ☐ Manufacturer's instructions.

Technique: preparation
1 Ensure that consultation, record-keeping and prior preparation of

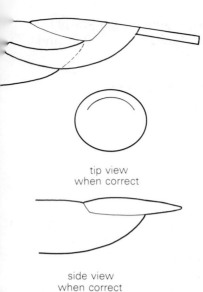

tip view
when correct

side view
when correct

FIGURE 20.3 *Placing the nail form (or tip) correctly: the line should follow the line of the nail plate*

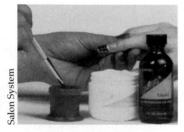

Salon System

FIGURE 20.4 *With the nail form in position, the brush is dipped in the liquid; excess liquid is wiped off against the side of the dish before dipping the brush into the powder*

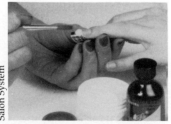

Salon System

FIGURE 20.5 *White tip powder being placed onto the nail form in front of the natural nail tip, and patted into place to form an extended nail tip*

the nails has been carried out as detailed on pages 194, 195 and 199.

2 Using a 600 grit file or finer, and light movements from the cuticle to the free edge, gently buff the nail plate to remove the surface shine and oils only, *without* causing mechanical damage to the nail.

3 Wipe excess dust away and apply a sanitiser to disinfect the nails and protect against infections (Figure 20.1).

4 Apply a thin coat of primer to the nail plate only, and allow it to dry naturally (Figure 20.2). Forced drying can cause contamination or lifting. Some primers dry the nail to a chalky-white finish, others (bonders rather than primers) leave a matt finish. *The nail surface must not be touched after this stage or contamination with body oils will cause subsequent lifting.* Should a client develop a reaction to the acid acrylic primer, this can be neutralised by rinsing with a solution of 60 ml (2 fl.oz.) of water and 15 ml (1 tablespoon) of baking soda, which is alkaline.

5 Apply the nail form by curving it and placing it under the free edge of the nail and attaching securely to the skin. Pinch the sides of the form together on the underside to ensure a deep curvature to the sculptured nail (Figure 20.3). Check that the form is extending the nail to follow a natural nail shape – look at the form from the side to ensure that it is not pointing up (ski-jump) or down (parrot's beak), but is forming a gentle, natural nail curvature.

Technique: nail sculpting

1 Place a small quantity of clear sculpting powder in one Dappen dish and a small quantity of liquid in the other Dappen dish. To achieve a realistic nail effect with a white free edge, a third Dappen dish should contain a small quantity of white sculpting powder.

2 To prime the brush, immerse it in the liquid, then wipe it clean on a paper towel. It is now ready for use.

   Dip the brush in the liquid and wipe the excess liquid on the side of the dish (Figure 20.4). Place the tip of the brush in the centre of the white sculpting powder and hold the brush until a small ball of powder, about the size of a small pea, adheres to the tip of the brush. Place this ball of powder onto the nail form in front of the natural nail tip (Figure 20.5). Shape and form the product into a tip shape, using patting movements of the sides of the brush. Keep the mixture within the natural nail line. Wipe the residue from the brush with a clean paper towel. This first ball of product is usually the biggest, subsequent balls being progressively smaller.

3 Dip the brush into the liquid and wipe the excess liquid on the side of the dish. Place the tip of the brush into the centre of the clear powder and hold the brush until a small ball of powder (only slightly smaller than the first) adheres to the tip. Place this ball of powder on the natural nail behind the white tip and pat it

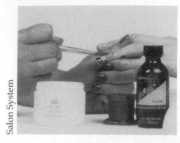

Salon System

FIGURE 20.6 *Progressively smaller and wetter balls of clear product are applied behind the tip and blended over the whole body of the nail*

level and side-by-side with the white tip, using the flat side of the brush. Dip the tip of the brush into the liquid (not too much) and blend the clear mixture gently over the tip.

4 Repeat this step with clear mixture and progressively smaller balls of product until the entire nail surface is covered up to the cuticle, making sure that the product does not come into actual contact with the cuticle (Figure 20.6). While applying the product, look constantly at the nail from all angles to ensure that a natural and aesthetic shape and curvature is being created. Too much product drawn to the tip of the nail creates a thick 'toucan's beak' effect. Too much product at the sides with not enough in the centre gives rise to a 'duck's bill' shape. Too much product in the centre leaves the nail looking like a claw. For the last application in the cuticle area, the smallest ball of product should be used, gently pushing it towards the cuticle until it is about 1.5 mm ($\frac{1}{16}$ in.) away. Then pull the brush towards the tip to blend any excess acrylic over the body of the nail.

Be careful to apply the product sparingly (more can always be added) and evenly over the surface of the nail. Taking an extra ten minutes a set in the application time can save up to an hour on filing time once the product has set.

5 In general, the mixture should be slightly wetter at the lunula area to give strong adhesion and comparatively drier at the tip to give strength. All powders lose their adhesive properties within a few seconds of being picked up on the brush so work must be done quickly for best adhesion. The product must be patted into shape, not brushed. 'Think thin' at the lunula in order to create a flexible nail plate which has no ridge when the natural nail grows out. Ideally, the product should be no thicker than nail varnish in this area. Too much product in this area gives a 'hump' shape to the nail and can cause lifting.

6 When learning, it helps to keep a dry, clean brush nearby which can be used to wipe away any acrylic which may flow into the cuticle or sidewall area where it would cause lifting if not removed.

7 Note that a clean, well cared-for brush makes it much easier to apply smooth nails. After each nail – for a beginner; two or three for the more experienced – dip the brush into the liquid and stroke it backwards and forwards across a paper towel to keep it clean. Always completely clean the brush *immediately* after the full application has been finished.

Technique: finishing the nail

1 After the recommended drying time, test for dryness by tapping the acrylic. It should sound hard and solid. Remove the nail form. Shape and clean the tops and sides of the sculptured nail, using the grades of file recommended by the manufacturers, possibly 100 grit for shaping but certainly no coarser than a 240–260 grit for starting to smooth the surface (Figure 20.7). *Do not apply too much*

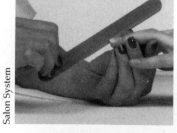

Salon System

FIGURE 20.7 *The acrylic having set and the nail form having been peeled away, the acrylic nail is filed into a neat shape*

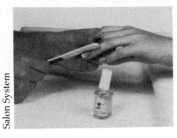

Salon System

FIGURE 20.8 *Fine-graded buffer files are used to smooth and buff the surface to a high gloss*

pressure to the surface when filing (see 'Lifting' and 'Filing', page 219). Continue gently to file smooth the tops of the nail using progressively finer grades of buffer files (Figure 20.8).

2　Ask the client to wash and thoroughly dry her hands, during which time the manicure station can be cleaned and fresh, dust-free towels can be brought out. These steps help prevent allergies to the acrylic dust and also prevent the dust from spoiling the varnish application. (If washing facilities are not available, the filing dust should be wiped away using a damp pad, or a bowl of water and a towel can be brought to the client so that she can rinse her hands.)

3　Apply nail varnish as usual (one base, two colour, one top), allowing each coat to dry.

4　Apply a fine cuticle oil (brush or spray) over the surface of the varnish to prevent smudging, and around the cuticles to moisturise and condition the cuticles.

Alternative 2–4 (if no basin is available):

2　Remove the dust and apply a cuticle oil to condition the cuticles and give extra shine to the nail plate. (Some manicurists increase the gloss of the nails still further by more buffing with the oil on the surface of the nail.)

3　Wipe over the nail surface using a non-acetone remover to remove the oil in readiness for varnishing.

4　Apply nail varnish in the usual way. Use of a base coat is essential on most products, as some varnishes, especially frosted ones, can cause yellowing of the product.

A full set of acrylic nails should take between one and two hours to apply, depending on experience.

Acrylic overlays or 'floaters'

These are terms given to a thin layer of acrylic coated over the natural nails in order to reinforce them.

Technique

1　The instructions given above should be followed for these too, except that nail forms are unnecessary. The first ball of acrylic should be applied to the stress line of the nail as this is the weakest part and needs most reinforcement – press down on the free edge of the nail: the stress line is the start of the whiteness in the nail bed, level with where the nail begins to bend at the sides.

2　Fill-ins need to be carried out in the same way as for true nail extensions.

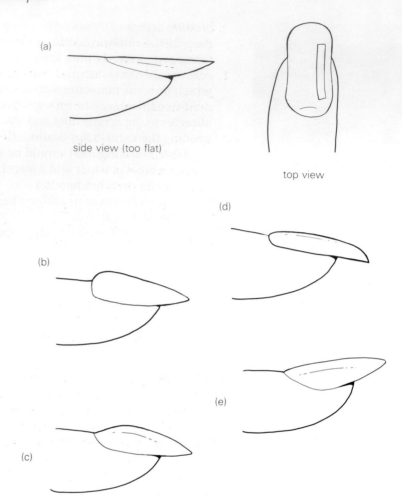

FIGURE 20.9 *Common faults in acrylic nail-shaping: (a) The 'duck's bill' – too much product at the sides, especially on the tip, and not enough in the middle, giving a flat, wide shape. (b) The 'hump' – too much product at the base. (c) The 'claw' – too much product in the middle. (d) The 'toucan's beak' – too much product at the tip. (e) The 'ski jump' – the nail form (or tip) was placed pointing upwards. (f) The 'parrot's beak' – the nail form (or tip) was placed pointing downwards*

Nail tip overlays

This is a method whereby plastic nail tips are used to extend the natural nail instead of using the nail forms. The whole is then coated with acrylic to reinforce the extension.

Additional materials

☐ Assorted sizes of nail tips with a short, concave well.
☐ Tip nippers or scissors.
☐ Nail glue.

Technique

1 Prepare the natural nail following steps 1–3 from the acrylic nail technique (pages 228–9).
2 Select, apply and shape the nail tip following all the instructions given in the section on nail tips (steps 3–10, page 238). The ridge need not be buffed completely smooth, just smoothed away a little.
3 Continue with the acrylic application technique (from step 4, page 229), making sure to roughen the plastic nail tip as well as the natural nail surface. However, the natural nail area only need be primed, not the plastic nail tips.

Obviously, there is no need for a form, nor for white powder to create a white tip (the white of the plastic serves this purpose). The first ball of acrylic should be placed onto the ledge at the base of the nail tip.

Nail tips and nail forms

The use of a nail tip as opposed to a nail form is a matter of personal preference.

1 When using tips the added preparation involved takes longer, but time is saved for the novice on the acrylic application, as the shape and length are already there.
2 A slightly out-of-place nail form can leave an irritating and dirt-catching ridge underneath the sculptured nail where the acrylic joins the nail. If the manicurist has a drill, this can be filed away using a fine cone-shaped attachment. The use of a tip avoids such a ridge.
3 Use of tips slightly increases material costs.
4 Achieving ten beautifully shaped and matched nails using nail forms demands a high level of skill. Once this skill is mastered, however, corrective treatments for misshapen nails are much easier when using nail forms; indeed such corrections may not be possible with nail tips. An extreme example of this would be rebuilding a damaged big-toe nail.

Acrylic nail fill-ins

As is explained to the client before acrylic nails are fitted, regular two-weekly fill-ins are essential (Figure 20.10). The wise manicurist will not do such work for clients unless they are prepared to fulfil this obligation, as clients who will not will give problems later (see pages 194–5).

Materials

The materials needed are the same as those needed to create a set of acrylic nails, with the addition of a pair of small-headed acrylic nippers.

Technique

1 Remove the nail varnish using a gentle, non-acetone nail varnish remover. During this procedure, carefully check each nail for irregularities such as lifting, cracks, chips, infections, or damage to the cuticle and surrounding area. Make a mental note of any problems.

2 Gently push back and neaten the cuticle. If the cuticles are bad, it will be necessary to use a non-oily cuticle remover to facilitate neatening. Bear in mind that the nail plate is porous: if moisture is absorbed prior to acrylic application, the product may lift. Apply as little as possible to the nail surface prior to acrylic, and certainly do not *soak* the nails in anything. Ensure complete drying with the aid of a dryer before the acrylic is applied.

    Also, do not apply too much pressure to the nail plate. Acrylic is fairly rigid, whereas the nail plate is very flexible – especially at the base. Downward pressure will cause the nail plate to bend and therefore be pushed away from the acrylic. This will lead to a poor-quality fill-in treatment which will not last long before it lifts away.

3 If there is any lifted acrylic, carefully clip it away using the acrylic nippers. If clipping is itself causing further lifting, then file the lifted acrylic away instead: this forced lifting (due to the flexibility of the nail plate) will be breaking apart the natural nail layers, causing the nail to become thin and weak. *During this stage, protective spectacles must be worn by both the client and the nail technician.*

4 Ask the client to scrub her nails with an antiseptic soap, to remove any dirt or chemicals from the nail and help to prevent any infection. (During this time the manicure station can be cleaned and products made ready for the next stage of the treatment.) The hands should be dried on a disposable towel or with a hot-air dryer. When she returns to the desk, dry the nails still further using a hand dryer.

5 If there are ridges where the acrylic has been clipped away, file these smooth to the nail surface using a medium (240–260 grit) file. Also at this stage, check the shape of the nail from the side. If acrylic has been used to build an aesthetically pleasing tip-to-base curve, this shape may have moved forward with the growth of the nail and need surface filing to re-balance the shape. If length has been taken off the nail, the free edge will need thinning to give a natural look.

6 Using a 600 grit file, gently take the shine off the regrowth area of the natural nail plate.

7 Remove any dust from the nail surface, apply sanitiser to the

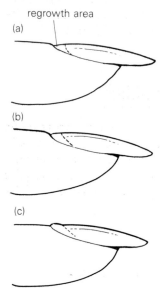

regrowth area

(a)

(b)

(c)

FIGURE 20.10 *The fill-in:*
(a) The nail extension after two or three weeks – the base needs to be filled in. (b) The same nail after correct treatment. (c) The same nail after incorrect treatment – too much acrylic has been used for the fill-in, leaving a thick and visible base

regrowth area, and let dry completely.

8 Apply primer *to the regrowth area only* and let dry. (Primer on old acrylic can cause discoloration.)

9 Apply the acrylic using a small brush (e.g. size 4) and one or two tiny balls of product, depending on the size of the nail. Place and work these as if they were the last application on a full nail – that is, push them into the cuticle area (1.5 mm ($\frac{1}{16}$ in.), away) and draw the excess over the nail body.

10 File and buff to a high gloss shine in the same way as for a full nail application.

A complete nail fill-in will take up to one and a half hours.

As new acrylic naturally bonds to old acrylic, it is easy to repair cracks and chips and to re-extend broken nails during a fill-in. At the end of either stage 5 or 6 these problem areas should be identified and prepared for repair. A shallow hairline crack can be surface-filed in readiness for the application of more acrylic over the area to repair the crack. A chip on the free edge, or a lifted free edge, can be clipped back and filed down a little in readiness for the application of a nail form and more acrylic to build a new nail tip. (This is sometimes done to renew the white tips as they grow forward, thus renewing the natural white-tipped look.) Always overlap new and old acrylic with clear acrylic in order to strengthen the junction area. A chip at the side can be filed down a little, then rebuilt over a nail form.

Renewing the natural look: the backfill

When white acrylic has been used to create a French manicure effect white-tipped nail, the growth of the natural nail causes the clearly defined free-edge line to move forward, and after about six weeks the desired effect is lost. It can be regained by renewing the acrylics completely; by clipping back the free edge and replacing it; or (if the manicurist has a drill) by backfilling the nails.

Materials
□ A manicurist's hand drill with a slow-speed control and a cylinder bit made of medium-grit sandpaper.
□ Protective glasses for the client and the manicurist to wear during the drilling work.

Technique
The backfill (Figure 20.11) can be carried out during a normal filling-in process when it will add about 20 minutes to the time needed. It can be carried out at the end of stage 5 or stage 6 (page 234).

1 Holding the drill so that the bit lies parallel to the surface of the free edge of the nail, slowly drill the acrylic away, moving the drill

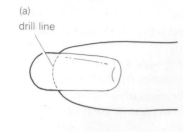

(a)

drill line

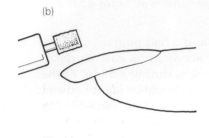

(b)

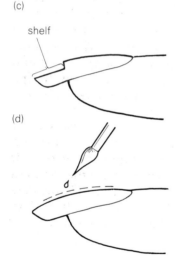

(c)

shelf

(d)

FIGURE 20.11 *The backfill:*
(a) The drill line to create a
new white tip is visualised.
(b) The old acrylic is drilled
away, up to the drill line.
(c) New, white acrylic is
added to the shelf thereby
created. (d) The junction is
reinforced with clear acrylic

bit from side to side and up to the start of the nail bed. Do this until a shelf is created to hold an application of new white acrylic. Do not drill down to the nail plate (if this is inadvertently exposed then the plate must be re-primed) and ensure that the drill line creates an aesthetically pleasing curve at the start of the free edge.

2 Brush away all the dust.

3 Now working with one nail at a time, wet the shelf with acrylic liquid and then fill the area drilled away with new, white acrylic.

4 Strengthen the stress point by applying a small amount of clear acrylic over the junction between the tip and the body of the nail.

5 Continue to complete the nail fill at the base of the nail.

6 File and buff to finish in the normal way.

This replacement of the white tip need only be done every three or four fills.

This method is also useful when the client has problems with her tip areas (e.g. lifting or cracks) but the base is still perfectly firm.

Odourless acrylics

The new-system odourless products have a chemical make-up completely different from that of the original acrylic products. Any odour is caused by the evaporation of the liquid from the product; products which dry quickly and completely (the original acrylics) tend to have a strong odour. Products with a low or no odour do not dry quickly and in fact do not dry out completely during the salon application but remain sticky on their surface. This feature changes their method of application slightly. (Note that low-odour products dry more quickly than no-odour products.)

1 Because the liquid does not evaporate quickly, the mix of powder and liquid should be kept very dry. To facilitate this, a tighter, shorter-bristled brush is best as it will pick up less liquid.

2 The sculpted nail has to be left to dry for up to 4 minutes (depending on the product). At the end of this time, it is still coated with a sticky layer.

3 This sticky layer is gently 'rolled' away, using a file in one direction only across the surface of the nail.

4 To take into account that this sticky layer will be removed, the initial product application has to be slightly thicker.

5 The surface of the nail is buffed in the usual way, although less buffing than normal is needed to obtain a good finish.

Removing acrylic nails

A solvent will be recommended for each acrylic system and the nails will dissolve and be removed using the method detailed on pages

226–7. Some older products are more difficult to remove, requiring filing away instead of, or as well as, the use of solvents. (The method may then be to soften in solvent, file away the softened area, then soften again and file again, until all the product has been removed.)

It is difficult (and time-consuming) to remove these products without inflicting damage to the natural nail plate. Many of the new-generation acrylics are much easier to remove, and enquiries must be made about this when first selecting a product to use in the salon.

NAIL TIPS

Nail tips are an extension method in their own right. Carefully blended in, they look quite natural and can be worn with or without nail varnish. With care, they will grow out with the natural nail, and no damage is done to the rest of the natural nail plate. Their only disadvantage is that they are so weak that most clients would break them off within a few days. It must be stressed that this method is unsuitable for full sets of nails where the client is going from short to long nails instantly and is not used to handling them. The only time that their use can be recommended successfully is for the careful client with long nails when she accidentally breaks a nail. In this instance, as she is used to handling her own nails with care, she will automatically be gentle with the new nail extension.

Nail tips can be reinforced and made very strong by the use of other products to overlay them. Acrylic, gel and fibreglass nail extension techniques commonly use tips instead of nail forms to create their basic shape. In such instances, there are deviations from the standard nail tip technique and these must be carefully followed if the finished product is to be effective. In these methods, the tips are left in place and help to create a well-formed, thin and light nail extension.

Materials
In addition to the usual manicure station:

☐ A selection of nail tips in a variety of sizes, curvatures and well depths.
☐ Quick-setting nail glue.
☐ Various grades of file, from buffers to 100 grit.
☐ Tip nippers.
☐ Methylated spirits (70 per cent alcohol).

Technique
1 Ensure that consultation, record-keeping and prior preparation of the nails have been carried out (pages 294, 295 and 299).
2 Wipe over the surface of the nail with methylated spirits (70 per cent alcohol) to ensure the total removal of surface oils and moisture.

3   Select the tip (see pages 212–13). This is all-important: the tip should fit from side to side of the nail and not leave a notch when growing up. If the nail is between widths, select the larger one and file down the sides to fit exactly. Some clients have flat nail beds, others have curved nail beds. If a flat tip is placed onto a curve, it will not stick properly at the sides but will 'wing up' and leave gaps. If a curved tip is placed onto a flat nail, stresses are created as the nail tries to pop back up, and the life of the completed tip will be diminished. Because of this, the nail technician really needs to keep both flat and curved nail tips.

When it comes to choosing a nail with or without a well, do remember that a nail with a well can always have the well cut away; there is no real need to keep stocks of nails *without* wells. However, nails without wells can give a better finish to tips as the ridge is graduated instead of cut, and the curvature of the nail is not as important. Choice of tip is largely a matter of personal preference.

4   Wipe over with methylated spirits (70 per cent alcohol) again.

5   Buff the shine gently off the area which the tip will cover, using a 600 grit file or finer. Do not touch the area, or body oils will be transferred to the nail plate and interfere with adhesion.

6   Apply a drop of glue to the centre of the well of the nail tip and spread it from side to side. Practice will show how much is needed to avoid flooding the nail or having insufficient glue and so creating air bubbles. With the former, have a tissue ready to mop up the excess; with the latter, take the tip off and start again.

7   Apply the ridge of the well of the tip to the edge of the nail plate at a 45° angle: rock the tip firmly into place so that the glue spreads over the whole of the join and makes a perfect seal. Hold the tip firmly until the glue has set. (Different glues have different setting times – read the instruction leaflets.)

8   Apply a thin layer of glue to the ledge at the junction of the tip and the natural nail. Allow this to set firmly.

9   Cut the tip to length and file it to the desired shape.

10 Buff the ledge level with the natural nail, taking care not to file the natural nail. To assist in this process, each time sufficient dust has been created, brush the dust into the ledge and apply more glue: this makes a stronger seal. If a large-welled tip has been used for extra strength, then the surface of the tip can be partially buffed away over the top and down the centre of the nail to take away the thickness, and therefore the whiteness, in this area. This gives a more natural-looking tip but leaves the strength and added stability at the sides.

11 When the ledge is level, continue to finish in the usual way with different grades of buffer files to create a high gloss finish. Apply oil to re-moisturise the cuticle.

12 Wipe over with a non-acetone nail varnish remover and apply nail varnish in the usual way (one ridge-filler base coat, two colour coats, one top coat).

Removing nail tips

Nail tips can be removed in the same way as temporary nail extensions (see page 206).

GEL NAILS

Gel nails, when set with a light source, have many advantages as a nail extension technique:

1 They are relatively strong, with good adhesion qualities (there is little lifting of the product).
2 The smooth nature of the gels means that there is little finishing-off filing to do to get them to a good finish. This means that they are very quick to apply in full sets and fill-ins.

However, there are disadvantages too:

1 Many varieties are not quite as strong as acrylic nails and so would not be suitable for a heavy-handed client. Light-setting fibreglass resin and fibreglass gauze 'sandwiches' are now being marketed to increase the strength factor of light-setting extensions; these also help to overcome allergy factors and the use of spray-setting agents.
2 The long curing time under the lamp – 1–2 minutes, repeated three or four times, is a long time in a busy schedule – does not make gel nails the ideal candidate for quick single repairs or extensions. Acrylic or spray-set fibreglass are much quicker on individual nails.
3 The stickiness of the gels, coupled with their long curing times, lead to more allergies arising from this method than from any other method. However, chemical formulations are improving all the time and this problem will probably be overcome in the near future.
4 The cost of a light source could be prohibitive to some individual manicurists or small salons. Two such light sources are needed, ideally, or work ceases if the only lamp in the salon breaks down!
5 The product is not easy to remove, although solvents are available.

The lightless gels are quicker for single nails and repairs, and are easier to remove. They share the same advantages as the light-cured gels, but also the same disadvantages in that they too are usually not as strong as acrylics and can cause allergic reactions, especially to the manicurist. The sprays used can be toxic and must only be used in a well ventilated area. They may be unpopular with clients if the clients have to breathe the fumes while sitting at the desk.

Light-setting and spray-setting gels are really two entirely different chemical products (see pages 214–15).

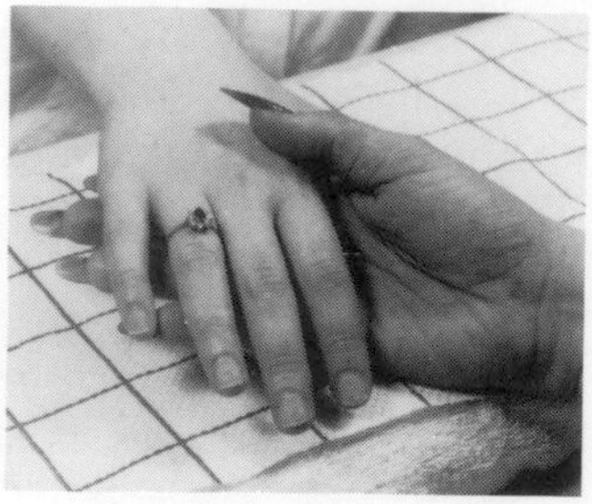

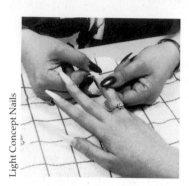

FIGURE 20.12 *Inspecting the nails for contra-indications before pre-manicuring*

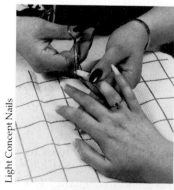

FIGURE 20.13 *After gently buffing away surface gloss and sanitising the nails, nail tips are applied*

FIGURE 20.14 *Cutting (and later filing) the nail tip to shape; the seam is then blended in and the gloss removed from its surface*

Light-cured gel nails

Materials

In addition to the usual manicure station:

- The gels, often three: a foundation gel, a builder gel, and a sealer gel. (Some systems use the same gel for all three layers.)
- Three separate brushes, one for each gel.
- A curing lamp with built-in timer.
- A primer.
- A sanitiser.
- Buffer and shaping files.
- A cuticle conditioner.
- Assorted nail tips, if the product is not to be sculpted.
- Gel remover and brush cleaner.

Technique

Some products can be sculpted over a nail form in the same way as acrylics in order to achieve a natural-looking white tip. Alternatively, the product is applied over a nail tip as a strengthening cover. Both techniques are detailed below.

Keep the pots of gel away from sunlight or the light source, or the gel will set. Try also to keep the gels away from any fluffy items such as mohair jumpers or cottonwool as the fibres get into the gel and complicate the treatment.

1 Ensure that consultation (Figure 20.12), record-keeping and prior preparation of the nails is carried out, as detailed on pages 194, 195 and 199.

2 Using a 600 grit file or finer, lightly buff the natural nail in the direction of nail growth to remove the shine from the surface of the nails.

3 Brush away the dust from the surface of the nails and wipe the nails with sanitiser. *Do not touch the nail surface* after this stage.

4 Select and apply a tip (Figure 20.13), following instructions 3–10 inclusive on page 238 (Figure 20.14). At stage 10, the ridge need not be buffed completely smooth as the gel will cover it; however, it does need to be blended in thoroughly as the gel systems are transparent and it will be seen. When the tip is complete, roughen the surface; brush away the dust; and, if the product being used requires a primer, apply the primer to the whole of the nail.

5 Apply a coat of foundation (bonder) gel to the whole of the nail and set it under the lamp.

6 Leaving the sticky residue on the surface, apply a coat of builder (sculpture) gel over the whole of the surface of the nail and set it with the lamp (Figure 20.15).

7 Repeat stage 6 with the sealant gel.

8 Wipe the sticky residue from the surface of the nail using a

non-acetone nail varnish remover. Buff the surface in the usual way to smooth it, seal the edges and give a high gloss shine (Figure 20.16). (Even though the surface will be glossy after the residue has been wiped away, this buffing still needs to be done to seal the edges of the product to the nail and prevent lifting.)

9 Some manufacturers advocate the use of a final thin coat of product and setting to achieve a final high gloss and save time on buffing.

Alternative from stage 4 to give a sculptured gel nail:

4 Apply the primer to the nail, if needed, followed by a coat of foundation (bonder) gel. Set this coat under the lamp. Apply a nail form, taking care not to touch the sticky surface, followed by a white gel sculpted to form a tip and overlap onto the natural nail plate. Set this under the lamp. Remove the nail form and clip the extension to shape if necessary. Apply the second gel quite thickly over the whole nail and set it under the lamp. Apply a coat of sealant and set it. Now wipe the sticky residue from the surface of the nail, and shape and finish with buffer files and sealant coat in the usual way.

When working it is important to make the best of the time available by doing a number of fingers at once. The routine to follow should be as follows:

1 Prepare all nails equally, up to the application of the product.
2 Apply product to four fingers of the left hand and put under the lamp.
3 Apply product to four fingers of the right hand while the left hand is curing, then put these under the lamp. Return to work on the left hand whilst the right hand is curing.

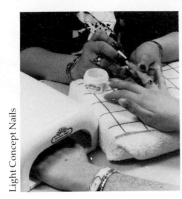

FIGURE 20.15 *Bonder, sculpture and sealant gels are applied in turn, each being set under the lamp*

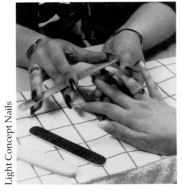

FIGURE 20.16 *After wiping away the sticky residue the nail surface is buffed or filed smooth*

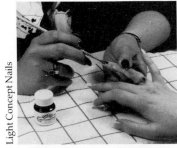

FIGURE 20.17 *Finally, the nail surface is coated with a high-gloss sealant*

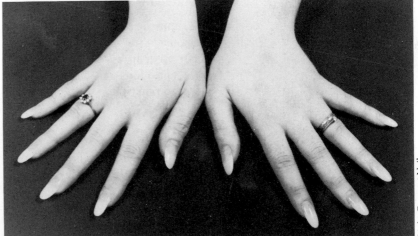

FIGURE 20.18 *The completed nails*

4 Alternate in this way until all three coats have been applied and cured. Remove the sticky residue.
5 Turn to the thumbs; work on and set both thumbs together until all three coats have been applied, set and the residue removed.
6 File in the usual way.

Gel nail fill-ins

These should be carried out every two weeks, as normal.

1 Remove the nail varnish and check the nails for any irregularities or contra-indications. Send the client to wash her hands in antiseptic soap and hot water.
2 Shorten and shape the nail, then gently buff out the ridge line and the whole surface of the nail (base to tip) using a 600 grit file. Continue until all the shine has been removed.
3 Brush away all the powder and wipe with a sanitiser. Prime the nail if a primer is included with the product in use.
4 Coat the nails with the three gels in succession, setting between coats and working in a routine as detailed earlier.
5 Wipe clean; buff; and smooth and varnish in the usual way.

Gel nail overlays

The fill-in technique can be used to form a strengthening overlay on natural nails. This overlay would have to be filled-in every two weeks like a normal extension.

Lightless gel nails

Materials

In addition to the usual manicure station:

☐ Nail sanitiser.
☐ Nail gel.
☐ Brush-on or spray-on activator.
☐ Buffers and files.
☐ Assorted nail tips.

Technique

1 Prepare the nails in the same way as for the light-setting gel system, right up to applying the gel.
2 *For the systems set with a brush-on activator*: Apply the gel starting about 1.5 mm ($\frac{1}{16}$ in.) away from the cuticle and in a line about 1.5 mm ($\frac{1}{16}$ in.) wide down the centre of the nail plate, ending at the free edge. Using a brush very wet with the activator, spread the gel over the entire surface of the nail plate as if it were nail

varnish. The activator will set the gel in about 20 seconds. Always wipe the brush clean before returning it to the activator bottle.

Repeat this stage until the recommended number of coats have been applied and set.

For the systems set with a spray-on activator: Brush the gel over the surface of the nail as if it were nail varnish. *With all the gel systems, gel should be applied as close to the cuticle as would be bright red nail varnish.* Holding the setting spray no less than 20 cm (8 in.) away from the nail surface, gently mist the surface of the gel. Spraying too closely or too hard will cause pitting on the surface of the gel. The setting reaction will create some warmth on the surface of the nail. If the product has been applied too thickly or misted too closely and the heat is enough to burn, quickly blow on the surface of the nail to cool it down.

Repeat this stage until the recommended number of coats have been applied and set. To save spray product, coat and spray two nails at once.

3 Finish the nails by buffing and varnishing in the usual way.

Lightless gel nail fill-ins

These should be carried out every two weeks, as normal. Preparations are made in the same way as for light-setting gels. The nails are coated with two or more coats of product, as detailed above; then buffed and varnished in the usual way.

Removing gel nails

A solvent will be recommended for each gel system and the nails will dissolve and be removed using the method detailed on pages 226–7. Lightless gels are generally easier to remove and leave less residue than do light-cured gels.

NAIL WRAPS

Although not a method of extension, knowledge of this technique of nail strengthening is needed if one is fully to understand the fibreglassing method of nail extension.

Nail wraps have been around in various forms since the advent of modern nail varnishes in the 1920s. The first wraps utilised tissue paper, which was torn and not cut (to give a more easily blended edge) to shape, and stuck onto the nail plate with an overlapping edge which was tucked underneath the free edge. The whole was secured using clear varnishes (succeeded by varnish-type glues applied with a brush). This method, often known as the Juliette wrap, was commonly used to patch and repair broken nails. Wraps were not very durable, often having to be replaced each time the varnish was removed. Neither were they very strong (paper not being ideal for the purpose), and even with efficient buffing in the repair could still be seen without varnish over the top, and often even after varnish had been applied. Another drawback was that clients detest the feel of anything underneath the free edge of the nail plate and the area is difficult to keep clean.

The Juliette wrap is still taught in colleges throughout the world and the technique holds valuable lessons for the manicurist. However, modern advances in wrapping techniques and materials have led to a wide variety of options for the nail technician wishing to repair a broken nail, strengthen a weak nail, or cover and protect a brittle flaking nail.

There are four fabrics available for nail wrapping techniques: paper, silk, fibreglass and linen.

Paper

Paper is cheap and easy to master. However, it is not very strong, and can be bulky in use, and it is visible on the nail surface. Nail varnish must be worn to cover it. It is most often seen in retail shops, where it is sold to the public to patch split or broken nails.

Silk

Silk is popular as a wrapping material simply because its name gives an initial positive response. It is virtually invisible when applied properly, so a nail varnish application is unnecessary. It is stronger than paper, but weaker than fibreglass or linen.

Fibreglass

This wrapping material is likewise popular because of its name, which in this case gives the impression of strength. In use, it is invisible and reasonably strong – stronger than silk but weaker than linen. Its main disadvantage, from the operator's point of view, is that the fabric has a tendency to fray, making it a little difficult to work with, a drawback which is easily overcome with a little practice. However, modern manufacturing techniques are overcoming this and fibreglass is the fabric to choose for the client needing an invisible wrap which is reasonably strong.

Linen

Linen is the strongest of the nail wrapping fabrics. It is not invisible when applied, so nail varnish has to be worn. Linen is the fabric to choose for the client who has weak or damaged nails and who requires a strong, durable nail wrap.

Not only must the nail technician choose her fabric, she must also choose whether or not it is backed with adhesive to ease placement on the surface of the nail; she must choose glues with or without accelerated-setting sprays; and she must choose whether the fabric is pre-cut to size, in bulk or in 2.5 cm × 1 m (1 in. × 1 yd.) long strips, with or without a plastic backing. The options can be endless. Accelerated-setting sprays are an optional expense; and the fabric, although dearer, is more economical of time and short-term expense in 2.5 cm (1 in.) wide strips. Although it is said that the self-adhesive fabric does not adhere quite as well in the long term as the non-adhesive fabrics (because the adhesive prevents the total penetration of the wrapping glue), it is the most frequently chosen because of speed and ease of application. Some nail technicians 'base' the natural nail surface with a layer of adhesive before applying the self-adhesive fabric, as this helps to strengthen the nail and improve adhesion. Modern methods of production are improving products all the time.

Materials

In addition to the usual manicure station:

- A 240–260 grit file.
- A 600 grit file plus buffing grade files.
- 70 per cent alcohol or acetone.
- Fabric, adhesive or non-adhesive.
- Fabric cutting scissors.
- Nail glue (or glues of differing consistencies – optional).
- Clear plastic film (e.g. a cut-up plastic bag).
- Accelerator spray (optional).
- Cuticle oil.

Technique

Although there are numerous variations of the nail wrapping technique, there are certain basic steps which most techniques have in common.

1 *Lightly* file the top of the nail plate using the roughest side of a three-sided buffer file (600 grit or finer). This removes the natural oils and makes the nail plate more porous to the glues. *Do not over-file.*
2 Remove the filings with 70 per cent alcohol or acetone. This will both disinfect the nail and remove any moisture or oils which can cause lifting of the wrap.
3 Cut the fabric to the correct size to fit the nail plate leaving at least 1.5 mm ($\frac{1}{16}$ in.) gap between the fabric and the edge of the nail plate. This trimming will need to be done even with pre-cut wraps.
4 Assuming that the fabric is non-adhesive, apply a thin layer of nail glue to the entire nail plate. It is not necessary to change the consistencies of the glues used for each coat, but some manicurists claim better results by using a thicker glue for the first application, followed by a thinner glue, and then an even thinner

glue to finish off with. Certainly the choice of a thicker glue for this first coat prevents it running into the cuticle and nail-wall areas. If the fabric is self-adhesive, stage 4 can be carried out and the glue allowed to dry before the next stage, to provide a 'base' which will give extra strength to the nail plate. If the fabric is non-adhesive, it can be easier for handling if it is left longer than the nail, secured with adhesive as instructed, and the extra length trimmed and filed away later.

If the glue being used is a very rapid-drying variety, it may be easier to apply it in a straight line down the centre of the nail plate. The tissue and plastic will spread it at the next stage.

5   Apply the fabric to the nail surface.

6   Smooth out the fabric. Too *much* glue will cause the fabric to slide around and if the glue gets onto the cuticle or skin it can cause the finished wrap to lift. Too *little* glue will cause dry places under the fabric, but these can usually be rectified later. To help, use a piece of plain, clean plastic (a cut-up plastic bag): when the fabric is in place, place the plastic over the nail and rub it to smooth the wrap, remove the excess glue, and dry the glue more quickly. Remove the plastic quickly.

7   Apply another thin layer of glue on top of the wrap. This is best done by running a line of glue down the centre of the nail plate over the fabric, then using the side of the glue nozzle to smooth the glue from side to side. A smooth finish is achieved in this way.

8   Allow the glue to dry naturally or use an accelerator. The accelerator dries and hardens the glue more rapidly. There are two types, brush-on and spray. Each can cause a heat reaction and burning, especially if applied too liberally. This, coupled with the extra cost and the time needed for an extra step, often militates against the use of an accelerator.

9   Repeat stages 7 and 8 one more time (twice more if a self-adhesive fabric has been used) to give a total of three glue layers – enough to smooth over the fibres of the fabric and give a high gloss finish when buffed.

10   Blend the nail wrap seam area into the natural nail using a medium-grade file (240–260 grit). Do not file too strongly or the natural nail may be damaged.

11   Buff and smooth the entire surface of the nail using a medium-grade file followed by a three-sided buffer file (600 grit and below). If silk or fibreglass fabric has been used, the client should be able to go without nail varnish and the nail look completely natural.

12   Apply oil to the nail surface and surrounding nail wall and cuticle to eliminate any dryness.

13   Wipe over with non-acetone nail varnish remover and apply nail varnish as usual.

As with any nail treatment which has progressed beyond the bounds of a straightforward manicure, the 'right' way to apply a wrap is highly subjective. All the above steps and options (and many lesser variations which have not been included) are mixed and matched by manicurists until they have devised the way that works best for them individually.

Removing nail wraps

There are many proprietory brands or nail-glue solvents now available. Single wraps are best soaked off in specially designed single-finger pots containing gently abrasive sponges and solvent fluids. More numerous wraps are best soaked off in pottery or glass bowls containing the relevant solvent (see pages 226–7).

After removal, the nails should be manicured and buffed to return them to a high gloss shine, and oil should be applied to counteract any dryness.

FIBREGLASS NAILS

Fibreglass is the most recent contender in the nail extension market. It has many advantages.

1 Having been developed from applications in the medical profession, it has few allergy problems.
2 It is a strong and flexible material, weaker than acrylic (so clients who are very heavy on their nails may be better with acrylics) but more flexible than most other materials. Its flexibility gives it a strength of its own, and the nails created by this method can be very thin and natural-looking.
3 It is easy to remove at any time and the underlying nail plate suffers no damage from continuous wear. Fibreglass nails are therefore ideal for clients wishing to protect their own nails whilst growing them, with the intention of removing the product once their own nails have reached a good length.
4 Fibreglass is an extremely versatile product and all manner of repairs and reinforcements can be easily and quickly carried out with this product.

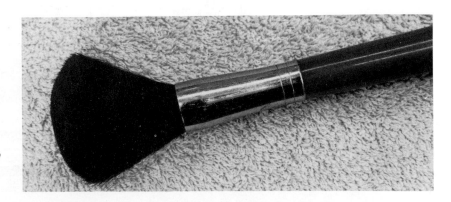

FIGURE 20.19 *A large make-up brush, used to remove nail dust*

5   Prior basing of the nail with fibreglass resin helps to protect the natural nail from filing damage when the tip is being blended into the natural nail during application.

Disadvantages include:

1   The toxicity of the sprays involved. Work must be carried out in a *very* well-ventilated area. Light-setting products are now available which make sprays unnecessary but increase the time of application (see page 239).
2   Client distaste for the sprays involved.
3   The cost of the product is higher than those of other products.
4   The fibreglass is applied over tips, and once the tip has grown out problems can occur with lifting of the product in the free-edge area. There seems little to do about this but replace the tips (i.e. the whole nail) once they have been filed out. A deeper well in the tip makes them last longer. (A lot of other products from all categories seem to experience this problem also, so it is by no means unique to this method.)
5   It takes time to build up speed with this technique as it is totally different from other methods. However, it is very fast for individual nails and repairs.

Although fibreglass has a unique method of application, it is advisable to read the sections on nail tip application (pages 237–9) and nail wrapping (pages 243–7) in conjunction with this section.

Materials
In addition to the usual manicure station (Figure 20.20):

☐   Product-compatible antiseptic cleansing wash (pH 5.5).
☐   Bonder resin with extender nozzle applicator.

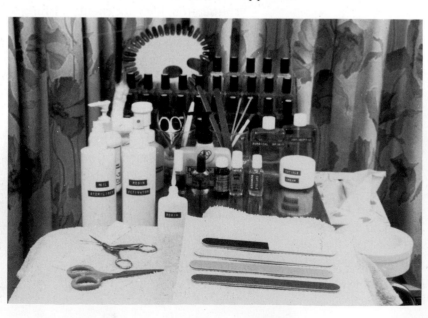

FIGURE 20.20 *Materials needed in the application of fibreglass nails*

□ Catalyst (resin activator) with pump spray applicator.
□ Fibreglass webbing.
□ 100 grit and 240 grit files, plus a 3- or 4-way buffer file.
□ Cuticle oil.
□ Fine fabric scissors (e.g. stork scissors).
□ Tip nippers.

Technique

1 Ensure that consultation, record-keeping and prior preparation of the nail has been carried out as detailed on pages 194, 195 and 199. Cleansing of the nails must be done using the product-compatible antiseptic cleansing wash, which will sanitise the nails and bring the nail surface to a natural pH of 5.5. This is important to ensure correct adhesion of the product without having to use a primer or file away the shine of the surface of the nails.

2 Apply the first base coat to the nail plate. When using the resin bottle, always hold it in a horizontal position so that the flow of the very fluid resin can be controlled (Figure 20.21). If the bottle is tipped upside down, too much resin will flood out onto the nail.

   Apply a line of resin to the nail surface and spread it over the plate using the side of the applicator nozzle (Figure 20.22). Do not allow the resin to go onto the cuticle or nail wall or it could cause lifting later. If it does, remove it immediately using a cuticle stick.

   Also, do not apply too much resin. This is because if too much product is applied the heat from the setting reaction, once the resin is activated, can burn the nail plate. A thin covering, similar to the thickness of a coat of base coat varnish, is sufficient.

   Each time the resin has been used, hold the bottle upright and gently squeeze the sides at the edges to create suction in the bottle and cause the resin to flow back into the bottle. If this is not done, the fine extender nozzle will block up as the resin sets at the end.

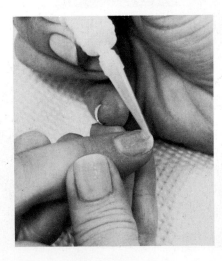 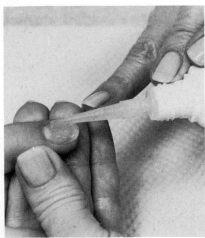

FIGURE 20.21 *The bottle is held horizontal while applying a line of resin down the cleansed surface of the nail*

FIGURE 20.22 *Using the nozzle of the applicator to spread the resin to each side*

3   Mist the nail with the catalyst spray (Figure 20.23). The bottle must be held *no less than* 40–45 cm (16–18 in.) away from the nail surface and the pump depressed once in a positive action to achieve a fine, even spray. If the pump is only half depressed, or depressed too cautiously, the catalyst will 'spit' out instead of misting. This will cause pitting of the resin on the nail, and the excess product can also cause overheating. Spraying too closely will also cause the same problems.

4   Apply a second base coat by repeating steps 2 and 3.

5   Select a nail tip in the same way as detailed on page 238 (Figure 20.24). Select for well depth as well as size, depending on the required finished effect.

6   Lightly buff the natural nail on the area where the nail tip is to be applied. Buff just sufficiently to remove the gloss from the surface (Figure 20.25). The dust can be left in place for increased bonding.

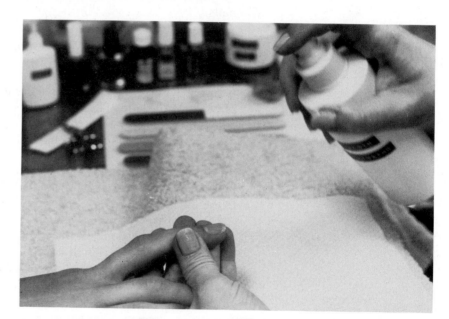

FIGURE 20.23 *Misting the nail with catalyst spray*

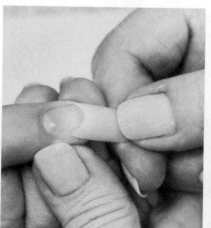
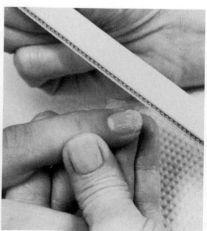

FIGURE 20.24 *Selecting a nail tip*

FIGURE 20.25 *Buffing the nail to remove the gloss from the surface*

7   Apply the nail tip. Apply a small drop of resin to the well of the tip (Figure 20.26) and spread it over the well with the nozzle. Firmly rock the tip onto the nail in the usual way (Figure 20.27; see page 238), pushing out any air pockets. As resins take a lot

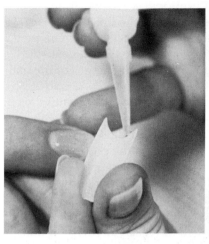
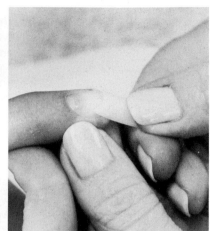

FIGURE 20.26 *Applying resin to the well of the tip*

FIGURE 20.27 *Rocking the tip firmly onto the nail*

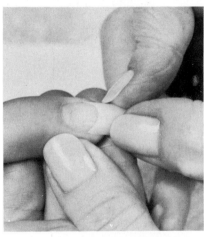
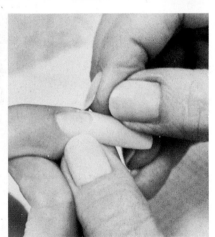

FIGURE 20.28 *Pressure is applied until the tip is secure*

FIGURE 20.29 *It may be necessary to hold down the sides*

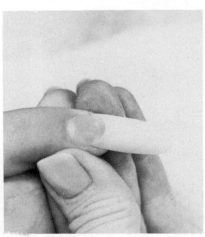
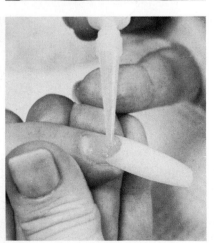

FIGURE 20.30 *The tip firmly stuck in place*

FIGURE 20.31 *Applying more resin to the seam and slightly behind the tip*

longer to dry than do quick-set glues, pressure needs to be applied for 10–15 seconds before the tip will be firmly fixed into place (Figures 20.28–20.30). Apply more resin to the seam and slightly behind the tip (Figure 20.31) – this gives added protection when filing – and mist with catalyst.

Resins will set without the aid of the catalyst, which is why they can stick the tips to the nail. However, allowed to set in this way on the surface of the nail, they will be porous and not as hard as when set with the catalyst spray.

8 Cut and shape the length of the nail tip using tip nippers and a 100 grit file (Figures 20.32 and 20.33). Take care to remove frills.

9 Blend the seam of the tip into the natural nail, starting with a 100 grit file and finishing with a 240 grit file (Figures 20.34 and 20.35). Do not file the ridge *completely* away as this could result in over-filing and the product being worn down to the natural nail surface. Care taken in blending the tip in properly will save time later and give a better and longer-lasting end result.

10 Brush away the dust.

11 Apply fibreglass webbing to the stress area (Figure 20.36). Cut a strip of fibreglass about 3–4 mm ($\frac{1}{8}$ in.) wide (wider on a large nail)

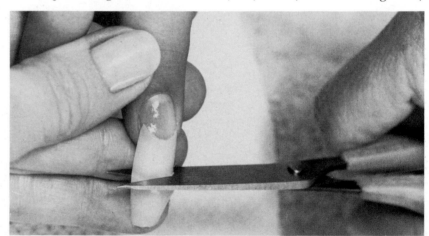

FIGURE 20.32 *Cutting the nail tip to the required length*

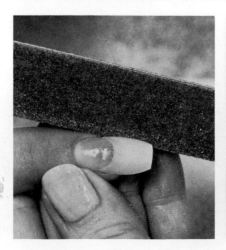

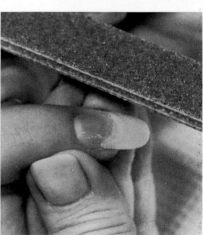

FIGURE 20.33 *Filing the nail tip to the required shape*

FIGURE 20.34 *Blending the seam of the tip into the natural nail, starting with a 100 grit file*

and apply along the stress line of the nail plate. Trim it so that it lies 1.5 mm ($\frac{1}{16}$ in.) away from the edges of the nail.

12 Apply a small drop of resin to the fibreglass and spread to wet and seal it completely (Figure 20.37). Mist with catalyst.

13 If extra strength is required, repeat stage 12.

14 Apply fibreglass webbing to the whole of the nail (Figure 20.38). Cut the webbing to the width of the nail and place it onto the nail surface, leaving a 1.5 mm ($\frac{1}{16}$ in.) gap at the cuticle and nail wall edges. Cut the length of the webbing to leave the same gap around the edge of the tip. This gap allows the resin to seal the edges of the webbing to the nail, which is vital if subsequent lifting is to be avoided.

15 Apply a small but long drop of resin down the centre of the nail and work it from side to side with the extender nozzle, starting at the base of the nail (Figure 20.39). Continue working from side to side, down the nail towards the tip and off the free edge, making sure that all the fibreglass is saturated just sufficiently to leave it clear instead of white. It does not take a lot of resin to obtain this effect and the resin must not be applied too thickly.

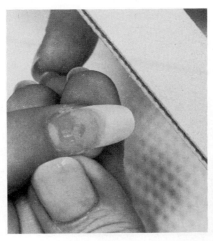
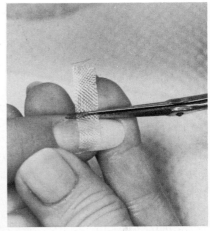

FIGURE 20.35 *Finishing the blending with a finer file so as not to file into the natural nail surface*

FIGURE 20.36 *Applying fibreglass webbing to the stress area*

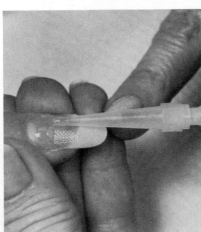
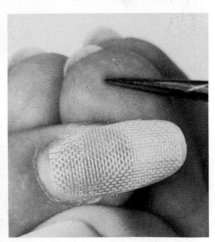

FIGURE 20.37 *Applying resin to the fibreglass and spreading it to wet and seal the webbing completely*

FIGURE 20.38 *Applying fibreglass webbing to the whole nail; note the gap around the edges*

16 Mist with catalyst, as before.

17 Repeat steps 15 and 16 twice more. Do not file between coats of resin, as this would break down the structure and strength of the nail, as well as creating harmful dust.

18 To finish off, start with a 240 grit file and gently, with no other pressure than the weight of the file, file the whole of the nail surface to dull the nail (Figure 20.40). If there are any shiny spots (low areas) fill them with resin – not too much at once – and mist the nail. Take extra care not to file into the natural nail plate when going around the edges of the nail with this medium-grade file. Continue filing smooth with a 600 grit file, then with the three sides of a buffer file to obtain a high gloss shine (Figure 20.41).

   If at any time during filing the fibreglass webbing is exposed (too much and too heavy filing) reapply one or two coats of resin and catalyst and continue to finish but with less pressure.

19 Apply a drop of cuticle oil and work it into the area (Figure 20.42).

20 If application has been done correctly, the finish should be totally natural: nail varnish is not required. If varnish is requested, a base coat is unnecessary as the product is not porous.

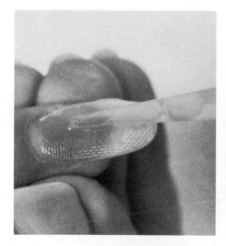
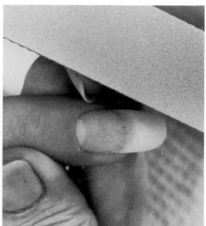

FIGURE 20.39 *Coating the webbing with resin*

FIGURE 20.40 *Filing the nail with a 240 grit file to dull the whole nail surface*

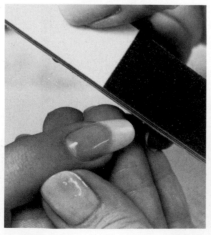
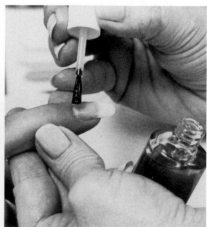

FIGURE 20.41 *Progressively finer buffer files are used to achieve a high gloss*

FIGURE 20.42 *A drop of cuticle oil removes any dryness in the cuticle area*

Maintenance

Fill-in treatments are of two types:

1 A first fill-in, in which only resin and catalyst are used.
2 A second fill-in, in which resin, catalyst and fibreglass mesh are used.

These fills are carried out alternately at two-week intervals. A first fill is quicker than a second fill and should be charged less accordingly. A full set of fibreglass nails takes approximately $1\frac{1}{2}$–2 hours; a first fill $\frac{3}{4}$ hour; and a second fill $1\frac{1}{4}$–$1\frac{1}{2}$ hours, including varnish application.

Fill-ins
A first fill-in:

1 This stage is the same as for the initial application.
2 Check the seams for any lifting product. Clip this away and file the seam level before proceeding. This product does not lift easily: if lifting occurs, look to the application technique for probable mistakes.
3 Apply a small amount of resin onto the regrowth area only. Spread it with the extender nozzle and mist with catalyst. (Repeat this stage if the client is hard on her nails.)
4 Apply a small amount of resin over the whole of the nail. Spread with the extender nozzle and mist with catalyst.
5 Very gently – as little additional product has been applied – file and buff the surface of the nail to a gloss finish, as detailed in the application technique.

A second fill-in:

1 Follow steps 1, 2 and 3 from the first fill-in.
2 Cut a small piece of fibreglass to cover the regrowth area and slightly overlap the previously meshed area. Keep the mesh 1.5 mm ($\frac{1}{16}$ in.) away from the cuticle and nail wall.
3 Apply a drop of resin to the centre of the fibreglass and spread it to cover and seal the edges of the mesh. Mist with catalyst. (Repeat this stage if the client is very hard on her nails.)
4 Repeat step 3, only carrying the resin forward a little way onto the rest of the extension.
5 Finish as in step 5 of the first fill-in.

Technique
When learning, one nail will have to be done at a time, but this is very wasteful of both product and time. Once speed allows, a routine should be established, for instance keeping both hands at the same stage in order to avoid wasting time in constantly picking up and putting down files, bottles, and so on. In addition, when applying resin and spray, work on the four fingers of one hand together, then

the four fingers of the other hand, then both thumbs together (as one would in working on gel nails). In this way wastage of product does not occur – one spray coats all four nails – and time is saved.

Removing fibreglass nails

A solvent will be recommended for each fibreglass system – often simply acetone with the addition of a teaspoonful of protective oil to each bowl. The false nail will dissolve and be worked off with a cuticle stick, using the method on pages 226–7. Fibreglass nails tend to come off easily and quickly, in a 15-minute soak, leaving no residue.

NAIL REPAIRS

Once the manicurist has started to work with any of the nail extension materials, she will quickly realise their potential for use as nail-repairing materials. Here are some simple examples.

Nail tips

A piece of plastic nail tip can be used to reinforce the side of a nail worn away through an occupational movement. The tip simply needs to be cut to the required shape and glued into position following all the rules for application of a nail tip. The raised edge of the plastic will be filed and buffed level with the nail plate in the usual way, and the repair will simply grow forwards and out with the natural nail plate.

This type of simple repair is visible unless nail varnish is worn, but it is very strong, simple and effective and does not encroach onto the rest of the nail surface.

Fibreglass

Fibreglass can be used to effect a clear and invisible repair which is very strong, and so durable and light that frequently it can stay in place until it has grown out. The nail must be prepared in the usual way (page 249), the crack or split being held together and resin and catalyst applied to the area to hold it in place. A layer of resin and catalyst is applied from 3 mm ($\frac{1}{8}$ in.) below the split to the end of the nail plate. A piece of fibreglass webbing is cut 3–6 mm ($\frac{1}{8}$–$\frac{1}{4}$ in.) wide (depending on the size of the nail and the severity of the split) and placed across the whole of the width of the nail plate over the top of the split. It is trimmed back 1–2 mm ($\frac{1}{16}$ in.) on the side without the split, but taken right to the edge of the side which *is* split. This is held in place by a layer of resin and catalyst. A second layer of webbing is placed over the top of this, a fraction to one side to avoid the edges of the two layers of webbing being immediately above one another and creating a ridge. This is coated with a layer of resin and catalyst. Two more coats of resin and catalyst are added over the repair, both extended to the end of the free edge and also slightly below the repair, to feather it into the natural nail tip. Finishing, filing and buffing are done in the usual way.

When nail growth allows the split to be filed out of the free edge, the remnants of the repair should be removed with acetone to prevent the tip from being tip-heavy and breaking off (see page 221).

Gels

Any of the gels could be used, with two coats applied to the area and set; followed by one coat over two-thirds or all of the nail to bond and strengthen the repair, the whole being finished in the usual way.

Acrylic

Acrylic too can be used to effect a repair. The crack or split should be glued first, then overlaid with acrylic in the usual way and buffed smooth. Acrylic is good for rebuilding missing areas of nail invisibly as it can be sculpted over a nail form. It would effect an invisible repair and reinforcement to the problem discussed above under 'Nail tips'.

General advice

One problem to be aware of when using extension materials for repairs is that of the tip becoming heavy and breaking off, as discussed in the general section on extensions (page 221). 'Feathering in' the product or removing the product before this happens are ways of avoiding this problem.

It can be seen that old methods of repair – using glues, paper wraps and strands of cotton, to name but a few – have been made obsolete by modern advances in nail products. The best way for a nail technician to master nail extension methods is to start using the materials to effect repairs in her standard manicuring work. In this way, she will rapidly gain product knowledge and an understanding of how the materials work.

PART VIII   Useful biology

21 HISTOLOGY, ANATOMY and PHYSIOLOGY

This chapter introduces some of the biology relevant to the work of the nail technician. Three branches of biology are relevant:

- ☐ *Histology* is the study of the groups of specialised cells called tissues. Histologists study the organisation of tissues at all levels, from the whole organ down to the molecular components of individual cells.
- ☐ *Anatomy* is that branch of biology concerned with the study of the structure of the body. Human anatomy is often studied by considering the individual systems that are made up of groups of tissues and organs.
- ☐ *Physiology* is the study of how the whole organism functions or works.

It is important for a manicurist to understand something of all three of these areas, especially in relation to the nails, skin, cells, hair, hands, arms, feet and legs:

1 To provide proper care, she needs to know the normal structure, the method of growth, and the factors affecting the growth of the areas she is working on, so that she can spot any disorders and understand what has caused them.
2 Background knowledge is invaluable when selecting products for use in the salon and for retail sale: it helps in understanding the effects substances will have on the nails and the skin.
3 Background knowledge is necessary if one is to understand the benefits of massage and give a correct massage.
4 Background knowledge enables the manicurist to have an answer ready for any question the client may ask, and thus promote her own image as a professional person.

THE CELL

The cell is the basic unit of all living things.

The human body develops from a single cell, which divides and subdivides many millions of times. Information stored in the DNA of the chromosomes in the nucleus of each cell allows the specialisation of cells; groups of adjacent cells may form tissues and organs, which

CELLS

are able to fulfil all the criteria of life,
but in a limited environment

TISSUES

comprise bone, connective tissue, nervous tissue, muscle,
blood, epithelial tissue, adipose tissue, and many others

ORGANS

comprise the heart, the lungs, the stomach, the kidneys, the skin,
the liver, the brain, the muscle blocks, and many others

SYSTEMS

comprise the nervous, digestive, respiratory, muscular, skeletal, cutaneous,
circulatory, lymphatic, endocrine, reproductive and urinary systems

THE COMPLETE ORGANISM

is able to fulfil all the criteria of life
in a much wider environment

FIGURE 21.1 *Levels of organisation in the human being*

together constitute the systems that collectively form the whole organism, the human being (Figure 21.1).

In this organism, each cell is to some extent protected from the outside world in a way that would not be possible on its own. The environment surrounding each cell provides it with the necessities of life – food, oxygen, water, removal of waste products, and a place in which to live, grow, reproduce, and die. However, each cell, like the whole organism of which it is a part, is sensitive to changes in its environment. Negative changes, such as a lack of oxygen, will lead to the poor health and maybe the death of the cell. Thus for example poor peripheral circulation results in the atrophy of the matrix and nails of the fingers and toes, severe cases resulting in the total loss of the nail tissue.

TABLE 21.1 *External environmental factors*

Bad	Good
Nail-biting	Manicures
Harsh detergents and chemicals	Use of rubber gloves
Mechanical trauma and repeated soaking	Care in the use of the hands
	Luxury treatments: hot oil baths, creams, etc.

Each cell is contained in the environment of the human body, and we are responsible for maintaining this environment correctly. A suitable diet, exercises, massage, and care as regards external factors all contribute towards looking after this environment. Understanding this will help the manicurist to advise her client about nail problems. A healthy cell environment leads to a healthy human body with healthy skin, hair and nails.

Cell structure

An average cell has a diameter of one hundredth of a millimetre. It is bounded by a partially permeable *cell* (or *plasma*) *membrane*; this encloses the *protoplasm*, the semi-fluid ground substance of the cell (Figure 21.2). Protoplasm is called *nucleoplasm* in the nucleus, and *cytoplasm* elsewhere.

Cytoplasm contains many granules and inclusions. Among these are *food granules*, such as starch grains; *mitochondria*, which are responsible for cellular respiration, in which energy is released to supply all the cell's needs; the *centrosome*, made of two *centrioles* which guide the division of the cell into two daughter cells at cell division; and *secretory granules*, which are involved in producing secretions. In fact, the cytoplasm is where most of the chemical reactions of the cell take place, building up materials and supplying energy for the cell's activities.

The *nucleus* is responsible for directing the activities and maintaining the life of the cell. It is bounded by a semi-permeable *nuclear membrane*. As well as nucleoplasm, it contains *chromatin granules*: these granules include the genetic material which condenses into chromosomes immediately prior to cell division. The *nucleolus* is a dense area within the nucleus.

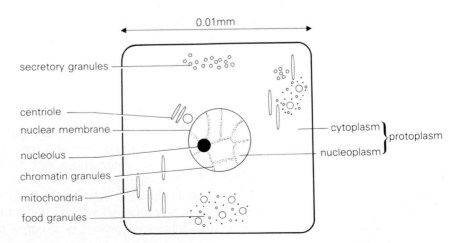

FIGURE 21.2 *The structure of the cell*

THE SKIN

The skin is the largest organ of the body, weighing around 3.5 kg (7 lb.) and with a surface area of about 2 m² (2 sq.yd.) in an average-sized person. It is an extremely flexible, thin, elastic covering for the body, and fulfils many essential metabolic and protective functions. A person who loses a lot of skin, for instance through extensive burns, will die. Scar tissue cannot fulfil these functions in the same way that healthy skin can.

The skin over the whole of the human body has basically the same structure (Figure 21.3), with local variations in thickness, strength, the amount of keratinisation, the sizes and numbers of hairs, the number and type of glands, colour, blood and nerve supply, and so on. Nails and hair are made of modified skin cells, so an understanding of the structure, function and formation of the skin helps the manicurist to understand normal and abnormal growth patterns of nails.

There are two major classes of skin; each covers large areas of the body but the two show important differences in structure and function.

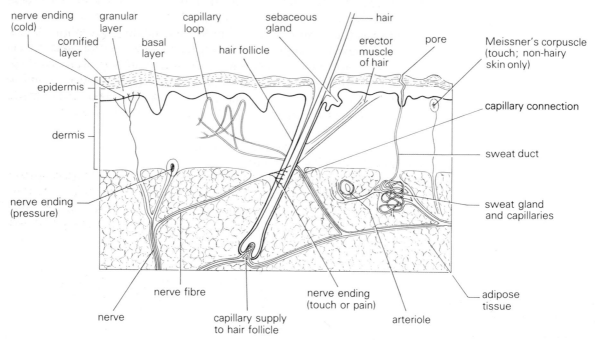

FIGURE 21.3 *A section through the skin*

Thick, hairless skin

This covers the palms of the hands, the soles of the feet, and the gripping surfaces of the fingers and toes. It has a complex pattern of friction ridges (e.g. fingerprints), not seen elsewhere on the body, which give a non-slip surface to aid in manipulation and movement. Thick, hairless skin has extra strength in the form of an additional layer, the *stratum lucidum*, which allows for the increased wear and tear in the areas in which it is situated (Figure 21.4). The *stratum*

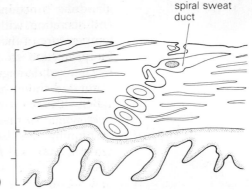

spiral sweat duct

stratum lucidum
and stratum
corneum
(cornified zone)

stratum basale,
stratum spinosum
and stratum
granulosum
(germinative zone)

FIGURE 21.4 *A section through thick, hairless skin from the sole of the foot, showing the comparative thickness of the epidermal layers – note the spiral duct from the sweat gland (×150)*

corneum (surface horny layer) is thicker than in hairy skin, being up to fifty cells deep in hairless skin and only a few cells deep in hairy skin. Hairless skin also has many sweat glands – the sweat produced assists in gripping objects – and many sensory nerve endings which give heightened sensitivity, especially touch. Because there are no hairs present, there are no sebaceous (oil-producing) glands, so these areas are prone to dryness. The epidermal and dermal layers (see below) are of differing thicknesses in hairless and hairy skin, hairless skin having a thick epidermis for strength and replacement, and a thin dermis; whereas hairy skin has a thin epidermis but a thick dermis with all its extra glands, follicles, muscles and the rest.

Thin, hairy skin

This kind of skin (Figure 21.5) composes most of the body's covering and fulfils the general functions of temperature control, excretion, protection from bacterial and fungal growth, ultraviolet rays and mechanical damage, and preventing or controlling the entry and exit of substances such as water and chemicals.

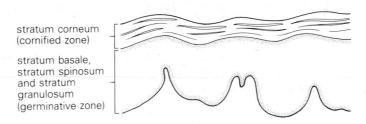

stratum corneum
(cornified zone)

stratum basale,
stratum spinosum
and stratum
granulosum
(germinative zone)

FIGURE 21.5 *A section through thin, hairy skin from the scalp (between hairs) – note how much thinner the keratinised layer is here compared with that in Figure 21.4 (×200)*

The microscopic structure of skin

Underneath a microscope, the skin can be seen to consist of many layers, but two distinct but closely held together layers are particularly obvious: the inner *dermis*, responsible for most sensory and all glandular functions of the skin, the nutrition of the area, excretion and secretion within the skin, and assisting in the control of the temperature of the body; and the outer *epidermis*, responsible mainly for protection from bacterial and fungal growth, ultraviolet rays, mechanical damage, and for the entry and exit of substances such as water and chemicals.

Beneath these two layers can be seen the underlying *adipose* or *fatty layer* which is responsible for heat insulation, energy storage and cushioning. The base of some of the skin structures, including the sweat glands and hair follicles, are found in the cushioning adipose tissue.

The dermis

Between 1 mm and 4 mm (0.04 in. and 0.16 in.) thick, the dermis is composed of connective tissue in which are embedded blood vessels, lymph ducts, sensory nerve endings, sweat and sebaceous glands, and hair follicles and their muscles. The soles of the feet and the palms of the hands, being made of thick, hairless skin, contain the highest concentration of sweat glands in the body and no hair follicles.

Connective tissue itself is a semi-solid gel with few cells. In the dermis it contains many strong and elastic collagen fibres which make the skin tough and elastic – so much so that when leather is being made the dermis and the epidermis are split from one another and each is chemically processed to make a different type of leather.

The dermis fulfils the important functions of heat regulation in the body (by means of regulation of the blood flow through the surface tissues); protection of underlying tissues and organs; originating the sensations of contact, heat and cold; sweat production; the production of sebum to prevent drying of the hair and surface skin and maintain an anti-bacterial acid pH; and supplying food and oxygen to the dividing and growing cells of the epidermis and taking away their waste products. This last function is carried out by the very good capillary blood supply in the dermis, especially in its uppermost layer where it joins with the actively dividing germinative zone of the epidermis above. This blood supply is even greater in the areas beneath the germinal matrix of the nail, where there is constant rapid, active cell division, and to the sterile matrix of the nail (nail bed) where it can be seen as the pink colour of the attached nail plate.

The epidermis

The epidermis is entirely protective in function, and is of special interest to the manicurist because nails are an evolutionary adaptation of this tough, keratinised cell-producing area, as too are hooves, horns, hairs, scales and feathers. An understanding of epidermal formation will lead to a greater understanding of the growth of the nail plate and its response to internal and external factors.

The *keratins* are a class of strong, fibrous, sulphur-rich protein molecules that serve as structural units for various tissues including nails, hair and skin. Cells capable of producing keratin are called *keratinocytes*, and the production of keratin within a cell, which eventually leads to the strengthening and later death of that cell, is known as *terminal keratinisation*.

The epidermis consists mainly of layers of keratinocytes, in various stages of growth, maturation and death (Figure 21.6). The purpose of the keratinocytes in the epidermis, in addition to their protective function, is that of constant renewal of the skin surface through

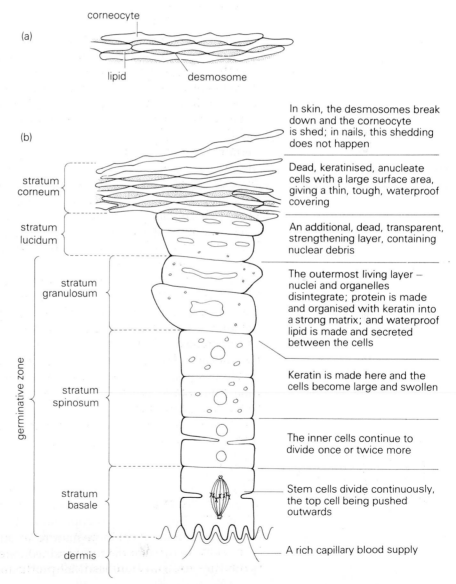

FIGURE 21.6 *The growth of the epidermis: (a) the stratum corneum; (b) the epidermis as a whole*

replacement of the surface cells. This is effected by the presence of a layer of actively dividing cells at the base which constantly replace the cells worn away at the surface. As the cells move away from the base of the epidermis, they undergo progressive changes in shape and content, eventually changing from polygonal living cells to dead flattened cells full of keratin.

Other cells, which stay where they are and do not take place in this constant process of renewal, are present in the basal layer of the epidermis. *Melanocytes*, for example, form the colour pigment granule melanin and pass this pigment on to other cells. Melanin absorbs ultraviolet radiation, protecting the cellular layers below from damage. Melanin production, usually genetically determined, is stimulated by the presence of ultraviolet rays. There are no melanocytes in the palms of the hands or the soles of the feet.

For ease of description, it is usual to divide the epidermis into a number of layers representing different stages in keratinocyte maturation, from the deepest to the most superficial layers. These layers (strata) are known as the *stratum basale, stratum spinosum, stratum granulosum, stratum lucidum* and *stratum corneum*. The strata basale, spinosum and granulosum together form the *germinative zone* (sometimes called the *stratum malpighii*), where all the cells are alive and the process of cell division takes place to varying degrees. The strata lucidum and corneum together form the *cornified zone*, where terminal keratinisation has already taken place and all the cells are dead.

The stratum basale

The stratum basale or base layer lies on a basement membrane which is highly folded to give a large surface area for the passage of materials through to the actively dividing cells. The basement membrane has a good blood supply to transport these materials. To the basement membrane is attached a single layer of dividing cells which are known as *stem cells*. These stay where they are, constantly dividing to form keratinocytes which move upwards and in turn divide again two or three times in the deeper layers of the stratum spinosum before ceasing to divide. The stratum basale is therefore made up of stem cells, keratinocytes in very early stages of maturation, and some non-keratinocytes including the pigment-forming melanocytes which pass the pigment to the immature keratinocytes.

The stratum spinosum

The stratum spinosum or *prickle-cell layer* is so named because the cell wall, when seen under the microscope, looks as if it has spiny prickles. The 'prickles' are in fact just areas where the cells are joined firmly together with microscopic structures called *desmosomes*.

This layer consists of more mature keratinocytes several cells deep. The cells both manufacture and contain many keratin filaments joined together in bundles. Many of these bundles are attached to desmosomes at the cell's surface; these join the cells together and give the tissue great strength. Melanin granules, which have been produced by melanocytes deeper in the basal layer, are gradually degraded by the keratinocytes so that they are absent in the surface layers of the skin which are finally shed as clear flakes. Because of all the manufacturing which goes on in the cell at this stage, the cells here are swollen and at their largest.

The stratum granulosum

The stratum granulosum or granular layer is the outermost living layer of the skin. Here various changes already begun in the lower stratum spinosum accelerate dramatically and a drastic change in keratinocyte structure occurs. The cells flatten and manufacture and accumulate dense protein granules of *keratohyalin* and *filaggrin*. The nuclei begin to disintegrate and the microscopic organs within the cell (the *organelles*) degenerate. The keratin filament bundles become enclosed in keratohyalin and filaggrin, and *disulphide bonds* stabilise the whole into a mass of chemically resistant, tough parallel fibres embedded in a tough protein matrix. Fats (lipids) are formed and secreted into the spaces between the cells to form a thick waterproof layer between the cells of what will become the stratum corneum. These lipid layers are not so thick in nails, hence nails absorb up to ten times more water than skin.

The stratum lucidum

The stratum lucidum or *clear layer* is only found in thick hairless skin. It is a poorly understood stage in keratinisation. The cells here often contain nuclear debris and are more transparent, but they otherwise resemble those of the stratum corneum.

The stratum corneum

The stratum corneum or cornified layer consists of closely packed layers of flattened, dead keratinocytes, sometimes now referred to as *corneocytes*. Because they are flattened they have a large, protective surface area, forming a thin but tough and waterproof covering for the body. In thin skin, as on the scalp, this layer is only a few cells thick. In thick skin, as on the soles of the feet, it can be up to fifty cells thick. The cells are compact with lots of keratin fibres formed into horizontal bundles, embedded in a tough protein matrix and stabilised by disulphide bonds. The intercellular spaces are filled with a lipid-based cement. The cells are still held together by desmosomes.

In skin, these desmosomes finally break down and the cell is shed from the surface of the skin. The average replacement time for a skin cell has been estimated at between 45 and 75 days, although the process can be much more rapid in very thin skin.

In nails, there are many more desmosomes and they do not break down, so the cells stay strongly bonded together to form a hard, protective plate. The keratin produced for nail formation is also of a stronger and harder variety than that produced for skin.

Environmental factors, such as constant abrasion or exposure to high levels of sunshine, will lead to a thickening of the whole epidermis, especially the cornified layer: examples are the corns that result from tight shoes and the calluses on the palms of manual workers.

The *nail plate* is formed in a flat, slit-like invagination of the germinative zone (the *nail fold*) by a series of changes similar to keratinisation in the epidermis – swelling, with subsequent breakdown of the nucleus, followed by flattening and shrinkage of the cell. This produces a plate of tough, keratinised cells (the nail) which is continually pushed forward by new growth.

THE NAIL AND SURROUNDING STRUCTURES

The human nail is the horny, semi-transparent, flattish and almost rectangular plate found on the top surface of the end of the last segment of each finger and toe. Nails are usually, although not always, convex (curved outwards) to varying degrees, both lengthwise and from side to side. They vary in thickness from about 0.5 mm to 0.75 mm ($\frac{1}{50}$ in. to $\frac{1}{35}$ in.) when healthy.

All species of primate have nails similar to these; they appear to be linked with the evolution of manipulative hands and feet. Other, less advanced, four-limbed animals possess much simpler horny (keratinised) claws.

The functions of the nail

The functions of the primate nail are these:

1 To aid manipulation, such as picking up small objects.
2 To heighten the sense of touch, both by providing an area with numerous nerve endings and by protecting the finger ends to give greater sensitivity to the tips.
3 To give a rigid support to the end of the finger to enable it to press on things without the flesh splaying up and out, as it does in severe nail-biters. (This helps with points 1 and 2 above.)
4 To protect the end of the finger or toe bone (the phalanx) from damage.
5 To allow the primate to scratch and groom itself and others.

The formation of the nail

Human nails begin to appear as the foetus is being formed in the womb. At about eight or nine weeks' gestation, the epidermis in the area where the nail is to form starts to differentiate and is known as the *nail anlage*.

At about ten weeks the two lateral, one distal and one proximal *nail grooves* become visible and represent the borders of the area where the nail plate is going to form. This area is called the *primary nail field*. The epidermis at the proximal nail groove folds inwards (invaginates). The germinative layer of the epidermis in this fold is then modified to form the germinal matrix.

At about eleven weeks the germinal matrix has grown down as a wedge of cells which attaches itself to the phalanx. Its function is to produce hard keratinised cells which stick together more firmly and are harder than the usual skin cells: this fold goes on to produce nail plate tissue instead of normal skin. Also at this time a ridge of keratinised tissue, the *distal nail ridge*, is formed on the proximal side of the distal nail groove. This ridge later flattens out and the nail plate grows forward over it. At this stage it becomes known as the *hyponychium*.

The formation of the area responsible for the growth of the nails and where the nail plate is going to be (the *nail field*) is complete by about the twelfth or thirteenth week of gestation. At about fourteen weeks the nail plate can be seen growing out from under the proximal nail fold.

The subsequent speed of growth of the nail plate depends on many factors which influence the speed of growth of the foetus as a whole, such as nutritional levels; but by the seventeenth to the twentieth weeks of gestation, fully grown fingernail plates, complete with tiny, fragile free edges, can be seen. At birth, the free edges are seen to be safely bent forward over the finger.

As in later life, the growth of the toenails in the foetus is slower than that of the fingernails, and their formation starts about ten days behind that of the fingernails.

The structure of the nail

There are three main regions to the nail: the *root*, the *body* and the *border* (Figure 21.7).

The root (radix)

This is the very base of the nail. It is not visible because it lies within a curved fold of epidermis (the *proximal nail fold*) which is approximately 5 mm ($\frac{1}{5}$ in.) deep (Figure 21.8). The cornified layer (stratum corneum) of the epidermis on the top layer of this fold extends onto the body of the nail to provide a seal against the outside environment, protecting it from bacteria, fluids, dirt and the like. The greater part of this seal is known as the *cuticle*, whilst that part of it which is in immediate contact with the nail body is known as the *eponychium*.

The cuticle is formed by the skin on the surface-folded part (apex)

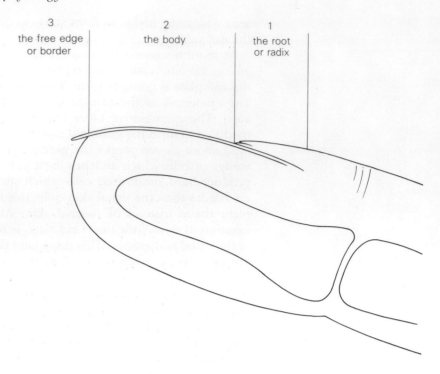

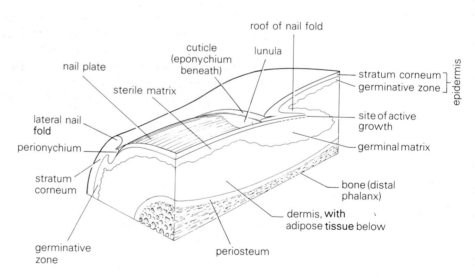

FIGURE 21.7 *The three main regions of the nail*

FIGURE 21.8 *The root of the nail (longitudinal section)*

and the top of the nail fold. The eponychium is formed by the undersurface of the roof of the nail fold immediately next to the apex and cuticle. The eponychium sticks closely to, and moves forward with, the newly formed nail plate. It can be seen as a very thin sheet of cornified cells which are shed a short distance along the nail plate. The protective seal of the eponychium is more difficult to remove from the surface of the nail plate than is the cuticle.

The root of the nail rests on and grows from a thick and specially adapted area of germinative zone epidermal cells known as the *germinal matrix.* This is closely bound to the top surface of the underlying phalangeal bone by fibrous dermal tissue.

The body

This is the visible portion of the nail plate that is attached to underlying tissues (Figure 21.8). The majority of the nail body is attached to the underlying tissues of the *sterile matrix* (nail bed). In its proximal part, however, in the area of the lunula, it is attached to the underlying tissues of the germinal matrix; and in its distal part it is attached to the underlying tissues of the hyponychium (see below).

The sterile matrix is made of a layer of germinative zone epidermal cells in which the surface layer is only partly keratinised, retaining their nuclei. The dead, cornified or horny zone (stratum corneum and stratum lucidum) is absent, as is the stratum granulosum.

The nail bed is highly corrugated longitudinally from base to tip on both its upper junction with the overlying nail plate and its lower junction with the dermis. The dermis at this lower junction contains an extensive blood supply which gives a pink colour to the translucent nail plate (Figure 21.9). These corrugations are deeper next to the lateral nail walls and play an extensive part in anchoring the nail plate to the nail bed. They are similar in formation to fingerprints and are known as the *epidermal rete.*

The germinal matrix extends underneath the nail body to the fingertip (distal) side of the *lunula*, a pale crescent-shaped area at the base of the nail. The lunula is not visible on all nails. Some people do not display any lunulae at all, while in others the lunula is largest on the thumb and is increasingly covered by the proximal nail fold on fingers 1–4 until it is almost or completely covered on the little finger.

FIGURE 21.9 *The mid nail plate (transverse section) – the junction between the epidermis and the dermis of the nail bed, when viewed across the finger, appears highly serrated: the dermis comprises many longitudinal grooves and ridges, which have an excellent blood supply*

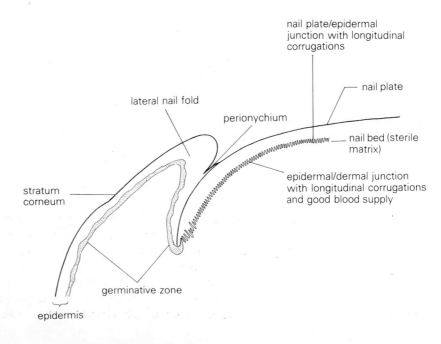

The pale appearance of the lunula is caused by a combination of three main factors.

1   The germinal matrix present beneath the lunula is thicker than the sterile matrix present beneath the rest of the nail plate. This prevents the red colour of the blood beneath the nail from showing through as well in the lunular area as it does through the rest of the nail plate.
2   If a nail is removed, a cloudy, crescent-shaped lunula can still be seen at the base of the plate. This is caused by the lack of maturity of the nail cells and the still incomplete deposition of keratin in this still forming area of nail plate.
3   The attachment of the nail plate to the nail bed is less firm in the lunular area of the nail, reflecting more light at the nail plate/nail bed junction in this area than from the rest of the nail plate.

The corrugations helping to attach the nail plate to the sterile matrix do not extend onto the germinal matrix. The nail plate/germinal matrix junction is linked together by numerous *papillae* (finger-shaped projections), which allow for the exchange of materials in this still growing area.

The sides of the body of the nail are bordered by a curved fold of epidermis known as the *lateral nail fold* (or nail wall). The cornified layer of the lateral nail fold extends fractionally onto the nail plate, forming a seal against the environment. This seal, similar to the eponychium under the cuticle, is sometimes known as the *perionychium*. The grooves that the sides of the nail plate move along, next to the lateral nail fold, are known as the *lateral nail grooves*.

Where the body of the nail leaves the nail bed and passes onto the epidermis of the hyponychium (Figure 21.10) there can often be seen

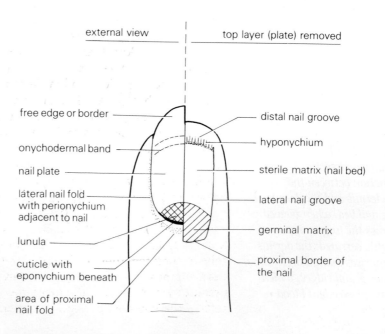

FIGURE 21.10 *The nail, viewed from above*

a faint yellow band visible through the nail plate. This is called the *onychodermal band* and is probably caused by the microscopic changes and the development of cornified layers under the nail plate in this area concealing the red or pink colour of the blood underneath.

The *hyponychium* itself is a narrow, crescent-shaped zone of epidermis to be found between the nail bed and the distal nail groove. At the start of the free edge there is a tiny forward extension of cornified tissue from the hyponychium onto the undersurface of the nail. The cornification and the extra-deep rete pegs in the hyponychium make an efficient seal against the outside environment, preventing any penetration of the nail plate/epidermal junction under normal circumstances.

The shallow *distal nail groove* separates the hyponychium and other structures of the nail from the epidermis of the fingertip. Small and inconspicuous in humans (except during gestation and at birth), it is large and well defined in other primates.

The border (free edge)

This is that part of the visible portion of the nail plate which is no longer attached to the nail bed. The shape of the free edge is determined by the shape of the distal edge of the germinal matrix (the edge of the lunula).

The microscopic structure of the nail

The cells of the nail can be thought of as similar to the cornified layer of the epidermis. They consist of flattened, dead, keratin-filled cells with no nuclei. They are originally formed in the germinal matrix, which extends round to include the very deepest layers of the underside of the proximal nail fold (sometimes known as the roof of the nail fold). Both these areas possess actively dividing cells (stem cells) which produce keratinocytes (keratin-producing cells) capable of undergoing rapid terminal keratinisation with a variety of hard keratin which is extremely resilient.

The keratinocytes of the nail are filled with very many closely-packed keratin fibres which lie at right angles to the direction of growth of the nail. These fibres are embedded in a dense protein matrix and make the nail hard. To give extra strength, immediately inside the cell wall lie bands of an even more dense protein which are linked up with many strong disulphide bonds.

Desmosomes are microscopic structures found on the outside of cell walls and linked up with the internal keratin fibres. Their function is to form links with desmosomes from surrounding cells, causing the cells to stick together. The cells of the nail possess more and stronger desmosomes than skin, and they are not programmed ultimately to break down as are the desmosomes of skin cells. Consequently the cells of the nail are not shed in the same manner as the outer layer of skin cells, but stick firmly together to form a solid nail plate. Unlike skin cells, there is very little lipid (fat) between the keratinised cells of the nail plate. This could account for the fact that nails are ten times more permeable to water than skin, although in their normal state they have a very low water content.

The underside of the nail develops from the germinal matrix, while the thin top surface of the nail is formed by the very deepest layers of the underside of the proximal nail fold and the most proximal portion of the germinal matrix. There is a distinction between these two layers, the dorsal (top) layer being much harder and more brittle than the thicker intermediate (lower) layer, which is more pliable (see page 315).

As new cells are formed, they are keratinised, become part of the substance of the nail plate, and are then steadily pushed forward by the force of the growth of more new cells behind them. They move along the top of the germinal matrix and onto the nail bed (sterile matrix), growing in a horizontal, lengthwise direction relative to the finger. This horizontal growth is due partly to the fact that the cells of the matrix are all aligned in that direction and partly to the pressure of the proximal nail fold above them.

Growth occurs only in the root and the area of the lunula, so the thickness of the growing base of the nail steadily increases until the end of the lunula, after which it stays the same.

The nail bed is structurally similar to normal skin with an upper epidermis and an inner dermis, except that it has no cornified zone (stratum corneum or lucidum), no stratum granulosum and no secretory or sebaceous glands. The epidermis of the nail bed is therefore only partly keratinised, the cells retaining their nuclei. The surface cells become firmly attached to the undersurface of the nail and move towards the tip of the finger at the same rate as the nail plate, providing a gliding surface for its growth. Like all epidermal cells, they are continually being replaced from below. Some writers refer to these cells as the third and inner layer of the nail, the ventral layer, but they are not part of the proper nail plate and the cells are shed at the free edge.

The firm attachment of the nail plate to the bed is largely a result of the tiny and numerous longitudinal corrugations (the epidermal rete) at the nail plate/epidermal junction. So strong is this bond that if the nail plate is torn off, the epidermis of the nail bed will be torn away with it.

There is growing evidence that the nail bed can pass materials, including mineral salts, into the nail plate as it grows forward; recent medical research has shown that some drugs pass freely into the nail plate through this zone. This helps to account both for the great adhesion of the plate to the nail bed and for the changes which can be seen in the nails of clients over short periods of three to four weeks when, for example, a healthy diet is started or an illness strikes.

The hyponychium is an area of epidermis, situated between the nail bed and the distal nail groove, which has granular and cornified layers. It produces cornified material which is shed under the free edge of the nail. The hyponychium has much larger corrugations penetrating deeper into the dermis than those of the nail bed. These corrugations are no longer longitudinal but polygonal (rete pegs). The cornification, together with the different configuration of the corrugations, gives extra adhesion of the end of the nail plate to the finger and increased protection against the environment in this potentially easily breached area of the body.

Under some circumstances the hyponychium will add a horny (cornified) substance to the underside of the nail plate, making it thick. The hyponychium can also become bigger and more active with bodily illness, leading to the deposit of excess horny material under the end of the nail (this is often seen in elderly arthritics and most frequently in toenails: see pages 317 and 319).

The dermis underneath the nail bed has a very rich blood supply which is at its most extensive underneath the germinal matrix at the base of the nail. The fingertips have a good blood supply, stemming from the superficial and deep palmar arches coming from the radial and ulnar arteries. There are two main vascular plexuses in the nail bed, one under the lunula, the *proximal vascular plexus*, and one at the tip of the finger, the *distal vascular plexus* (Figure 21.11). These plexuses give rise to shorter vessels which run between the collagen bundles and from which the subepidermal capillary loops arise. These loops are numerous under the longitudinal grooves of the nail bed. The subepidermal layers of the lunula do not have a good blood supply, which is why the nail plate cells die and undergo terminal keratinisation, but the deeper layers here are the site of the proximal vascular plexus.

The nail bed has a rich supply of lymphatic ducts.

site of distal vascular plexus

site of proximal vascular plexus

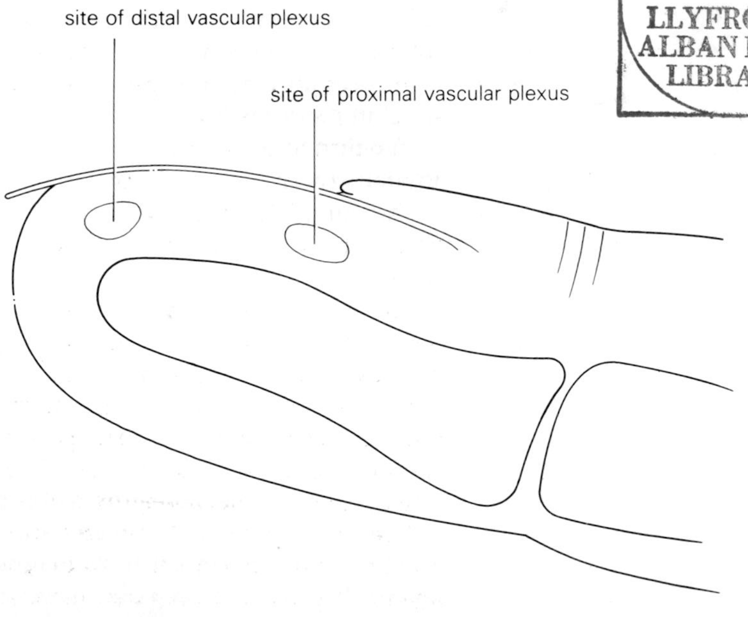

FIGURE 21.11 *The sites of the two major arterial groupings under the nail plate (longitudinal section) – capillaries taking blood to the sterile matrix and germinative matrix have their origins here*

The dermis beneath the nail contains numerous sensory nerve endings, including *Merkel terminals.* These serve an important tactile (touch) function and aid in the manipulation of objects.

The epidermis and dermis under the nail bed is attached to the *periosteum* (the membrane surrounding the bone) of the end finger bone (distal phalanx) by collagen fibres which radiate from the periosteum to the epidermis of the nail bed. These fibres bind the structures closely together to form a distinct, confined compartment. If the nail bed becomes bruised or infected, pressure can build up in this compartment making it extremely painful due to the restricted space between the bone and the nail plate. Doctors often have to release such pressures by piercing the nail plate to prevent the plate from being forced away from the bed and shed. Care must be taken that any local infections do not spread to the bone itself, which is close to the nail bed.

Nail growth

The rate of nail growth varies from digit to digit and individual to individual, with age, environmental temperature and other factors, even with the time of day! The speed of growth is directly related to the length of the digit: the longer the finger, the faster the nail growth. This is probably due to the blood supply and activity of the area. Consequently, on the hand the nail of the middle (second) finger is the fastest-growing and that of the little finger is the slowest-growing, growth ranging from 0.5 mm to 1.2 mm ($\frac{1}{50}$ in. to $\frac{1}{20}$ in) per week. It takes from 4 to 6 months (on average $5\frac{1}{2}$) for a fingernail to grow from the matrix to the free edge. The nails on the most frequently used hand – the right hand in right-handed people – grow more quickly than those on the other hand. A nail on an inflamed finger will grow more quickly than normal. These effects are linked to the increased blood supply. Nail growth can be speeded up (e.g. in psoriasis) or slowed down (e.g. in measles) by illness.

Fingernails grow approximately two to three times more quickly than toenails. Nails grow faster in the summer than in the winter; and faster in young people than in old people. The speed and strength of nail growth is not linked to any one dietary factor but is improved when a well-balanced diet is followed (see the dietary advice for the manicurist, page 10).

The composition of the nail plate

The nail plate, as a protein, is composed mostly of carbon, oxygen, nitrogen, sulphur, hydrogen, and tiny quantities of many trace elements, including calcium, magnesium, copper, manganese, zinc and iron.

THE CIRCULATION OF BLOOD TO THE HANDS AND FEET

Blood and the vessels that it is carried in form the essential internal transport system of the body, linking every part with every other part. The blood carries food in the form of nutrients in solution from the digestive system, and oxygen from the lungs, to the living tissues. Here the food and oxygen are used to release energy and to make new tissues. The waste products are excreted into the blood to be transported away – carbon dioxide to the lungs and nitrogenous wastes to the liver and kidneys. Blood also carries chemical messengers (*hormones*), and *antibodies* and *leucocytes* to fight bacterial invasion at any part of the body.

The heart is the central pumping mechanism which keeps the blood circulating. The arteries, veins and capillaries are the vessels along which the blood flows.

Arteries

Arteries carry bright red oxygenated blood, under pressure, away from the heart. They have muscular walls to contain the blood and maintain the pressure which causes the blood to move. If arteries are cut, the blood spurts out with each heart beat; most are usually buried deep under muscles which give some protection against damage.

The hand and lower arm
The *brachial artery* runs down the inner middle of the upper arm, through the front of the elbow. About 1 cm ($\frac{1}{2}$ in.) below the elbow joint it branches to form the radial and ulnar arteries (Figure 21.12):

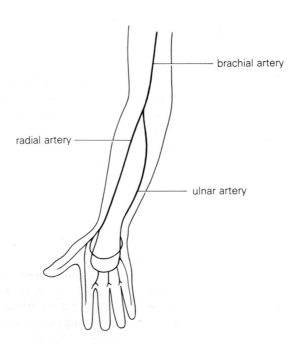

brachial artery

radial artery

ulnar artery

FIGURE 21.12 *Main arteries of the right lower arm*

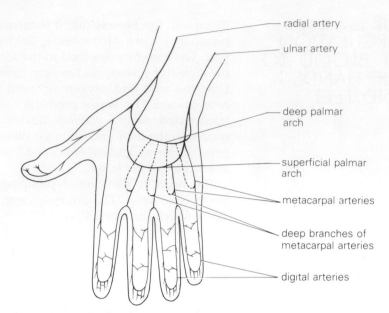

radial artery
ulnar artery
deep palmar arch
superficial palmar arch
metacarpal arteries
deep branches of metacarpal arteries
digital arteries

FIGURE 21.13 *Main arteries of the right hand*

□ The *radial artery* passes down the thumb side of the forearm (near the radius bone) to the wrist (Figure 21.13). This is the artery which provides the most commonly known and used pulse point, the radial pulse point, just above the wrist. It then passes between the first and second metacarpal bones and enters the palm of the hand. In general terms, blood from the radial artery and its branches supplies the thumb side of the arm and hand, and the back of the hand.

□ The *ulnar artery* passes down the little-finger side of the forearm (near the ulna bone), crosses the wrist and passes into the hand. In general terms, blood from the ulnar artery and its branches supplies the little-finger side of the arm and hand, and the palm of the hand.

The *deep* and *superficial palmar arches* are interconnections between the radial and ulnar arteries. Branches arise from these which supply the hands and fingers – the *metacarpal arteries*, which supply the main area of the hand, and the *digital arteries*, which supply the fingers. Branches of the digital arteries form the two vascular plexuses which are to be found underneath each nail.

Each of these arteries of the hands may be prefixed with the terms 'dorsal' and 'palmar', 'dorsal' meaning on the back of the hand and 'palmar' meaning on the underneath (palm) of the hand.

The foot and lower leg

The *femoral artery* from the top of the leg goes behind the knee and becomes the *popliteal artery*, branches of which supply blood to the knee joint (Figure 21.14). Just below the knee, the popliteal artery divides into the anterior and posterior tibial arteries:

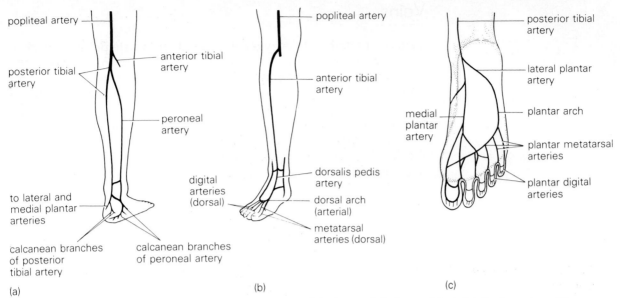

FIGURE 21.14 *Arteries of the lower right leg and foot: (a) the leg, viewed from the back; (b) the leg, viewed from the front; (c) the sole of the foot*

□ The *anterior tibial artery* passes between the tibia and fibula bones to the front of the leg where it follows the tibia down. It then runs in front of the ankle joint and over the top of the foot where it is then called the *dorsalis pedis artery*. Branches from this feed the top of the foot and form the dorsal arterial arch and the dorsal digital arteries. The dorsalis pedis artery then passes between the first and second metatarsal bones into the sole of the foot, where it joins with and becomes part of the *plantar arch*.

□ The *posterior tibial artery* runs down the middle of the back of the leg, behind the ankle joint and round to the inside of the underneath of the foot where it divides to form the lateral and medial plantar arteries. It also forms some *calcanean branches*, which take blood to the heel.

The *lateral plantar artery* curves along the outside edge of the underneath of the foot and forms the plantar arch. The dorsalis pedis artery joins with the plantar arch as it approaches the toes. The *plantar digital* and *metatarsal arteries* arise from the plantar arch.

The *medial plantar artery* runs down the foot near to the inside edge and divides up to form some of the plantar digital arteries to the toes.

The posterior tibial artery branches near the knee to form the *peroneal artery* which runs down the outside of the leg, over the ankle bone and divides up to form further calcanean branches.

Veins

Veins carry dark red deoxygenated blood and waste products back to the heart. This blood is under very little pressure from behind; the vein walls, instead of being muscular, contain a system of valves to prevent the backflow of blood under gravity. When the vessels are squeezed by the natural movement of body muscles around them, the blood is forced forward and the valves stop it from flowing back when the muscle pressure is released. In this way the blood is returned to the heart. This is why movement and exercises are important to maintain the circulation and thus the health of the body. There are more veins than arteries, collecting the blood and returning it to the heart.

If cut, the blood in veins does not spurt out but wells out steadily. Not needing as much protection, veins often run parallel with arteries but not as deep within the tissues, and they often take their name from the nearest artery.

The hand and lower arm

These veins can be roughly classed into those which lie near to the surface of the skin (superficial) and those which lie much deeper within the limb (deep).

The deep veins follow the course of the arteries and have the same names – the *digital veins*, the *metacarpal veins*, the *deep palmar venous arch*, and the *ulnar* and *radial veins*.

The superficial veins begin in the hand with networks of veins on the front and back of the hands called the *palmar venous plexus* and the *dorsal venous network* respectively. These receive blood from some of the digital veins and lead into the cephalic, basilic and median veins (Figure 21.15):

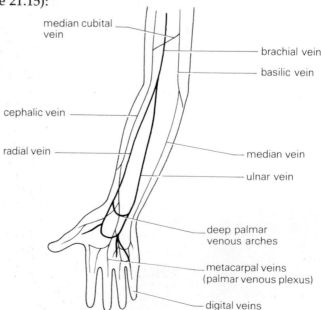

FIGURE 21.15 *Deep and superficial veins of the right hand*

☐ The *cephalic vein* begins at the back of the hand as the dorsal venous network, much of which can be seen by the naked eye. It goes round the back of the thumb to the inside of the forearm and up to the elbow where it crosses in front of the elbow joint and branches shortly after. Throughout its length it receives blood from the superficial tissues on the thumb side of the hand, forearm and arm.

☐ The *basilic vein* begins at the back of the hand on the little-finger side. It goes up the middle of the forearm and upper arm and receives blood from the middle regions of the hand, forearm and arm. There are many small veins which link the cephalic and basilic veins together.

☐ The *median vein* begins at the palmar surface of the hand and passes up the front of the forearm, ending in the basilic vein.

The foot and lower leg

There are both deep and superficial veins in the lower leg and foot. The superficial veins receive less support from surrounding tissues than do deep veins. This, coupled with weight and the force of gravity, can slow the passage of blood through them. There are communicating veins between the superficial and deep veins through which blood passes from the superficial to the deep vessels.

The deep veins accompany the arteries and their branches and have the same names – *digital* and *metatarsal veins*, *plantar venous arch*, *posterior* and *anterior tibial veins*, and the *popliteal vein*.

There are two main superficial veins, the short and long saphenous veins (Figure 21.16):

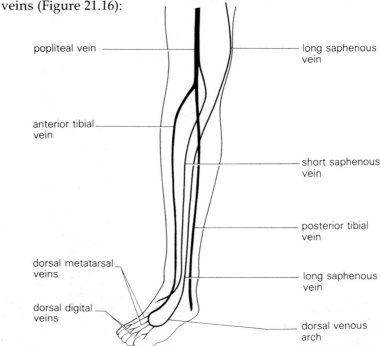

popliteal vein

anterior tibial vein

dorsal metatarsal veins

dorsal digital veins

long saphenous vein

short saphenous vein

posterior tibial vein

long saphenous vein

dorsal venous arch

FIGURE 21.16 *Deep and superficial veins of the foot and lower leg*

☐ The *long saphenous vein* is the longest vein in the body, beginning at the *dorsal venous arch* on the top of the foot, and running up the inner side of the lower leg and thigh until it joins the femoral vein at the top of the leg.

☐ The *short saphenous vein* begins behind the ankle joint, where its many subsidiaries drain the area from the top of the foot, and travels up the back of the lower leg where it joins the deep popliteal vein in the popliteal space behind the knee. Many small veins drain from the surface tissues of the feet and legs into these veins.

Capillaries

Capillaries form the link between arteries and veins. They are tiny vessels which thread through the body tissues. Each cell in the body is no more than one or two cells away from the nearest capillary. They have walls of only one cell's thickness; blood plasma containing nutrients, oxygen and other materials (collectively called *tissue fluid*) can seep through them, being forced out under pressure from the arteries behind (Figure 21.17). Tissue fluid bathes all the spaces in between the body cells. The cells take from it what they need for their functioning and excrete their waste products into it. The tissue fluid flows constantly around the cells, and some of it returns to the capillaries at the venous end where the pressure is low and allows its

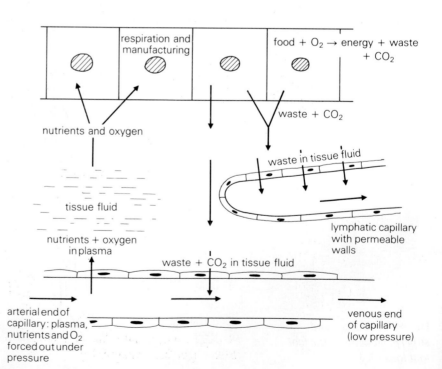

FIGURE 21.17 *The exchange of nutrients, gases and waste between capillaries, tissue fluid, cells and lymphatics*

return. The capillaries then converge together to form veins, which return the blood to the heart.

Not all tissue fluid returns immediately into the blood circulation; some has insufficient pressure behind it to push it back into the capillaries. The rest of the fluid, along with larger cell debris and microbes which are unable to pass through the walls of the capillaries, passes through the more permeable walls of the lymphatic ducts to enter the lymphatic system.

THE LYMPHATIC SYSTEM

The lymphatic system starts off as a series of thin-walled, blind-ending tubes (*lymphatic ducts*), containing valves which prevent the backflow of fluid within them. These ducts, with the same wall structure as capillaries, only more permeable, thread between the cells of the body in the same way as capillaries. Any tissue fluid which is not returned to the circulation via the capillaries seeps into these ducts, where it becomes known as lymph. When the ducts are squeezed by the natural movement of the surrounding muscles, the lymph is forced along them.

The lymphatic ducts progressively join together and at intervals along their length there are lymph nodes through which the lymph has to pass (Figure 21.18). These nodes clean the lymph of debris and

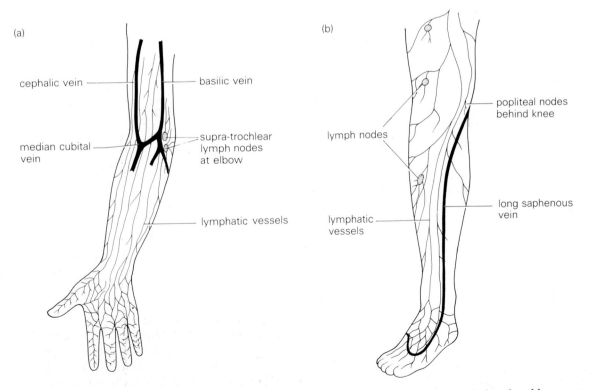

FIGURE 21.18 *Lymphatic ducts and nodes: (a) the right hand and lower arm; (b) the right foot and lower leg*

microbes before it is returned to the general blood circulation. The lymph vessels become larger as they join together, and eventually form the thoracic duct and the right lymphatic duct which discharge their contents into the general blood circulation at the left and right subclavian veins respectively. These veins represent an area of low pressure in the blood circulatory system, immediately before the vena cava and the heart.

The lymphatic system as a whole also has other components which play a vital part in the functioning of the immune system of the body, the system responsible for disease control.

THE NERVOUS SYSTEM OF THE HANDS AND FEET

The nerve supply to the hands and feet is part of the *peripheral nervous system*. It comprises *sensory* nerve fibres, which carry impulses from sensory end organs (nerve endings), for example in the skin, via the spinal cord, to the brain; and *motor* nerve fibres, which carry impulses from the brain, via the spinal cord, to the effector organs (such as muscles). There are also *autonomic* nerve fibres which control the automatic (subconscious) functions, including temperature control.

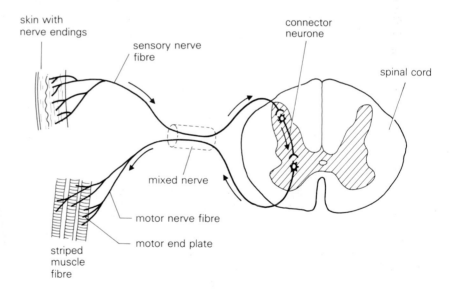

skin with nerve endings

sensory nerve fibre

connector neurone

spinal cord

mixed nerve

motor nerve fibre

motor end plate

striped muscle fibre

FIGURE 21.19 *A single reflex arc using the spinal cord only (e.g. a knee jerk): most nerve impulses travel to the brain and back via the cord instead of passing through the simple connector neurone – because of this, the brain can perceive a stimulus and formulate an adequate response almost instantaneously*

Hands and arms

The nerve fibres relating to the hands and arms exit from the spinal column between the lower cervical and upper thoracic vertebrae. This group of nerve fibres gather and intermix under the arms and above and behind the subclavian vessels to form the *brachial plexus*. From this plexus arise the nerves which actually lead to the arms and hands. Because of this grouping in the brachial plexus, these nerves are a combination of sensory, motor and autonomic fibres. The nerves

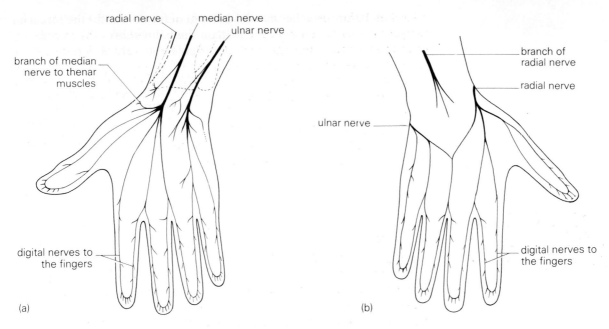

FIGURE 21.20 *Nerves supplying the right hand: (a) the palm; (b) the back*

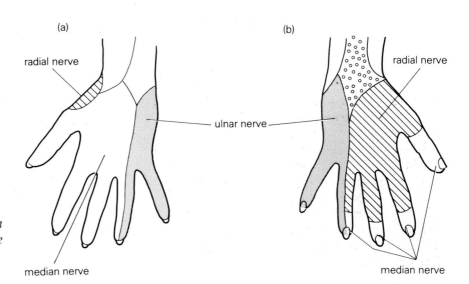

FIGURE 21.21 *The distribution of the cutaneous nerves of the right hand: (a) the palm; (b) the back*

of the brachial plexus which supply the hand and lower arm (Figure 21.20) are as follows:

☐ The *radial nerve* winds down the arm roughly on the thumb side (the side of the radius bone). It supplies the extensors of the wrist and finger joints, in the back of the forearm, and the skin on the back side of the thumb, the first two fingers and half of the side of the third finger.

☐ The *median nerve* is so called because it runs down the midline of the arm, close to the brachial artery and in front of the elbow joint. It supplies the muscles in front of (underneath) the forearm, and the small muscles and skin on the palm side of the thumb, the first two fingers and half of the side of the third finger.

☐ The *ulnar nerve* passes down the arm on the side of the little finger (the side of the ulna bone). It supplies the muscles on the ulnar side of the forearm, the muscles in the palm of the hand, and the skin on the whole of the little finger and the adjacent half of the third finger.

Feet and legs

The nerve fibres relating to the legs and feet exit from the spinal column between the lower lumbar and upper sacral vertebrae. This group of nerve fibres gather and intermix at the back of the pelvis to form the *sacral plexus*. From this plexus arise the nerves which actually lead to the legs and feet. Because of this grouping in the sacral plexus, these nerves are a combination of sensory, motor and autonomic fibres. The nerves of the sacral plexus which supply the foot and lower leg are as follows:

☐ The *sciatic nerve* is the largest nerve in the body. It passes through the buttocks and down the back of the thigh where it divides about halfway down the femur to form the *tibial* and *common peroneal nerves* (Figure 21.22).

☐ The *tibial nerve* continues down the back of the leg to supply the muscles and skin at the back of the lower leg, and the muscles and skin of the sole of the foot and toes.

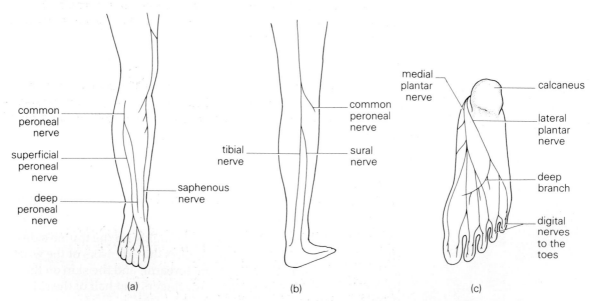

FIGURE 21.22 *Nerves supplying the right leg and foot: (a) main nerves of the leg, viewed from the front; (b) main nerves of the leg, viewed from the back; (c) plantar nerves of the foot*

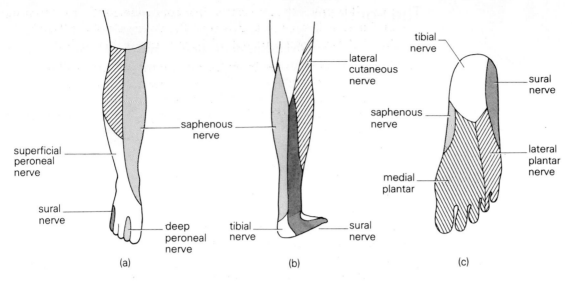

FIGURE 21.23 *The distribution of the cutaneous nerves: (a) the leg, viewed from the front; (b) the leg, viewed from the back; (c) the sole of the foot*

- ☐ The *sural nerve* is a branch off the tibial nerve and supplies the tissues in the area of the heel, the outside of the ankle, and part of the top of the foot.
- ☐ The *common peroneal nerve* bends to the front of the leg below the knee, where it divides into two branches, the *deep* and *superficial peroneal nerves*. The deep peroneal nerve, sometimes known as the *anterior tibial* (front of the tibia) nerve, and the superficial peroneal nerve, sometimes known as the *musculocutaneous nerve*, both supply the skin and muscles of the front part of the lower leg and the top of the foot and toes.

THE MUSCULAR SYSTEM OF THE HANDS AND FEET

There are so many layers of muscles, tendons and ligaments in the hands and feet – approximately 135 in each foot alone, for instance – that only a few of the main ones are discussed below, by way of examples.

Terms used

- ☐ *Extension* Straightening or bending backwards.
- ☐ *Flexion* Bending forward.
- ☐ *Abduction* Movement away from the midline of the body.
- ☐ *Adduction* Movement towards the midline of the body.
- ☐ *Pronation* Turning the palm of the hand down.
- ☐ *Supination* Turning the palm of the hand up.
- ☐ *Inversion* Turning the sole of the foot inwards.
- ☐ *Eversion* Turning the sole of the foot outwards.
- ☐ *Plantarflexion* Extending the foot to point the toes.
- ☐ *Dorsiflexion* Bending back the foot and toes.

The hand

Many of the finer movements of the fingers and thumbs are produced by numerous small muscles in the hand, including the thenar and hypothenar muscles (Figure 21.24).

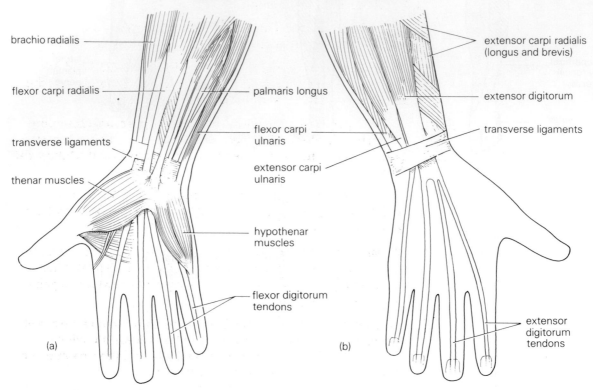

FIGURE 21.24 *Some muscles and tendons of the lower right arm and hand: (a) the palm; (b) the back*

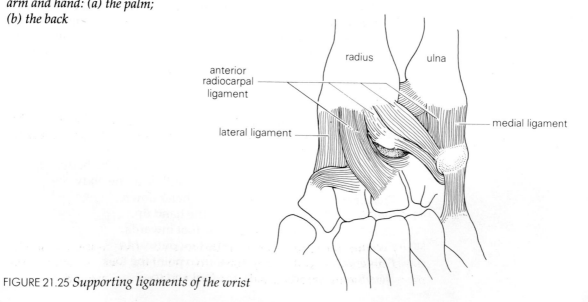

FIGURE 21.25 *Supporting ligaments of the wrist*

Muscles in the forearm with tendons extending into the hand are responsible for all the powerful movements that occur in the wrists and hands. The tendons passing over the wrists are encased in tubes of synovial membrane to allow them to move smoothly, and they are held close to the wrist bones by strong transverse ligaments (Figure 21.25). These are some examples:

- □ *Extensor carpi ulnaris* Origin – humerus; insertion – 5th metacarpal bone; function – extends and adducts the wrist.

- □ *Flexor carpi radialis* Origin – humerus; insertion – 2nd and 3rd metacarpal bones; function – flexes the wrist joint and helps the extensor carpi radialis to abduct the wrist joint.

- □ *Flexor carpi ulnaris* Origin – humerus and upper ulna; insertion – pisiform, hamate and 5th metacarpal bones; function – flexes the wrist joint and helps the extensor carpi ulnaris to adduct the wrist joint.

- □ *Extensor carpi radialis (longus and brevis)* Origin – humerus; insertion – 2nd and 3rd metacarpal bones; function – extends and abducts the wrist.

- □ *Pronator teres* Origin – the base of the humerus and the top of the ulna; insertion – the shaft of the radius; function – rotates the radioulnar joints to move the hand from palm upwards to palm downwards (i.e. pronation).

- □ *Supinator muscle* Origin – the base of the humerus and the top of the ulna; insertion – the upper shaft of the radius; function – rotates the radioulnar joints to move the hand from a palm down to a palm upwards position (i.e. supination).

- □ *Extensor digitorum tendons* These run down the back of the digits to extend them when contracted.

- □ *Flexor digitorum tendons* These run down the front of the digits to flex them when contracted.

The wrist

There are four important ligaments which strengthen this joint: the *medial* and *lateral ligaments* and the *anterior* and *posterior radiocarpal ligaments.*

The feet

Many of the finer movements of the toes and feet, more obvious in those disabled people who have to use their feet as hands, are produced by numerous small muscles in the feet and around the toes,

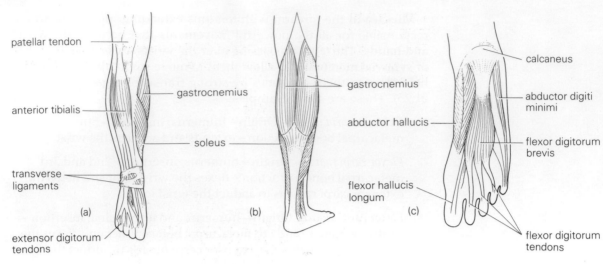

FIGURE 21.26 *Muscles of the right leg and foot: (a) main muscles of the leg, viewed from the front; (b) main muscles of the leg, viewed from the back; (c) some plantar muscles of the foot*

including the *abductor hallucis*, the *flexor digitorum brevis* and the *abductor digiti minimi* (Figure 21.26).

Muscles in the lower leg with tendons extending over the ankle joint and into the foot are responsible for all the powerful movements that occur in the ankles and feet. They also help to support the arches of the feet and maintain the balance of the body. In the same way as in the wrist, the tendons passing over the ankle are protected by synovial sheaths which allow them to move smoothly, and they are held closely against the ankle joint with strong transverse ligaments. These are some of the main muscles causing movement of the feet and ankles:

☐ *Gastrocnemius* Origin – femur; insertion – calcaneus, via the calcanean tendon (Achilles tendon); function – plantarflexion of the ankle joint to straighten the foot.

☐ *Anterior tibialis muscle* Origin – upper tibia; insertion – middle cuneiform; function – dorsiflexion of the foot to bend it up towards the body.

☐ *Soleus* Origin – upper tibia and fibula; insertion – joins with the calcanean tendon of the gastrocnemius; function – plantarflexion of the ankle and stabilising the joint when standing.

☐ *Extensor digitorum tendons* These run down the tops of the toes to straighten them when the associated muscle is contracted.

☐ *Flexor digitorum tendons* These run underneath the length of the toes to bend them when the associated muscle is contracted.

The ankle

There are four important ligaments which strengthen this joint: the *anterior, posterior* and *lateral ligaments* (not shown in Figure 21.27), and the *deltoid ligament*.

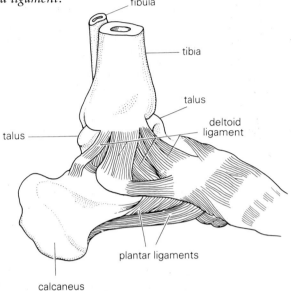

FIGURE 21.27 *Supporting ligaments of the left ankle joint*

THE BONES OF THE HANDS AND FEET

The forearms

The *radius* and the *ulna* are the two bones of the forearm (Figure 21.28). They articulate (form a movable joint) with the *humerus* at the elbow and the *carpals* at the wrist, as well as with each other at each end (the *radioulnar joints)*.

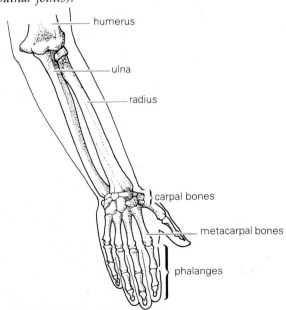

FIGURE 21.28 *Bones of the lower arm and hand*

The hands

There are 27 bones in the hands and wrists (Figure 21.29), made up as follows:

☐ 8 *carpal* (wrist) *bones*, arranged in two rows of four from the thumb side outwards: a proximal row (nearest to the body), *scaphoid, lunate, triquetral, pisiform*; and a distal row, *trapezium, trapezoid, capitate, hamate*. These bones are fitted closely together and held in place by ligaments which allow controlled movement between them. Tendons of muscles from the forearm cross the wrist and produce movement in the fingers. They are held close to the bones by strong, fibrous bands called transverse ligaments.

☐ 5 *metacarpal bones*, which can be felt along the back of the hand between the wrist and the fingers. They are numbered from the thumb outwards.

☐ 14 *phalanges* or finger bones, two in the thumb and three in each finger.

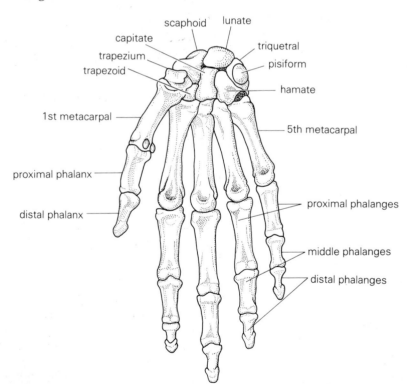

FIGURE 21.29 *Bones of the hand, viewed from the palm*

The lower leg

The *tibia* (shin bone) and *fibula* are the two bones of the lower leg (Figure 21.30). They articulate with each other at either end. The tibia also articulates with the *femur* (thigh bone) at the top to form the knee,

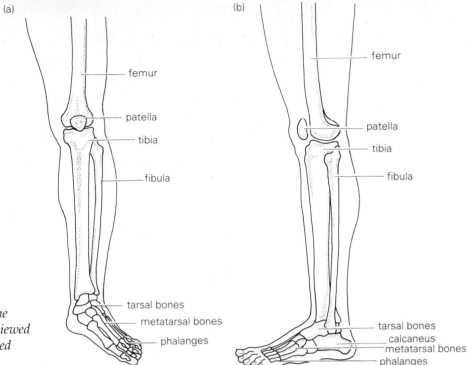

FIGURE 21.30 *Bones of the lower leg and foot: (a) viewed from the front; (b) viewed from the side*

and with the *talus* at the bottom to form the ankle joint. The fibula also articulates with the talus at the ankle joint.

The foot

There are 26 bones in the ankle and foot (Figure 21.31), in a similar arrangement to those in the hands; these bones, though, are bound together more rigidly by ligaments. The bones are arranged as follows:

☐   7 *tarsal* (ankle) *bones*, at the back of the foot: the *talus, calcaneus, cuboid, navicular, lateral cuneiform, intermediate cuneiform* and *medial cuneiform bones.* The talus articulates with the tibia and fibula to form the ankle joint. Strong transverse ligaments encircle the ankle to hold muscle tendons which pass underneath from the leg to the foot closely against the bones. The calcaneus is the largest of the tarsal bones and disperses and transmits a great deal of the weight of the body into the ground. The other bones articulate with each other and with the metatarsal bones in such a way as to help to form four arches.

☐   5 *metatarsal bones*, which form most of the length of the foot and can be felt along the top of the foot between the ankle and the toes. They are numbered from the medial side (big-toe side) of the foot outwards.

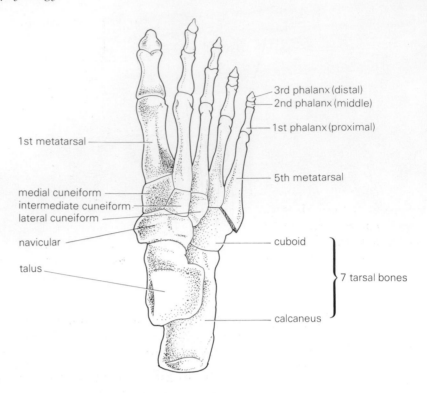

1st metatarsal

3rd phalanx (distal)
2nd phalanx (middle)
1st phalanx (proximal)

5th metatarsal

medial cuneiform
intermediate cuneiform
lateral cuneiform

navicular

cuboid

talus

7 tarsal bones

calcaneus

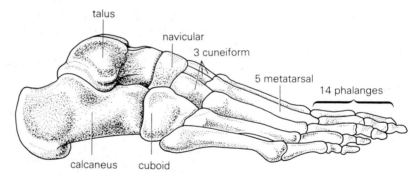

talus

navicular

3 cuneiform

5 metatarsal

14 phalanges

calcaneus   cuboid

FIGURE 21.31 *Bones of the right foot: (a) viewed from the top; (b) viewed from the side*

☐   14 *phalanges* or toe bones, two in the big toe and three in each of the other toes.

The arches of the foot

The foot is not a rigid structure, but a series of strong, flexible arches formed and supported by bones and very strong muscles and ligaments (Figure 21.32). This structure enables it to support the weight of the body when standing and move it in any direction for walking, running and jumping, whether it is on an even or uneven surface. It also leaves room for blood vessels and nerves in the sole of the foot, preventing pressure on them from the body weight.

There are four arches, two running the length of the foot, the

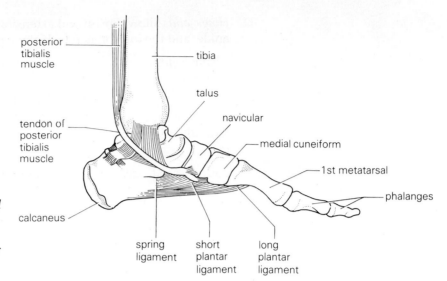

FIGURE 21.32 *The tendons and ligaments supporting the arches of the foot (the view is of a cut through the middle of the foot)*

medial and lateral longitudinal arches, and two running across the foot, the transverse arches. All are supported by plantar ligaments and various muscles.

☐ The *medial longitudinal arch*, on the big-toe side of the foot, is the highest of the arches and is formed by the first three metatarsal bones, the three cuneiform, the navicular and the calcaneus bones. Its primary support comes from the posterior tibialis muscle, whose tendon passes through the ankle and inserts into the navicular, cuboid, metatarsal and medial cuneiform bones, and the spring ligament, which stretches from the calcaneus to the navicular bone. In a well-formed foot, only the calcaneus and the distal ends of the metatarsal bones should connect with the ground.

☐ The *lateral longitudinal arch* is less prominent than the medial arch. It is formed from the calcaneus, the cuboid and the 4th and 5th metatarsal bones, supported by the short muscles of the foot which make up the fleshy parts. Only the calcaneus and the metatarsals should touch the ground.

☐ The *transverse arches* are supported by the short muscles of the foot. They are not easy to see, but run across the foot at the level of the three cuneiform and the cuboid bones.

Joints

All the joints between the bones of the hands and feet are *synovial joints* (freely-moving joints) with capsules. They move in different ways to give the extensive range of movements possible. The classification of these synovial joints is as follows:

☐ *Hinge joints* allow flexion and extension only – examples are the ankle, and the interphalangeal joints of fingers and toes.

☐ *Gliding joints* allow the surfaces to glide over one another – examples are the joints between the carpal (wrist) bones and the tarsal (ankle) bones.

☐ *Pivot joints* allow rotation around an axis – an example is the radioulnar joints between the ends of the radius and ulna bones in the forearm.

☐ *Condyloid and saddle joints* allow rotation around two axes to allow flexion, extension, abduction, adduction, and combinations of all these – examples of these joints are the wrist, the metacarpophalangeal (hand and finger junction) and the metatarsophalangeal (foot and toe junction) joints.

PART IX   # Nail disorders and diseases

22 DISORDERS and DISEASES

DIAGNOSING PROBLEMS

The terms 'dis-order' and 'dis-ease', when applied to the living world, literally mean the same thing: a derangement or disturbance in the usual structure or function, or both, of something. Modern usage of these words, however, tends towards the use of 'disease' as meaning a derangement or disturbance caused by an infectious or contagious condition and 'disorder' as meaning a derangement or disturbance caused by a physical problem. Under this terminology, nail-biting would be classed as a disorder, whereas athlete's foot would be classed as a disease.

Terms used
- □   *Onyx* The Latin word for nail.
- □   *Onychosis* Any disorder of the nail.
- □   *Onychia* Inflammation of the bed of the nail.
- □   *Paronychia* Inflammation of the tissues surrounding the nail.
- □   *Periungual* Around the nail.
- □   *Subungual* Under the nail.

The manicurist's responsibilities
Onychophagy (nail-biting), hangnails, poor nail plate conditions (e.g. ridges, furrows, pitting, flaking, splitting, softness or brittleness) and paronychia, taken in that order of frequency, are probably the most common disorders that the manicurist will find in her work. Others that she will find only occasionally – but often enough to need a thorough knowledge of them – are fungal and bacterial infections, onychia, warts, pterygium (severely overgrown cuticle), habit tics, bruises, allergies, and nail loss or replacement. Many other nail disorders exist, some due to external causes, still others caused by problems in the body as a whole (e.g. poor blood circulation). Doctors often use the condition of the nails to help them diagnose physical problems.

The manicurist does not *need* to know about many of these complaints, but extra knowledge often proves useful in understanding unusual problems. *The manicurist is not a doctor*, but must be able to recognise when and when not to treat a nail. Nails and surrounding tissues showing signs of inflammation, pus formation, pain or fungal infection, *must* be referred to a doctor.

As a professional person, the manicurist must be able to make a valid judgement: if she feels that it is wrong to carry out a service on a client, she must not carry it out, however insistent the client. The refusal to carry out a service when it is inappropriate will protect the manicurist and other clients from disease, and the manicurist from costly legal battles in the event of ineffective treatment.

Management options: a checklist

The following options relate to the table of disorders given below:

1 Manicure as normal.

2 Manicure as normal, perhaps taking care to be extra gentle. The client should already know about this condition and should be having, or will already have had, treatment for it from a doctor. If no treatment has been given then she must be advised to consult a doctor.

3 Manicure as normal, but extra treatments are indicated. Advice should be given about extra salon and home treatments to improve the condition of the nails, such as hot oil or nutritive baths and home-care creams to moisturise; nail caps to smooth furrows or pits or mend splits; extensions to lengthen; buffing; thinning; use of ridge-filler base coats; hardeners for home use; and the padding of ingrowing nails. If the condition gives any cause for concern, the client must be asked to see her doctor before her next visit to the manicurist.

4 Do not manicure at all, but refer the client to the doctor.

TABLE 22.1 *Disorders and diseases: a table for quick reference*

Technical name (common name)	Description	Causes	Appearance	Management option
Beau's lines or ridges	Horizontal shallow or deep ridges across the nail plate	Systemic changes, for example due to illness, drugs or pregnancy, injury, psoriasis, dermatitis, paronychia, false nails, excessive dieting		3
Blue nails	Nails with a bluish tinge to their colouring around the lunula	Lack of oxygen in the bloodstream, usually resulting from poor circulation or heart disease		2

Technical name (common name)	Description	Causes	Appearance	Management option
Bruised nails	Dark purplish spots of congealed blood beneath the nail plate	An injury		2
Eggshell nails	Thin, white, extremely fragile nails, usually curving under at the free edge	Chronic illness		2
Furrows – longitudinal (corrugated nails)	Ridged lines running from base to tip of the nail	Single furrows: congenital defect, injury to matrix. Multiple furrows: psoriasis, systemic unbalance, minor illness, arthritis		3
Habit tic	Numerous horizontal ridges in a band down the centre of the nail	The damage is caused by a nervous habit of picking at or scratching one nail with another at the proximal nail fold		3
Hangnail (agnail)	A small tear or split in the cuticle	Nail-biting; injury; frequent immersion in water; over-exposure to drying agents (e.g. cold or detergents)		3 (4 if infected)
Koilonychia (spoon nails)	Flat or spoon-shaped nails, often thin and soft	Iron-deficiency anaemia, excessive exposure to oils and soaps; congenital: transitory in children for no apparent cause		2
Lamellar dystrophy (lamellar splitting)	Flaking and peeling back of the nail layers at the nail tip	Mechanical trauma; repeated wetting and drying of the nail; use of detergents and solvents; external drying factors		3
Leukonychia	White spots or lines within the nail plate	Cause not really known: variously attributed to trauma, illness or mineral deficiencies; often spontaneous		1 (2 if causing concern)
Malignant melanoma	A painless spreading brown pigmentation beneath or around the nail (uncommon)	A cancer of the nail area: early medical treatment could save the person's life		2

Technical name (common name)	Description	Causes	Appearance	Management option
Onychatrophia (atrophy)	Degeneration: thin, fragile nails which split easily, lose shine, smell, and separate	Injury to matrix; systemic problem (e.g. poor circulation, diabetes, chronic infection)		2
Onychauxis (hypertrophy)	A thickening or overgrowth of the nail plate	Psoriasis; trauma; fungal infection; old age; pressure on nail (esp. toes)		4 (1 if no fungus present)
Onychoclasis (broken nail)	The breaking of the free edge of the nail	Mechanical trauma		3 (4 if below flesh line and infected)
Onychocryptosis (unguis incarnatus, ingrowing nail)	Nail growth into the surrounding tissue pain; sometimes inflammation	Incorrect shaping of the nail (i.e. taking plate away at the sides), pressure from ill-fitting shoes		3 (4 if infected)
Onychogryphosis (claw nail)	Thick, excessively curved, grainy fibrous tissue below: usually seen in toes; ram's horn if not kept short	Injury – usually the repeated trauma of pressure from incorrect footwear		3
Onycholysis	Lifting of the nail plate from its bed, seen as a white area	Fungal or bacterial infection; trauma; adverse reaction to drugs; psoriasis		4
Onychomadesis (defluvium unguium)	The nail loosens at the base and the old nail is pushed off as the new nail grows forward	Mechanical trauma (e.g. the large toenails of squash players); illness creating a Beau's line penetrating all through the plate		4
Onychomycosis	Any fungal infection of the nail plate; lifting; discoloration; rotting of the plate	A fungal infection which has entered through a break in the body's defences (e.g. a lifted area) or which has spread from a surrounding skin infection		4
Onychophagy (nail-biting)	Ragged and bitten-back free edge; often the skin around the nail is bitten; sometimes the nail plate is torn back	Frequent in children, often persists into adult life; once thought to be linked with tension and insecurity but recent studies have undermined this theory: no known cause		3

Technical name (common name)	Description	Causes	Appearance	Management option
Onychorrhexis	Longitudinal splitting in conjunction with furrows (see above)	Trauma on furrows or as a natural result of the furrows		3
Onychotillomania (trichofellomania)	The habit of causing damage to the nail plate (e.g. with scissors)	Self-inflicted damage done deliberately, usually to draw attention to some other psychological or psychiatric problem		4
Panaritium (whitlow)	A localised red, swollen and painful area at the side or base of the nail plate; infection (pus) is often present	Result of bacterial infection that has been allowed to enter via a break in the skin (e.g. biting or accidental)		4
Paronychia (felon)	An infectious and inflammatory condition of the tissues surrounding the nail	As panaritium: acute form – injury; chronic form – dermatitis or repeated immersion in water; often complicated by fungal infection		4
Pitting	Tiny pits over the surface of the nail plate	Psoriasis; dermatitis; alopecia areata; chronic paronychia		3
Platonychia	An increase in curvature across the long axis of the nail plate	Cause not really known: could be due to pressure on toenails		2
Pterygium, simple	A manicurist's term for the overgrowth of cuticle which sticks to the nail plate	Neglect; congenital		3
Pterygium unguis	A scarring loss of the nail matrix: the proximal nail fold and cuticle are drawn over the nail bed; the true plate degenerates	Fusion of proximal nail fold with nail bed, seen in elderly clients, linked with poor blood circulation, blood vessel disease lichen planus		2
Splinter haemorrhage	Tiny, longitudinal streaks of blood under the nail plate	Minor trauma, both systemic (e.g. psoriasis or rheumatoid arthritis) and external (e.g. fungal infection or dermatitis)		1

Technical name (common name)	Description	Causes	Appearance	Management option
Trachyonychia (rough nails)	Extreme roughness of the surface of the nails (sandpaper)	Psoriasis, alopecia, and other systemic disorders		2
Verruca vulgaris (common warts)	Raised lumps of horny tissue; in areas of pressure (feet) they turn in	A viral infection		4

A SURVEY OF NAIL DISORDERS AND DISEASES

Allergy

An allergy is an adverse reaction directed mistakenly by the body's immune defence system to an externally applied or ingested foreign substance. Any or all of the following symptoms can be present with an allergic reaction towards substances applied to the fingernail area. The finger pads become tender, hot, red and sensitive to the touch. The finger pads and the area around the nails become itchy and swollen. The tissues around the edge of the nail plate become dry, peeling away at the sides as in contact dermatitis conditions. Sometimes blisters or sores appear in this area, especially when the itching has driven the client to scratch the area, with consequent scab formation. If allowed to progress, infection and pus formation around the cuticle and nail wall can ensue.

Allergies to nail products can sometimes appear on the face in the form of red weals or rashes on the cheeks, chin or eyelids. These are due to the client touching her face with her nails when these are covered with the sensitising product.

The most common sensitisers in the nail profession are:

□ acrylic monomers (e.g. methyl, butyl and ethyl methacrylate);
□ ethyl cyanoacrylate (used in nail glues);
□ epoxy monomers;
□ formaldehyde.

Certain colourants used to present a major problem, but these are not now permitted in European and American products. Nail varnishes rarely cause allergies, but base coats can due to their adhesive resin content.

During sculptured nail application, the acrylic monomer liquids are mixed with polymer powders and catalysts to create a reaction (polymerisation) which forms a hard acrylic substance suitable for a nail extension. An allergy arises when incomplete polymerisation of the monomer takes place, leaving uncured monomer to sensitise the client. Such reactions usually develop from two to twelve months after commencement of the treatment. Gel systems are notorious for sensitising the manicurist as it is virtually impossible to work with the sticky product without coming into repeated contact with the un-cured monomer.

Nail wraps using ethyl cyanoacrylate glues are frequent sensitisers. The dust created during their filing goes onto the surrounding skin and other areas such as the eyelids if the client brushes her eyes. This can then cause an allergic reaction or rash, or both.

Formaldehyde is no longer used in many products as its potential for sensitisation has been recognised. Amounts as low as 3 per cent of formaldehyde in water are known to irritate the eyes and nose. This 3 per cent solution is often used to treat warts, but use must not continue longer than three weeks or sensitisation to formaldehyde can occur. A formaldehyde solution of 34 or 38 per cent formaldehyde in water (also known as formalin) is a powerful antiseptic and can harden tissues; formalin is used in nail hardeners. (If nail hardeners are allowed to go onto the tissues surrounding the nail, they can cause an inflammatory paronychia.)

Management

Of prime importance is to discontinue using the sensitiser immediately. Any suspect product (e.g. nail extensions) must be removed also. If infection is present, or any symptoms causing concern (e.g. severe swelling and irritation), then the client should be sent to the doctor with an explanatory letter. If, however, the symptoms are not a problem – simple symptoms include excessive dryness around the nail plate area – then gentle manicuring and the use of salon treatments to return moisture to the area (e.g. warm oil baths) should rectify the complaint. The client should be given an antiseptic moisturiser or cuticle cream for home use until all the dryness has healed. This should only take a few days.

Under no circumstances should the sensitising agent be used on that client again. Future reactions become more severe as the client has become more sensitive to that product than she was before. It is, therefore, important that this reaction be noted on her record card.

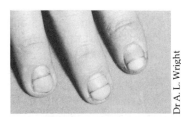

Dr A. L. Wright

Beau's lines

These horizontal shallow or deep ridges traversing the nail plate arise as a result of illness in the body. Generally, the deeper the ridges, the more serious the illness. A minor illness can sometimes leave a ridge in the thumbnail only, whilst more serious problems affect other nails, seeming to affect the index finger first after the thumb and then 'spreading' out along the other fingers to the little finger.

Being linked with the formation of the nail, Beau's lines are only noticeable two to three weeks *after* a period of illness; they progress forward with the nail growth until they grow out. This takes 4–6 months in fingernails and 8–18 months in toenails. As they reach the free edge, they are often found to be lines of weakness that snap off with minor trauma.

They indicate a time when the body's resources were being channelled elsewhere at the expense of the nail plate. A very severe illness can actually result in a cessation of nail plate growth altogether for a short time, resulting in the termination of the existing nail plate and the regrowth of a new nail plate. This grows forward like a normal Beau's line, but there is an actual break in the nail.

Any systemic illness, from measles to malnutrition, from heat stroke to heart attacks, may result in the formation of a Beau's line. Such lines are also seen when the blood flow to the fingers is reduced. A common cause of this is Raynaud's phenomenon, where spasm of the digital arteries occurs. This may be precipitated by cold and is seen in connection with a number of systemic illnesses.

Beau's lines do not cause any long-term damage to the nail.

Multiple small horizontal ridges may occur with hand dermatitis or any inflammatory condition affecting the soft tissues around the nail. A single horizontal ridge can also be caused by the wearing of stick-on gold or plastic false nails. Here the indentation is caused by pressure at the base of the false nail.

Careless filing around the base during the application or filling-in of false nail extensions can also result in the formation of single horizontal ridges if the natural nail is filed into by mistake.

Management

This can be by lessening the visibility of the ridges by buffing or by using ridge-filler base coats. If the ridges are deep, however, the hollows can be filled in using most nail extension materials (e.g. acrylic, gels or fibreglass) to give a smooth surface. This latter course is sometimes necessary to add strength to the free edge as the weak ridge reaches this area.

A Beau's line forming a break all the way through the nail is best left alone apart from keeping the free edge short so that it does not catch and tear off too soon. Sometimes a protective dressing is necessary, but the client will be (or should be) seeing a doctor if the condition is so pronounced. The new growing nail will push the old nail forward and take its place, with natural shedding of the old nail as time progresses. This natural progression should be encouraged in order to avoid the new nail from becoming deformed in any way.

Blue nails

The blue colour shows itself as a blue tint to the lunula at the base of the nail and this indicates impaired circulation or heart disease. (A person must not wear nail varnish or coverings during an operation, so that the anaesthetist can use the possible appearance of this blue tinge as a first warning of insufficient oxygen reaching the tissues of the body.) Oxygenated blood is bright red and appears pink through the nail plate. Deoxygenated blood is darker with a bluish tinge, and appears blue when seen through the nail plate. Poor circulation leads to less oxygen in the blood, hence the blue tinge at the base of the nail plate.

Management

This is a medical complaint and a doctor should be seen. However, it does not contra-indicate manicures. Additional care should be taken, however, during the massage procedure. Poor circulation, resulting in lack of oxygen and nutrients to the nail bed, will result in other problems arising in the nails, such as Beau's lines, fragility, and in extreme cases (frequently seen in elderly clients) nail atrophy and possibly pterygium formation.

Brittle nails

This is a condition in which the nail plate is so hard (and usually thick) that mechanical trauma to the nail will cause the free edge to snap or shatter. This condition is most often seen in middle-aged and older people, simply because the nail plate generally becomes more brittle and thicker with age.

Management

Regular manicures, coupled with the use of cuticle and hand creams, should produce lovely long nails. In a manual occupation (and for toenails) it is best to keep the nails short to avoid damage. Use of nail clippers or scissors must definitely be avoided as these will shatter and split the nail plate. Length must be reduced by means of real or synthetic emery boards. Most problems arise through clients cutting the free edge themselves at home.

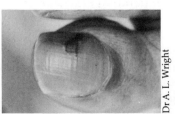

Dr A. L. Wright

Bruised nails

Exactly as the name suggests, bruised nails display dark purplish (sometimes almost black or brown) spots of congealed blood through the transparent nail plate. These are due to injury (e.g. a blow), and bleeding between the nail bed and nail plate. Sometimes the blow has been severe enough for the client to have seen a doctor, who may have had to pierce the nail plate in order to release the blood before pressure caused the nail plate to lift. The dried blood attaches itself to the underside of the nail plate and grows out with it.

Management

If the nail plate has been pierced, then a letter from the doctor authorising a manicure and the application of nail varnish must be obtained. Frequently such clients will be wearing a dressing anyway, so that finger is missed from the manicure.

If the nail has not been pierced, then manicure as normal but be extra gentle and avoid pressure over the bruised area. Cover the nail plate with a dark-coloured nail varnish to hide the dark patch.

Eggshell nails

Here the nail plate is noticeably thin, white and more flexible than the normal nail. These nails are very fragile, and usually curve under at the free edge. (Softness and opacity are signs of an increased water content in the nail plate, up to 30 per cent instead of the normal 18 per cent.)

Eggshell nails are caused by chronic illness stemming from a systemic (bodily) origin. The client should already be receiving medical treatment for this. If she is not, she must be advised to go to her doctor.

Management

There is no treatment that the manicurist can give to improve the condition, but manicures can be given as long as extra care is taken and pressure avoided near the cuticle area.

Fragilitas unguium

A term given to nails which are thin and weak but which are also very brittle, breaking off and splitting into layers very easily. This is a very common problem caused by the basic structure of the nail and its response to the abuses of the modern environment.

A normal nail plate contains about 15–18 per cent water but nail tissue is absorbent and so this percentage can increase to 30 per cent (when the nail is very soft and obviously expanded) or decrease to 10 per cent (when the nail is very brittle). A thin nail plate cannot stabilise its water content as easily as a thick nail plate as it has a larger surface area/volume ratio and more evaporation can take place. Repeated saturation (e.g. during washing-up) followed by dehydration (by central heating or drying products) means that the nail is constantly expanding and contracting, a process leading to the splitting apart of the nail layers. This splitting is made worse by the use of soaps and detergents which remove oils from the nail plate, thereby reducing still further the adhesion between the layers. Note that it is the dehydrated stage which is brittle.

Management
Dry atmospheres and frequent immersion in water should be avoided. The use of emollient creams to guard against moisture loss and to replace oils should be encouraged. The wearing of nail varnish can prevent the loss of moisture through the top surface of the nail (carry it below the free edge to help further), but the use of nail varnish remover (a drying agent) should be minimised. (Compare lamellar dystrophy.)

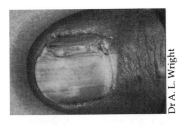

Dr A. L. Wright

Furrows (longitudinal)

Single longitudinal furrows
These are caused by damage to the nail matrix where the nail is being formed. For some clients this will have been a lifetime problem on one (quite common) or more (very uncommon) nails, due to a congenital defect: such people were simply born that way.

Other clients can trace the start of the problem back to an injury, for example being 'stabbed' at the base of the nail by a compass point while at school! This permanently damages that part of the matrix which will then forever grow a faulty nail plate in that area, resulting in a longitudinal furrow.

If a prominent longitudinal ridge is present which has only just arisen and which cannot be traced back to any injury, then a doctor should be seen – furrows can be caused by pressure from a benign or malignant tumour in the proximal nail fold. A manicurist should not treat this category of furrow until permission has been obtained from the doctor.

These single furrows usually present no problem until they reach the free edge, when the flaw can break apart to give a permanent split at the free edge. This is irritating in that it catches and snags on fabrics, and it can be dangerous in that such snags can result in the plate tearing to below the flesh line, thereby exposing it to infection.

Sometimes, however, the furrow is an actual split right through to the nail bed. The body adapts its localised tissues in such a way that skin is underneath this split, not bare nail bed, so there is no danger other than that of snagging, as above. It is, however, unsightly.

Management
Management used to be by buffing and keeping the nail very short. However, modern techniques of nail extension and repair have allowed the management to become more civilised and cosmetically acceptable. *As long as there is no open access to the nail tissues below*, a nail extension or cover (cap) will smooth the furrow, seal the free edge, and make the nail look like a normal nail. Regular fill-ins will of course have to be performed as this is a cosmetic cover, not a healing treatment.

It is important that there be no opening to the tissues below for two reasons. First, if a low-grade and therefore not obvious infection were present, it would be sealed into the tissues where it would develop and cause subsequent problems. Secondly, false nail products can be sensitisers: they must not be applied to living tissue, only to dead nail plate, or an allergic reaction could easily follow.

If the furrow is not very deep and is a line of weakness rather than a site of continual splitting at the free edge (if it just splits when knocked), then the constant use of a modern cellulose-film type of nail hardener can sometimes strengthen the nail sufficiently for the furrow to cease to be a problem.

Multiple longitudinal furrows

These are shallow ridges and furrows running from the base to the tip of the nail plate and covering all of the nails. They usually present no problems other than cosmetic ones. However, they can be more pronounced, in which case they can lead to a condition known as onychorrhexis (page 325).

Multiple longitudinal ridges may accompany psoriasis and alopecia areata, as well as other more serious illnesses which the manicurist will not see in her salon. More usually, these furrows are a sign of a systemic unbalance or minor illness, and they will grow out and disappear as normal health returns. In older people single longitudinal ridges may accompany arthritis. Some naturopaths link them with malabsorption from the digestive system.

Management

Gentle buffing can reduce the visibility of the furrows, as can the use of a ridge-filling base coat prior to varnish application. If the furrows are severe then a thin covering of a nail extension product (e.g. acrylic, gel or fibreglass) before buffing will fill the hollows.

Filing and shaping must be carried out with a fine emery board as the edges of these nails are often fragile. Use of a suitable nail hardener can help overcome fragility if the nails are soft, but often this type of nail is already hard and brittle, in which case hardeners must be avoided and oils and creams recommended instead.

When fragile, these nails need to be kept short. If they are strong, they can grow to the usual longer lengths with the aid of regular manicures.

In clients over thirty, a furrow can sometimes take on a beaded appearance – it looks like a row of tiny beads down the surface of the nail plate instead of a line. This is due to an intermittent disturbance in the growth of the plate in the matrix.

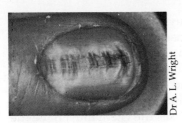

Dr A. L. Wright

Habit tic

This is the name given to damage caused to the surface of the nail by constantly picking at or playing with the nail.

It is most frequently seen on thumbnails, where it appears as a series of horizontal ridges in a band down the centre of the nail only (not completely from side to side). It is due to the client having a nervous habit of constantly picking at and scratching the surface of the nail with another nail, particularly at the proximal nail fold where the softer portion of recently formed nail is easily deformed.

Management

Although aware of her habit, the client is often unaware that it is that which is causing the damage, assuming instead that she is picking at it because it is rough, rather than making it rough through picking at it. Once this is pointed out to her, she may break the habit immediately, and a fibreglass cover (cap) could be put over the nail surface to smooth out the ridges for cosmetic purposes while new nail grows. Alternatively, a plaster could be worn over the nail to prevent and break the habit.

New nail growth will be smooth once the habit has been broken and the cuticle has recovered.

Hangnail (agnail)

These are splits and tears in the cuticle surrounding the nail. Frequently, there are small pieces of dried epidermis sticking up which have split away from the lateral nail fold. These catch and irritate, often leading to the client biting them away and tearing the skin still further.

Splits frequently extend as far as the underlying dermis, when they are painful and allow infection to enter the area. When this occurs, the condition can progress to paronychia (inflammation of the tissue surrounding the nail, also known as a felon) or a panaritium (an abscess at the side or base of the nail, also known as a whitlow).

Hangnails are common in nail-biters, but are also caused by injury, neglect or by over-exposure to drying agents such as detergents, extreme cold, frequent immersion in water, or not drying the hands properly. These cause the skin surrounding the nail to dry out and crack.

Management

A standard manicure, in which the skin is softened with cuticle creams, the cuticle eased back and the loose bits of skin gently cut away with cuticle clippers, is sufficient. An anti-bacterial nail soak during the manicure, and the use of an anti-bacterial cream at the end of the manicure, are added precautions which it is sensible to take.

The client should be encouraged to buy a rich cuticle oil or cream for nightly home application to moisturise the cuticle area, and the cause (e.g. biting or over-exposure to solvents) established and eradicated (e.g. by ceasing to bite the nails, or by wearing rubber gloves for protection when doing wet and 'messy' jobs).

The manicurist must not treat the nail if there is infection present (i.e. paronychia or panaritium). In such cases the client must have the condition explained to her and be referred to her doctor. Explain that she can return for a manicure once the infection has cleared up. To manicure with infection present could spread the infection to other nails and surrounding soft tissues and also make the existing infection worse.

Hapalonychia

Hapalonychia means soft nails. Softness at the base of the nail next to the cuticle is usually linked with a systemic disorder, such as a dermatitis or eczema – an inflammation of the skin related either to chronic skin irritation or to an allergy. A generalised soft nail condition could be due to the client's nails naturally retaining a lot of water (the nail plate is very soft after immersion in water), or it could simply be the way that her nails grow.

Management
Nail hardeners are formulated to harden soft nails and so correct usage of a good hardener should help alleviate the problem.

When the nails are soft, care must be taken not to exert a lot of pressure during cuticle work or damage could be done to the matrix, nail plate and nail bed.

Koilonychia

Here the nail shape is depressed so that it is flat, or concave (spoon-shaped). Some people have this shape of nail because they have inherited it and the shape will never change. Others develop it as a symptom of iron-deficiency anaemia, the shape returning to normal as the anaemia is treated. Others develop this change from working with oils and soaps (the condition is frequently seen in car mechanics), which soften the nails and cause them to curve upwards as they grow; avoidance of these products will let the nail shape return to normal. Children and infants often have this nail shape naturally and it changes to the normal shape as the child grows up.

Management
Manicures can be carried out as normal but the nails need to be kept

short as they will not only catch but look unsightly as they curve up at the end of the finger. The manicurist can do nothing to alter the shape, but can perhaps advise the client on the cause of the problem and recommend her to see a doctor if necessary.

Lamellar dystrophy (lamellar splitting)

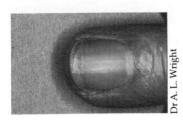

Dr A. L. Wright

The nail plate is made up of layers known as lamellae (page 276). When these layers break apart horizontally at the distal portion of the plate (the tip) and flake away or peel back, the condition is known as lamellar dystrophy. This condition can be caused by repeated small traumas to the nail tips. It is more frequently caused by the repeated saturation and drying out of the porous nail surface, which leads to expansion and contraction of the lamellae and their subsequent flaking apart (compare fragilitas unguium). The removal of natural oils from the nail plate by the use of solvents also reduces the adhesion between the nail layers.

Saturation (water uptake) occurs every time the nails are placed in water for any length of time, especially when the water is alkaline, as it is when washing. (Note that water uptake occurs at the same time as oils are being dissolved from the nail plate during washing-up.) Dehydration (drying out) and also the removal of oils from the nail plate can occur in a number of ways, including the following:

- ☐ frequent immersion in solvents such as soaps and detergents (housewives);
- ☐ soil (gardeners);
- ☐ chalk (teachers);
- ☐ paper (secretaries);
- ☐ nail varnish removers;
- ☐ central heating (laboratory assistants or production workers);
- ☐ chemicals (laboratory assistants or production workers).

From this list it is easy to see why lamellar dystrophy is more common in women than in men, and in winter rather than in summer.

Management
This condition is not easy to keep under control. Capping (covering) with extension products is unsuccessful because the capping breaks away from the tips with the nail flakes. Varnish applications will break away (chip) at the tip after one or two days, and the client must be instructed not to keep removing her nail varnish and replacing it with fresh as the constant use of varnish remover will only add to her problem; the correct procedure would be for her to simply touch in the flaked area with the same colour (cream varnishes are easier to touch in than pearlised) and remove the varnish only once a week at most. Nail extensions are a cosmetic answer for the desperate client but offer no permanent solution.

With perseverance, the following programme should work, but it does involve a lot of care and time:

☐ weekly manicures, possibly incorporating a hot oil or nutritive cream bath;
☐ frequent home use of rich hand creams, especially after immersion of the hands in water;
☐ nightly application of a good cuticle oil or cream over the whole of the nail area;
☐ regular use of a nail hardener that does not contain formaldehyde;
☐ the wearing of rubber gloves for all messy jobs (e.g. washing-up, polishing and gardening).

Leukonychia

This term refers to either localised (partial) or generalised (total) whiteness in the nail plate. The manicurist will probably never see nail plates which are totally white (*leukonychia totalis*), which is due to a congenital deformity, but will frequently see examples of partial leukonychia, including punctata and striata.

In *leukonychia punctata*, the whiteness appears as scattered dots within the nail plate. These can appear at the cuticle area or partially along the nail plate, get bigger or smaller or disappear altogether, or grow out with the nail plate. Their cause is unknown, though it could be trauma; some naturopaths relate them to zinc, iron, or calcium deficiencies but there is no scientific evidence for this.

In *leukonychia striata*, the whiteness appears as bands across the nail plate. They can be a result of illness, but are more often due to trauma, such as using too much pressure when pushing back the cuticle in a manicure. These lines will grow out with the nail. Leukonychia may also be a feature of onychomycosis.

It is not known exactly what causes the whiteness. It could be due to air bubbles between the nail plate layers, or to the incomplete keratinisation of the nail plate cells so that nuclear debris remains in the cells.

Management

There is nothing the manicurist can do to eliminate the white areas. She can advise the client not to apply pressure to the nail base area when manicuring at home, and work gently over this area herself when manicuring. The white marks can be covered, using a good-quality nail varnish.

Onychalgia nervosa

This is a term given to extremely sensitive nails.

Management

Nothing can be done to make these nails less sensitive, and such a client frequently finds any work in the cuticle area too painful to endure. Management of the cuticle must be by additional salon treatments (e.g. hot oil baths) and by encouraging the client into the nightly home use of cuticle oils, which will prevent the cuticles from growing up the nail plate and keep them in good condition so that they do not need to be clipped.

Onychatrophia (atrophy)

A degeneration of the nail plate, with symptoms ranging from decreasing size, thinning nail plate, excessive ridging, pterygium formation, to the occasional loss of the nail with scarring so that it cannot grow back. It can be caused by injury to the matrix, or by a systemic complaint such as a circulation problem, diabetes or chronic infection.

Management

There is nothing the nail technician can do except keep the nail short whilst a doctor is being consulted. The client should be advised to protect the weak nail as much as possible by avoiding soaps and detergents and by wearing rubber gloves for all dirty jobs.

Onychauxis (hypertrophy)

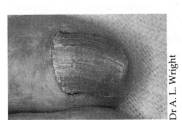

Dr A. L. Wright

This is a thickening or overgrowth of the nail plate and it is most commonly seen on one or more nails as a result of psoriasis or fungal infections. The hyponychium is often involved (page 277). It can also be seen on little-toe nails which often become thicker (sometimes even claw-like) as a result of pressure. Onychauxis is frequently seen in the large-toe nails of elderly clients and can be due to pressure on the nail (see onychogryphosis) or simply old age.

Management

On hands, because of the possible involvement of a fungal organism, any client with unusual thickening of the nails should be advised to go to the doctor for an accurate diagnosis. With medical permission, an experienced nail technician can file down some of the thickening, and buff and manicure the nails in the normal way.

On toenails, severe thickening is best referred to a chiropodist who is trained to file the nail away using electric files.

Onychia

Onychia is the name given to any inflammation of the nail bed. It can sometimes extend as far back as the matrix, where the nail is formed. It is usually accompanied by separation and disturbance of the nail plate from its bed. If pus forms and cannot escape, a doctor may have to pierce the nail plate in the affected area to release the pressure to prevent the nail from coming off.

Onychia can arise as a result of a mechanical trauma, such as shutting the fingertips in a door, or from paronychia (an infection of the tissues surrounding the nail) if the infection is left untreated and goes on to invade the nail bed.

Management

As onychia is an infection and the tissues will be inflamed, a manicure must not be given but the client must be referred to her doctor for correct diagnosis and treatment.

Onychoclasis (broken nail)

A complicated name for the simple breaking of the free edge of the nail. This is usually caused by a mechanical trauma – a bang or knock.

Management

If the nail is broken below the free edge so that raw flesh is exposed and the area is painful, do not manicure. Dress the area using an antiseptic cream and a plaster or a small, sterile dressing. Should infection occur, ask the client to see her doctor. When the area has healed it can be manicured or the nail plate artificially extended, as desired. *Do not put an extension over an open wound as infection could be sealed into the wound.*

For a normal break, the nail could simply be manicured and left short, or an extension could be fitted so that the nail matched in with the rest of the hand.

If the client has retained the piece of torn-off nail, or if the free edge is 'hanging by a thread', the free edge can be stuck back into place and reinforced to look natural by means of modern nail extension products.

Onychocryptosis (ingrowing nail)

This is the correct term for an ingrowing nail, also known as an *unguis incarnatus*. Although this condition may be found in the fingernails, it is more commonly found in the toenails. The symptoms, causes and management are the same for both toe- and fingernails, and this information is included in the section on common foot disorders (page 187).

Onychogryphosis (claw nail)

Here the nails become very thick and excessively curved. Quite often the plate has a lot of grainy fibrous tissue below it coming from the hyponychium (see page 277). This adds to the thickness and causes pain and bleeding if it is cut into in an effort to shorten and thin the nail. If not kept short, the curvature makes the nail look like a ram's horn.

This problem usually arises after an injury such as a severe knock. It is frequently seen on the toenails (especially the large toenail) of older clients, where it is probably due to repeated trauma in the form of pressure from footwear.

Management

These nails must be kept very short. Because of their thickness, they are difficult to cut; files and pliers are the easiest implements to use for this purpose. If the thickness is too great, or if there is a lot of granular tissue making it difficult to reduce the length easily, then the client should be referred to a doctor or a chiropodist who will have been trained to deal with the condition. There is no cure.

Onycholysis

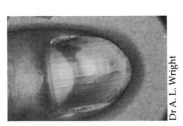

Dr A. L. Wright

This term encompasses any lifting of the nail plate from its bed. If the condition is left untreated, the lifting can spread until the whole nail comes loose and is shed. Nail plate lifting can be seen as a whitish or semi-translucent area of nail plate. As the contact with the nail bed is lost, so is the pink coloration usually gained from the blood within the nail bed.

If this lifted area discolours, a fungal or bacterial infection under the lifted area may be the culprit. Fungal infections are usually colourless, yellow-grey or white; bacterial or yeast infections may be dark.

Onycholysis can have many causes, including fungal or bacterial infections, trauma, adverse reactions to drugs, circulatory problems, psoriasis and systemic illness. It is of professional interest that it has been known to occur through the over-use (at home) of nail hardeners containing formaldehyde, through the over-zealous use of manicure tools (e.g. cuticle knives and sticks), and as an allergy reaction to the liquid monomers used in nail extensions. Phenol was used as a constituent of nail products until it was discovered that it caused onycholysis. Care must be taken with all chemicals applied to the nail plate.

Management

As there is the possibility of infection, all instances of onycholysis should be referred to a doctor for proper diagnosis and treatment. If the complaint is allowed to progress, the nail plate could be lost, temporarily or permanently (see onychomycosis).

Onychomadesis

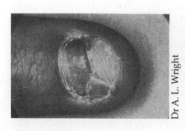

Dr A. L. Wright

As with onycholysis, this can lead to nails being shed. Here the nail loosens at the base and the old nail is 'pushed off' as the new nail grows forward. This can happen following a mechanical trauma (e.g. a knock), or through an illness which interrupts the nutrition to the nail (compare Beau's lines). It is frequently seen on the large toenails of squash players, who may have worn too-tight footwear or let their nails grow too long.

Management

A doctor should be seen to ensure that further damage does not occur. The manicurist can then help by keeping the nail plate very short so that it does not catch on anything and tear off too soon. (If this were to happen the new nail might become deformed.) If necessary, a dressing, finger stall or plaster may be worn to prevent this. Eventually, the new nail will push the old nail off as it grows up. This will take about 4–6 months in fingers and 8–18 months in toes.

Onychomycosis

This is a term used to refer to any infection of the nail area caused by a fungus. Some of these fungi are saprophytic – that is, they live on dead tissue. Others are dermatophytic – they invade the living tissue of the nail folds, bed and skin.

The manicurist will encounter fungal infections which can be related to two main causes: those which are related to trauma, and those which have spread to the nail area from a skin infection. Both can produce onycholysis and leukonychia, but fungi rarely produce dark discolorations, such colourings usually being due to bacterial infections.

Trauma

A client may lift the free edge of the nail slightly from its bed through a knock, gardening, or a splinter piercing the hyponychium. This lifted area must be observed weekly. Some reattach straight away. Most cases will grow out as new nail pushes forward. Still others will stay the same, due to keratinisation (thickening) of the nail bed; these must be observed indefinitely as they provide warm damp areas ideal for fungal establishment and growth. Sometimes, though, this lifted area begins to increase in size and this is often due to a fungal infection of the nail area inside the air space, which is invading the living nail bed and causing further onycholysis. This may or may not be accompanied by a colour change. In the majority of these cases, the only colour change the fungus causes is a whitening of the nail plate. This is often accompanied by a hardening or a softening of the nail plate from its usual state. If the lifting has spread to other nails, this is an almost certain indication of a fungal infection.

In some types of fungal infection, when it is in an advanced stage (a new client may present with this), the surface of the nail plate at the sides may appear 'rotten' or 'soggy'. This is because some fungi can feed on the keratin in the nail plate. This type of infection is not often seen by the manicurist.

Any unaccountable lifting, long-term lifting or increase in the size of a lifted area must be viewed with suspicion and referred to a doctor for correct diagnosis and treatment.

A variety of fungi and yeasts, all of which are free-living in soil and water, may be incriminated in such infections.

Dr A. L. Wright

☐ *Tinea pedis* commonly known as *ringworm of the foot* or *athlete's foot*, is a very common skin infection which, if neglected, can invade one or two toenails as well. The nail turns a yellowish-grey colour, becomes brittle, and separates from the nail bed. Treatment is lengthy once the nail is involved, involving the taking of tablets for up to 18 months. It has been found that the application of anti-fungal creams is ineffective against well-established fungal infections of the nails. (See page 183.)

☐ *Tinea unguium* is a ringworm infection of the fingernails. It is not common but when it occurs, usually several nails are affected, often asymmetrically. The infected areas go yellowish-grey in colour, become brittle, and separate from the nail bed. Treatment is the same as for tinea pedis.

☐ *Scopulariopsis brevicaulis* is a rare fungal infection, usually confined to the large toenails. The fungus is common outside the human body but only becomes invasive on damaged keratin, on which it can live. Infected nails have a chalky-white or yellow appearance and the fungus is extremely difficult to treat.

☐ Some species of the fungus *Candida*, growing in a yeast-like form, can occur in lifted areas of nail plate (as already described), or occur on the surface of the nail plate (when it looks like tinea unguium). Being common in the air all around us, *Candida* frequently invades a weak area in the body's defences – if the cuticle is lost through paronychia (a bacterial infection) or other damage, for example, the fungus can invade the space between the nail plate and the posterior nail fold. Here it causes chronic inflammation and occasionally pus formation. Being within the body tissues, it is difficult to eradicate and perpetuates the paronychia.

A doctor can take a sample of infected tissue and send it away for microscopic analysis and culture in order to determine the species present and treat accordingly. Treatment of an invasive fungal infection is slow (6–18 months) and not always successful. It is sufficient for the nail technician simply to recognise that there may be a fungal infection present: she can then refrain from treating the client and refer her to her doctor for help, and prevent the spread of the disease among her clients, in the salon and to herself. If the manicurist sees something unusual occurring in the nails of a client which perturbs her – such as an excess curvature, roughness or flatness, onycholysis with a colour change (white, brown or yellow-grey), a texture change, splinter haemorrhages or the like, occurring in one or more nails for no apparent reason – she should refer the client to her doctor for a correct diagnosis and treatment. Any of these changes could be caused by a fungal infection.

Bacterial infections usually take the form of paronychias. However, there is another type of non-invasive bacterial infection which is sometimes seen in the nail salon: this occurs as a green-black discoloration on the surface of the nail plate, but underneath a lifted section of nail covering or extension material. It is often incorrectly described as a 'mould' or fungal infection, when it is actually bacterial in origin and often caused by members of the *Pseudomonas* species (e.g. *Pseudomonas aeruginosa*). Most dark-coloured discolorations are formed by bacteria, not fungi.

The warm damp areas created by lifted areas of false nail are ideal for fungi and bacteria to establish themselves and grow. The difference with *Pseudomonas* is that the infection is on *top* of the nail plate and cannot easily penetrate through the hard shiny protective plate to obtain food. (This is one very good reason for not buffing the shine away during preparation for false nail application.) Fungi need an organic source of food, easily found in the debris under a lifted natural nail plate; bacteria seem able to survive in the more hardy environment of an air gap under a lifted false nail. In some cases, early in the development of false nail products, they even seemed able to metabolise the false nail and adhesive products themselves!

Early stages of this type of infection, within the first two weeks or so, are seen as an area of very dark green (sometimes almost black) discoloration beneath the lifted area of false nail. When the false nail is clipped back to show the area, the nail plate will look normal but simply be discoloured by the growth of the bacteria. This is the one example when a nail technician can treat the infection herself (because it is not invasive), by soaking the fingernail for 10 minutes in a container of surgical spirit, or antiseptic recommended by the manufacturers of the false nail: this will dry up the moisture and kill any surface bacteria. The nail can be allowed to dry, buffed lightly (discarding the buffer, to be sure), and painted with a recommended antiseptic primer (often called a thermolize solution); the nail fill treatment can then be continued. The discoloration will be left on the nail and will grow out.

If the nail is left free of covering, including nail varnish, the discoloration will fade and wear away. Application of diluted chlorine bleach can be used to help fade it, although most clients are happy simply to disguise the area with nail varnish. Obviously the area must be checked at future appointments to ensure that it has not increased in size. If it has, the covering must be removed and the client referred to the doctor straight away as this is a sign that complications have developed and the infection has re-established itself.

Some manicurists prefer to leave the covering off an infected area for a few days after treatment. This is the best option to follow as the conditions for growth have then been removed and the infection cannot re-establish itself. Some clients, however, 'need' their 'nails' for special occasions and would prefer them to be filled straight away. The manicurist must use her professional judgement as to the correct path to follow, depending on the severity of the infection. A client having regular two-weekly fills cannot have developed an invasive infection during that interval so sanitation and filling is an acceptable management procedure.

Occasionally, however, a client will present herself with nails which have not been seen or filled for several weeks. She may have been gluing them herself at home 'to save money'. (The use of cyanoacrylate glues seems, in some cases, to encourage bacterial growth, probably due to the trapping of minute air bubbles or even to the provision of nutrients.) In such a case a bacterial infection could be well-established, having penetrated the nail plate and caused potential lifting of the natural nail. The false nail material must be removed, the nails sanitised, and the client referred to her doctor with a covering letter. This situation should not happen in a salon because a manicurist must *insist* on two-weekly fills for her clients or refuse to take them as clients at all.

When a fungal or bacterial infection has been seen in the salon, all equipment, materials and the like should of course be dealt with by correct sanitary procedure – either disposed of or sterilised, as appropriate to each item.

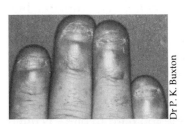

Dr P. K. Buxton

Onychophagy (biting the nail plate)

Nail-biting, often including the biting of the skin around the margin of the nail, is often seen in schoolchildren, most of whom give up the practice as they approach adolescence. Frequently, however, it persists in varying degrees into adult life, some people biting only when under pressure or tension (e.g. during a stressful event or while watching an exciting film), others biting continually and making an awful mess of their nails. Recent psychological studies have rebutted any link between insecurity and nail-biting; the cause is not known.

Biting can be simply around the free edge, or of the skin around the nail. When taken to extreme, the free edge is bitten back to expose the hyponychium and in very severe cases the biting can be over the surface of the nail, picking away the layers with the teeth to leave only hard skin and small spikes of nail with a tiny remnant of whole nail plate towards the base. Often people can be seen who bite nine nails and save one long one for scratching. Conversely, clients may stop biting up to nine nails and use one or more nails for their biting habit.

Minor nail-biting, although unsightly and often leading to panaritia (whitlows) if the skin is involved, does not do any long-term damage to the nail. Very severe nail-biting over a period of time reduces the length of the nail bed: the nail cannot reattach itself to the 'bed' if the bed has become scarred. When these nails are eventually allowed to grow, the free edge starts some considerable way down from the fingertip. Thus the free edge has to be quite long just to reach the end of the finger. As a consequence, these nails cannot often grow to any real lengths in the future: they are not supported sufficiently and will break off unless they are very strong. Often, too, the nail bed down the sides of the nail groove becomes scarred so that the free edge reaches deep down the sides of the nails. This is an area which will collect dirt and dry skin and prove to be a weak area, prone to splitting and flaking.

For some unknown reason, nails which have been badly bitten for a long time often (though not always) prove to be very strong when they are finally allowed to grow.

Management

Children often outgrow the habit naturally, or, for an older child, by appeal to a commonsense approach on the grounds of pride. This can be done by introducing children to professional manicures at around 8–10 years of age. Even a single visit for a manicure at this time alerts them to nail and hand care which they will then copy at home. Most children love to copy any adult behaviour in an attempt to appear grown-up.

The painting on of nasty-tasting compounds does not usually prove very successful as children frequently suck all the compound away at once so that they can then continue biting at their leisure! Compounds may work on adults who *want* to give up but bite unknowingly, as for example while watching television. The nasty taste as soon as the fingers go into the mouth serves to remind them of what they are doing. Adults are better treated by encouraging an alternative behaviour that keeps their hands otherwise occupied at a time when they usually bite their nails (e.g. knitting whilst watching television).

The wearing of false nails – nails that are too hard to bite – is often enough to break the habit, but it is important to undertake a nail care routine, complete with varnish application, after their removal or the habit quickly returns.

Regular manicures with the emphasis on removing any ragged edges of nail and cuticle, and the application of skin softening creams to the cuticle, followed by a varnish application, are often enough to break the habit. Not only have the irritating 'catching' bits been removed, but the client is paying for a service and will think twice before ruining the paid-for work. Varnish also serves as a reminder not to bite (although some clients bite the varnish off !).

Regular weekly manicures often instil the pride necessary to stop nail-biting, and these present the most successful approach. Nail hardeners, cuticle oils and hand creams can be sold for home use and all help the client to build up a care pattern which increases her pride and success rate. Files for home use are essential, here, so that if a snag occurs it can be filed smooth immediately before the temptation to bite off the rest becomes too great.

A person who used to bite her nails when under stress is likely to lapse back into the habit whenever she is placed in a stressful situation.

Onychophosis (subungual hyperkeratosis)

These are terms used for a growth of horny epithelium on the nail bed. The condition is a result of hyperplasia of the epidermis: an increase in the size and number of the cells of the epidermis. It is seen in severe nail-biters, under the tips of nails of people suffering from psoriasis and hand dermatitis, and sometimes under thickened and lifted toenails. (Compare onychogryphosis, page 319.)

Management
A manicurist cannot do anything to improve this condition, simply keep the area clean and moisturised for comfort.

Onychoptosis

This term refers to any shedding of the nails. Shedding can be whole or partial; can accompany diseases, such as syphilis; can occur spontaneously and periodically; can be as a result of a trauma (mechanical, chemical, or drug-induced); and can also be caused by many other reasons. (See also onycholysis, page 319.)

Management
The manicurist can do nothing here and the client must be referred to her doctor for correct diagnosis and treatment. Once the doctor has given permission, manicures may be resumed.

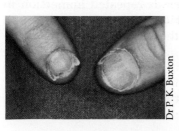
Dr P. K. Buxton

Onychorrhexis

This is a term given to an excess of longitudinal striations (stripes) along the nail plate. These stripes are known as furrows (see page

312). They are lines of weakness in the nail plate, and as such frequently break open when knocked, to produce longitudinal and parallel splits in the free edge.

Management
As for furrows.

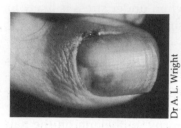

Dr A. L. Wright

Panaritium (whitlow)

A panaritium appears as a localised, red, swollen and painful area at the side or base of the nail plate. It often exudes pus and is the result of a bacterial infection which has entered through a break in the skin, usually caused by biting or by an accident, as for example a splinter or the clumsy use of a cuticle knife or clippers. It is commonly known as a whitlow and, being an inflammation of the tissues around the nail plate, it is also a localised form of paronychia.

Management
Panaritia are managed in the same way as is paronychia (see below).

Paronychia (felon)

Paronychia is an infectious, inflammatory condition of the tissues surrounding the nails. It is a very common condition and appears as a red, swollen and painful area in the tissues around the nail. There can also be pus present, which can exude from the junction with the nail plate or from the skin around the nail.

Commonly called a felon, paronychia is due to a bacterial infection which has been allowed to enter through a break in the body's defences around the nail plate. Acute (sudden and severe) paronychia usually occurs as a result of an injury (see panaritium, above) and so usually only affects one nail. A Beau's line may be caused on the nail plate as a result of this.

Chronic (long-term) paronychia usually affects several nails and is due to a more long-standing cause, such as repeated immersion in water (washing-up) or the presence of dermatitis. Paronychia can become chronic due to the invasion of the damaged tissue with the yeast *Candida albicans* (see onychomycosis). Chronic paronychia can give rise to pitting of the surface of the nail plate or multiple horizontal fissures.

Formaldehyde-based nail hardeners, if allowed to go onto the skin, can cause paronychia.

Management

Paronychia, as it is a bacterial infection, must not be treated by a manicurist. Manicure is contra-indicated and the client should be referred to her doctor for drainage of the area if necessary, and for antibiotic treatment.

Pitting

Here the surface of the nail plate is covered with tiny pits, like large pinpricks. They do not go all the way through the plate. There is evidence to show that they develop as tiny areas of incomplete keratinisation during the growth of the nail, which are then not as strong as the rest of the nail and slough away to leave pits as the nail plate grows forward. The pits can be scattered irregularly over the surface of a few nails, or formed in horizontal lines across the nails. They are seen as side-effects of psoriasis, dermatitis, alopecia, and chronic paronychia.

Management

Manicures can be carried out as normal. As long as the client knows the cause of the pits and is receiving treatment for the underlying problem, cosmetic repairs can be suggested. These can take the form of covering (capping) the nail plate with a harmless extension material such as fibreglass. This is easily carried out to smooth the surface of the nail. Fibreglass is cited here because of the ease of its removal (using acetone) if necessary without the nail plate being weakened further.

Platonychia

This is a term used for excessive curvature in the long axis of the nail. This means that the nail plate is curved round and down at the sides into the flesh of the finger or toe so that it acts like a pincer on the tissues. It can lead to ingrowing nails, or stop the blood from circulating through the finger tissues properly. The nails may come to resemble claws.

The cause is not known; in toenails it *could* be due to the surrounding pressure of shoes and socks.

Management

There is no treatment. The nails can be manicured and filed short to help prevent ingrowing nail edges. If the condition becomes too bad, the nail plate has to be surgically removed.

Pterygium unguis

Many manicurists refer to the simple overgrowth of neglected cuticle onto the nail plate as pterygium. The cuticle in this case can simply be softened, pushed back and clipped away as part of a normal manicure.

True pterygium, however, is an overgrowth of cuticle onto the nail due to a scarring loss of the nail matrix. It is often seen in elderly clients with very poor circulation.

A pterygium usually starts on one nail and spreads to others. The cuticle appears fused with the nail plate in the centre, so that cuticle work is impossible. It then grows forward, seeming to split the nail into two. Eventually the two halves of the nail become smaller and smaller as the pterygium becomes larger, until the true nail plate almost or entirely disappears.

What actually happens is that the proximal (dorsal) nail fold becomes fused with the nail matrix so that the true structure of the cuticle, nail fold, matrix, nail bed and nail plate is lost, being replaced with a tough scar tissue which grows forward in the same way as does a nail plate.

Management

Manicures can be continued as long as possible, but it is impossible to do any cuticle work. The emphasis is solely on trimming down the flakes of nail so that they do not catch on clothing. There is no cure, and the nail plate is eventually replaced with tough scar tissue.

Check that the client is seeing a doctor. If she is not, advise her to go to one.

Splinter haemorrhages

These are a type of subungual (under the nail) haematomata (bruises). They look like, and are, tiny short splinters of dried blood running lengthwise along the nail plate.

They are common, and are usually due to minor traumas, though they may also be seen in relation to a number of systemic illnesses.

Management

Splinter haemorrhages grow out with the nail plate and do not need any special attention. Manicure as normal and suggest a deeper shade of nail varnish to cover the discolorations.

Trachyonychia (rough nails)

This is a roughness of the surface of the nail plates such that they feel

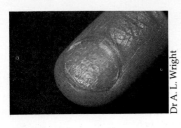

like fine sandpaper. It is linked with systemic problems, notably psoriasis and alopecia.

Management

Manicure can still be carried out, although this extreme roughness is a sign of ill-health in the client and if she is not already seeing a doctor she should be advised to do so. If her condition is known to her doctor, then buffing can be carried out to smooth the nails: this must not be done, however, before this symptom has been used by the doctor as an aid to diagnosis.

Verruca vulgaris (common warts)

The correct name for common warts. They are an outgrowth of the skin, usually circular, caused by an infection of the skin tissues by a virus. They are contagious and most common on the hands. They can disappear spontaneously, or persist for many years (between 2–15 years without treatment).

They are most painful on the soles of the feet (plantar warts, verruca plantaris – see page 188) when the pressure leads to them becoming depressed beneath the surface of the skin. Here they press on nerves in the soles of the feet and so cause pain.

Warts can grow beneath the nail plate, where they are forced to go down into the tissues as they would on the sole of the foot. The nail plate can be forced upwards by their presence. When growing around the nail plate, they look just like normal warts on other areas of the hand: round, raised and callused.

Nail-biters tend to spread the condition on themselves so that the warts run into one another and invade large portions of the nail fold. Sometimes the structure of the nail plate can be affected by their presence, although it is usually the nail-biting that does the damage.

Management

Warts are contagious: they are spread by contact. The manicurist should not perform any treatment on any area where there are warts. The client should be referred to a doctor, who will treat them with diathermy (burning them away), liquid nitrogen cryotherapy (freezing them away), or with creams and solutions.

Doctors may use a 3 per cent formalin solution to treat warts. Certain nail varnishes and nail hardeners contain small amounts of formalin, and it has been found that painting such a varnish over the surface of a wart will frequently eliminate it within two or three weeks. This must be tried only on minor warts, and must be discontinued after three weeks if it has not worked so that formalin sensitivity does not develop.

Infrequently used terms

- *Anonychia* The absence of a nail plate (usually from birth).

- *Macronychia* A condition in which the nail plate is larger than normal.

- *Micronychia* A condition in which the nail plate is smaller than normal.

- *Polyonychia* A condition in which there are two or more nails on one finger or toe.

- *Usere des ongles* Wearing away of the nails due to scratching.

NAIL PLATE COLOUR CHANGES

Colour changes in the nail plate can be due to external influences, or be a sign of a disorder of the nail plate or an internal change of some kind. The following are some examples:

- Longitudinal pigmented streaks appear normally in the nails of people with pigmented skins. In white people, however, they can be a sign of a systemic disorder such as Addison's disease; or, if recent in occurrence, a sign of a possible malignant melanoma of the nail.

- Yellow nail syndrome, where the nails turn a yellow or yellow-green colour, thicken and harden, and this is accompanied by a slowing or stopping of the growth of the nail: this is usually due to a disorder of the lymphatic system or the respiratory system. Poor circulation can also be involved.

- Blue nails, most noticeable at the lunula area, are due to a lack of oxygen in the blood (cyanosis), usually because of a heart or circulatory problem.

- Brown, white, green or black discolorations can be caused by bacterial infections, white or yellow-grey discolorations by fungal infections.

- Black nails can be caused by bruising.

- White nails, where the white is in the bed rather than the nails, and the pink area is reduced to a band near the nail tip, can be a sign of cirrhosis of the liver or anaemia (Terry's nails).

- Red half-moons can be seen with congestive heart failure.

- A white lower half of the nail and a pink tip half of the nail can be a sign of chronic kidney failure (Lindsay's nails).

- A yellow horizontal stripe can be due to intensive therapy with tetracycline (an antibiotic). Other drugs too can cause discoloration of the nail plate.

- Yellow and yellow-brown discolorations can be caused by external factors, including hair and other dyes; nicotine; iodine; potassium permanganate; nail varnish; photographic developers; artificial tan products; and ointments and medicaments, such as acne preparations and ammoniated mercury in psoriasis medications.

SKIN CONDITIONS

There are four main skin conditions with which the nail technician will come into contact which may affect the condition of the nails. These are psoriasis, impetigo, dermatitis and eczema.

Psoriasis

This is a disorder of the skin in which raised, rough, reddened areas appear, covered with fine silvery scales. The nails are involved in up to half of the cases.

Psoriasis is an inflammatory skin condition in which changes in the lower part of the skin (the dermis) result in an increased production of cells in the upper part of the skin (the epidermis). It is not infectious, but it *is* often hereditary. It may also be associated with arthritis.

In nails, psoriasis can cause pitting, mottling, onycholysis, Beau's lines, thickening, subungual haemorrhages, colour changes, excess curvature, degeneration, thickening of the distal nail bed, and conditions encouraging the invasion of fungal infections. Psoriasis is in fact the most important cause of nail disorders. Psoriasis may appear in the nails even though it is not apparent anywhere else in the body.

Impetigo

Impetigo is an infectious skin disease caused by bacteria (usually a species of *Staphylococcus*). It starts with the formation of vesicles on the skin; these later dry up, leaving yellow-brown scabs, the discharge from which is highly contagious. It is found particularly on the face, but the disease spreads from place to place over the skin. It does not affect the nails, but a manicurist *must not* perform a service on a client with impetigo because of its contagiousness.

Eczema and dermatitis

These two terms are used interchangeably as basically they have the same meaning. They are names given to an inflammation of the skin which may result from a variety of factors including both a hereditary disposition and environmental contacts. The environmental (or contact) factors include occupational contact with irritants such as soap and water, detergents, solvents, and the like; and allergic reactions to chemicals such as rubber or nickel.

All forms of eczema and dermatitis can give rise to nail changes, which include multiple irregular horizontal ridges, pitting, subungual haemorrhages, hypertrophy, chronic paronychia (often with associated candidal infection), onycholysis and nail shedding.

NAIL GROWTH

- □ *Genetic factors* Nail growth is partially dependent on inherited factors. Some people have a naturally slower or quicker rate of nail growth than others.

- □ *Vitamin supplements* These will not help nails to grow more rapidly. Vitamins have not been shown to be essential to nail growth at all.

- □ *Nutrition* Good nutrition is necessary for normal nail growth. In cases of malnutrition or anorexia nervosa the nail growth is slowed. Poor nutrition (as experienced by unhealthy dieters) also causes Beau's lines, brittleness and flaking.

- □ *Speed of growth* Fingernails grow an average of 0.5–1.2 mm ($\frac{1}{50}$–$\frac{1}{20}$ in.) per week and take 4–6 months (on average, $5\frac{1}{2}$ months) to grow from the matrix to the free edge. Toenails grow at a half to a third of the rate of fingernails, it taking 8–18 months to replace a large toenail.

- □ *Length of digit* The longer the digit, the faster the rate of growth of the nail.

- □ *Warmth* Heat accelerates nail growth. Nails grow faster in summer than in winter, and in warmer climates than in colder ones.

- □ *Daytime* Nails grow faster during the day than at night.

- □ *Use of hands* The hand which is in predominant use has a faster rate of nail growth than the less-used hand (thus the nails of the right hand grow faster than those of the left hand in right-handed people, and vice versa).

- □ *Infections* Acute viral infections, such as measles and mumps, slow and affect nail growth, sometimes causing conditions such as ridging, weakening, thinning, thickening, pitting, or lifting.

- □ *Medicines* Some medications likewise slow and affect nail growth.

- □ *Longest recorded nail* The longest nail on record belongs to an Indian man with a 37 inch (94 cm) thumbnail. It took 35 years to grow that long.

- □ *Gelatin* Contrary to popular belief, the eating of gelatin has never been scientifically shown to speed nail growth or to contribute to nail strength. Gelatin is simply a source of protein, and not as good a source as eggs, milk, meat and so on. It would help only if the client were suffering from protein deprivation.

- □ *Disorders* Nails suffering from psoriasis and onycholysis grow faster than normal nails.

- □ *Death* Nail growth continues throughout life and ceases at death. The apparent growth of nails for two or three days after death is actually due to shrinkage of the soft tissues around the nail.

Miscellaneous notes

- ☐   *Calcium* The nail plate contains only 2 parts per 1000 of calcium.

- ☐   *Iron* A shortage of iron is associated with flat or spoon-shaped nails, as well as thinning and brittleness of the nail plate.

- ☐   *Thickening* Nails gradually thicken with age.

- ☐   *Diet* Healthy nails are correlated with a healthy body and healthy hair. A normal and well-balanced diet is essential to all of these. A client who rigidly diets on black coffee and cottage cheese should not complain when her nails, skin and hair become dry, flaky and brittle, and her muscle tone becomes flaccid.

- ☐   *The nail bed* The pinker the nail bed, the better the blood circulation and hence the better the health of the nail.

- ☐   *Flying* Air hostesses and other people who fly a lot will suffer dry, flaking and brittle nails as a result of the dehydrating effects that flying has on the body as a whole.

- ☐   *Toughness* Along with bones and teeth, nails are amongst the toughest tissues in the body, partly because their water content is only around 18 per cent or below.

- ☐   *Absorbency* The nail plate is absorbent. When it is in water, it will absorb water, expand and become soft. As it dries out, it will contract again. It is this expansion and contraction that makes nail covers and capping rather unsuccessful in some clients – a movable nail and an immovable product together cause breaking away one from the other.

PART X Business management

23 CARE and CONTROL of STOCK

Terms used

'Stock' is a term used in businesses to encompass all the items kept by an organisation either to be used or to be sold at a later date. Stock can take many forms, depending on the type of organisation which is holding the items, but in general it falls into five main categories:

1 *Stock-in-trade* are ready-to-sell items which have been bought to be resold – for a manicurist, retail-sized nail varnishes, lipsticks, retail packs of emery boards and the like (Figure 23.1).

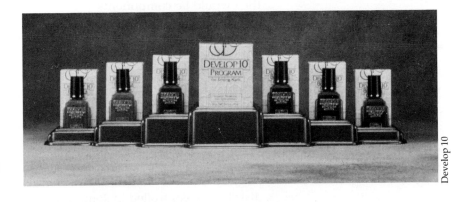

FIGURE 23.1 *Stock-in-trade: a retail display*

Develop 10

2 *Finished goods* are items which have been made and are now ready to sell – if a salon made its own hand cream and packaged it to sell to customers, this would be an example of finished goods.

   A manicurist works in a service industry: she is providing a service for the public, not manufacturing an item for sale. For the purpose of this section, the end product of her service, such as a completed set of sculptured nails or a completed manicure, can be considered to be 'finished goods'.

3 *Raw materials and components* are items which have been bought and are waiting to be turned into finished goods, such as the constituents of the salon's hand cream.

   If the end products of the services of the manicurist are considered as finished goods, then all the items used which are to be seen on the client at the completion of the manicurist's work – such as the tips, liquid and powder used in creating a set of sculptured nails, or the base coat, nail varnish and top coat used in producing a completed manicure – represent the raw materials and components.

4 *Spare parts* are items that are kept to replace others which may break down, become damaged or wear out in the salon – spare manicure bowls, drill heads for a manicure machine, brushes for nail sculpting, cuticle clippers, knives, and so on.

5 *Consumable items* are small and inexpensive everyday things which do not fall into any of the other categories but which are necessary for the running of the business: toilet and till rolls, office paper and envelopes, pens, pencils, rubbers, emery boards, tissues, cottonwool, cuticle sticks, cuticle cream and remover and cleaning materials.

The above examples of finished goods, stock-in-trade, raw materials, spare parts and consumable items are all related to a nail salon. However, what is classed as a consumable item, for example, in one trade may be classed as something else in another. Take emery boards, for instance: at their place of manufacture they would be finished goods; a wholesaler selling them would class them as stock-in-trade; to a nail salon they are consumable items; while to a firm including them in kits for manicuring or false nail application, they would be components.

THE NEED FOR STOCK CONTROL

All stock has a value, and it is valuable to a business in two ways:

1 All items have a *monetary* value, because they all cost money to obtain.

2 All items have a *utility* or *opportunity* value: in effect, the cost to the business of *not* having them – the delay incurred, or the inability to carry out a service, or the loss of a retail sale.

Because stock is valuable, it has to be cared for and its use and distribution controlled in some way.

Monetary value

Money has to be spent in order to buy stock in. Until this stock is sold, or used to perform a profit-making service, this money is tied up in the stock and cannot be used for anything else. Quite often, this money has had to be borrowed, from the bank in the case of a small firm or from the shareholders if it is a large firm. Both the bank and the shareholders will expect some return on their loan or investment in the form of interest or a share of the profits. This return can be thought of as a rent for the borrowed money.

In view of this 'rent' paid for borrowing money, it is unwise to borrow more than is necessary at any one time, or to tie money up in

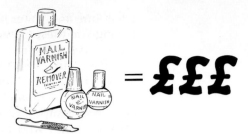

FIGURE 23.2 *Stock is money*

overstocking. Each promotional 'special offer' must be looked at sensibly. Is it worth tying money up in extra stock in order to buy in at a reduced price? If the item is something which is used a lot and will not deteriorate or go out of fashion (e.g. emery boards) then the answer may be 'yes'. Before a rational decision can be made, however, the savings have to be weighed against the interest charges on borrowed money, or the loss of potential interest on salon profits. There are arguments for paying more for buying in smaller quantities as well as for buying in bulk cheaply. Each item on offer must be judged on its own merit at the time.

Businesses need money for other things, too. Staff wages have to be paid; there will be rent and rates for the shop, and gas, electricity,

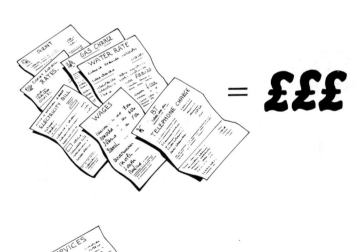

FIGURE 23.3 *Outgoings*

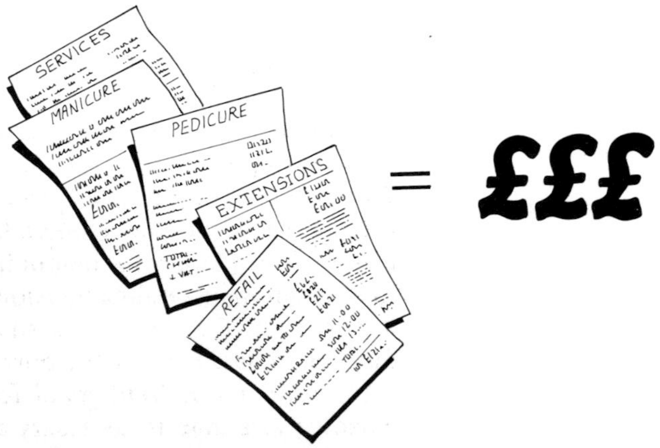

FIGURE 23.4 *Income*

telephone and water bills. Money tied up in stock cannot be used in paying for these. It is no use having overstocked shelves and no money to pay the rent.

If at any time a business finds that is has *more* money than it needs, it can 'lend' this money to a bank or building society and earn interest on it. This is incidental to the main business, but it does make sense to keep any temporary excess of money in an account where it is earning money whilst it is waiting to be used. Any permanent surplus of money should be used to pay off debts or be reinvested in the business; or it could be distributed as profits.

Some items of stock, such as cuticle sticks, emery boards and envelopes, are non-perishable and do not go out of fashion. Provided that they are kept clean and dry and continue to be required by the salon, their value does not decrease. Other items, though, lose value, or even become worthless, as time goes by, turning what appeared to be a bulk-buy saving into a long-term loss – coloured nail varnishes can 'separate', for example; creams may become rancid, or the new season's colours may make old ones obsolete. Retail packaging can become dirty or damaged, making the goods less saleable. Gaily-coloured Christmas packaging will not sell in January. New developments may make old treatments obsolete, for instance in false nail techniques. For an item such as plastic false nails for tipping or full coverage, new manufacturing advances may produce goods superior to those in stock.

Old stock can be very hard to sell at full price and it is impractical to go on using up old, inferior materials when superior new ones have been developed.

Utility or opportunity value

If a customer walks into the salon and asks for a retail item which is out of stock, or a service which cannot be performed because the necessary materials are out of stock, then one of three things will happen: the customer may be prepared to wait until the item or service is available; she may be persuaded to accept an alternative, if one is available; or she may go elsewhere. If she goes elsewhere, then the opportunity for a sale, either of goods or services, has been lost. What is more important for the future of the salon, however, is that if the client goes elsewhere this time and is satisfied, then she will go to the other salon the *next* time she requires a service to be performed or when she wants a retail product. This could mean a considerable financial loss to the salon in the long term, not only from that customer but from the potential customers amongst her social circle whom she might then recommend to go to the rival salon.

OBJECTIVES

It can be seen that there are two things to aim at as far as stock is concerned:

1 having enough stock to meet reasonable expectations (to satisfy all the expected customers until the next time that the stocks are replenished);
2 not having more stock than is needed, so that space and money are not tied up needlessly and stock does not become obsolete.

This difficult balancing act can be achieved with an adequate system of control and care of stock.

ADMINIS-
TRATION

Stock records

Stock records (Figure 23.5) are needed to show three things:

1 what stock the business has, and where it is;
2 how much stock there is, both present and on order;
3 where the stock has gone to and when.

Stock records should not be more complicated than necessary, nor should they need inconveniently frequent updating.

The keeping of records should not interfere with the actual business of looking after the client. The object of the salon is to provide a service: the client will not want to stand waiting whilst the assistant fills in forms which look as if they could be left until later. Sales or stock withdrawal details can be jotted down on a daily

FIGURE 23.5 *An example of a stock record*

STOCK RECORD

Accounting unit: *Single bottle*
How packed: *Boxes of 2 bottles*
Location: Shelf *1* Row *1*

Description: *Nail Varnish*
Type/Grade: *Professional* Colour: *Electric Red 116* Size: *14 ml* *prof. bottle*

Stock code: R M P 1 1 6

Stock levels — Maximum *6* Minimum *2* Re-order *4*

Record of receipts and issues						Record of orders			
Date	Ref	In	Out	Balance	Remarks	Date	Supplier	Qty	Received
1/4	stock taking			5	checked E.A.	6/4	Reuma	2	10/5 EA
6/4			1	4	order PR	10/5	"	4	8/6 EA
20/4			1	3	EA	12/6	"	2	
30/4			1	2	EA				
9/5			1	1	PR				
10/5		2		3	checked + order EA				
21/5			1	2	LG				
31/5			1	1	VS				
12/6		4	1	4	checked + order EA				

renewable sheet of paper kept for the purpose on the reception desk, and be transferred to the correct forms during a quiet period or at the end of the day. If the record is altered each time stock is used or received, so that it continues to show the current levels of stock, and if the salon knows how low stock levels can fall without running out, the record will make clear when it is time to order more stocks.

Occasionally, usually at the end of each financial year, it is necessary to work out the value of all the stocks which a business owns. Stock records can help in calculating the value of this stock; and comparison between the actual counted levels of stock and those shown on the records will show up any discrepancy caused by stock being withdrawn without being recorded.

Stock records can identify items which are not being used or which are being used less frequently. Based on this information items can be withdrawn from sale, or fewer of these items kept in stock, thus reducing the total amount of money tied up in stock.

It is advisable to include three levels in stock records:

1 the maximum amount of this item which should be held in stock;
2 the minimum amount of this item which should be held in stock;
3 the level at which an order for more of this stock should be placed, bearing in mind the length of time it takes for new stocks to be ordered and delivered.

These three levels can only be calculated from experience of how fast items are used, how long they take to get, and, sometimes, on how much they cost and how much space they take up. Inflammable chemicals such as acetone, for example, should never be held in large quantities due to the fire risk; these must be replenished by buying little and often. Very expensive items, such as gold and diamond false nails, need only be held at low stock levels (perhaps one of each design) provided that a reputable firm is dealt with which will deliver by return of post.

Records must also include, for stocktaking purposes, a comprehensive description of size, colour, quantity, and the unit of quantity. They should show how much there is in stock, what has been taken out from stock and when, what has gone into stock and when, what is on order at the present time, and when the actual stock was last checked against the records.

There are a number of different ways of keeping these records, from entries on blank sheets of paper through record cards such as the one shown, to computerisation. If a computer is used, it is often necessary to represent information in numeric form, so there are usually codes to identify different items.

Smaller shops may not be able to, or want to, keep such detailed records of all their stocks. Itemised records may only be used for the more valuable items, with the rest of the stock being assessed on monetary totals. (The total of the invoices for items coming in, and the total of the takings for items going out, can be regarded as totals of receipts and issues in monetary form.) This system works quite well where the profit margin for all the items sold is the same. Where it is not, then the goods must be divided into groups of like profit margin in order to obtain a fully comprehensive record for stock control. This division can be made at the till where codes can be given to each group.

A further distinction must be made in the salon between takings for goods and takings for services as the expected profit margins for each of these categories is totally different. The expected profit margin for goods is up to 100 per cent of cost, whilst that of services is at least 800 per cent of the cost of the materials used. Wages represent the largest item in the costing of a service, representing about one-third to one-half of the cost of each treatment. (The term 'profit margin' used here relates to gross profit: the mark-up or profit before any expenses have been taken into consideration.)

The requirements of Her Majesty's Customs and Excise for VAT (value-added tax) may mean that separate totals of sales are required for various classes of goods if the rate of tax varies. This does not apply when VAT is chargeable on all services and sales at a flat rate, but the VAT rate is changed from time to time, and VAT may be levied at different rates on different classes of items.

To reiterate, stock records can therefore be kept in the form of itemised records, or monetary totals, or a combination of these methods.

Stock documentation

The documents needed for the keeping of accurate stock records should be kept to a minimum and kept as simple as possible:

☐ *Record cards*, such as that in Figure 23.5, are ideal for itemised recording.

☐ A *blank sheet of paper*, renewed daily, is sufficient for the temporary jotting of notes about items which need further attention when there is time, such as a sale or stock withdrawal which needs proper recording, a repair which needs attending to, or an order which needs placing.

☐ A *stock list* recording every item kept in the salon can be used as a checklist when ordering stock, or to record levels of each item during stocktaking. It ensures that items are not overlooked.

☐ An *advice note* is sent by a supplier to a customer to confirm that goods have been sent. It acts as a warning that the goods are about to arrive, serves as a reminder if they do not (e.g. 'non-arrival after 14 days of receipt of this note *must* be notified to us *in writing*'), and usually says how they are being sent, such as by private carrier or by post.

☐ A *packing or delivery note* often contains the same information as the advice note but is packed with the goods and should be used to check that everything is complete and correct.

☐ A *'goods received' voucher* is often a copy of the packing note; sometimes it must be returned to the supplier as a receipt for the goods. In cases where the goods are delivered directly, by private carrier, this note is the one presented for signing before the goods are released, and is then returned to the carrier as a receipt.

☐ An *invoice* is a document that records the fact that the ownership of goods has passed from the supplier to the customer (Figure 23.6). It tells the customer how much is owed to the supplier and how much tax has been paid. Invoices should be carefully filed away for future inspection by accountants or VAT inspectors. They are tax-input documents for VAT purposes, as well as records of expenditure. Each business expenditure needs to be accounted for by the production of a receipt or a receipted invoice.

SALES INVOICE

BEAUTY SUPPLIES, BLYTHE AVENUE, LONDON, W1
Tel. No. 071 123 456

Invoice Address:

THE BEAUTY CLINIC
40 THORPE AVENUE
KENTON
MIDDLESEX

Invoice No:	501367
Customer A/C No:	DW71143X
Our Ref:	TGA 122
Customer Ref:	BC/JJ/12
Date:	24/4/92

Quantity	Description	Code	Unit Price	TOTAL PRICE
25	Nail Varnish	B234-1	2.70	67.50
1	Cuticle Knife	A078-2	3.95	3.95
1 box	Disposable Gloves	A114-9	5.95	5.95
6	Hand Towel	A342-0	2.50	15.00

PAYMENT SHOULD REACH US BY: 30/5/92

Total goods	92.40
V.A.T. @ 17.5%	16.17
Total amount due	108.57

VAT Reg No. 012 345 67   TERMS & CONDITIONS OF SALE OVERLEAF

FIGURE 23.6 *An invoice*

□ *A debit note* is similar to an invoice but is used when an additional charge has to be made after the invoice has been prepared and sent.

□ *A credit note* is an invoice in reverse – a note to show that the supplier owes the customer money. It is used when the original invoice has to be cancelled or reduced because goods have been sent back, or have not arrived, or have been damaged in transit, or because they have been overcharged, or because not enough were delivered.

Valuing stock

It is important to know the value of stock on the premises, for insurance, year-end accounts, reordering, and other reasons. Large or expensive items of stock are usually recorded manually on stock record cards. If any of the stock is being valued on a monetary basis (see above), divisions can be made on electronic tills in which different codes, programmed to represent different categories of retail goods or services, are fed in before the prices of the items: these code numbers are translated into product details which are printed on the receipts for the convenience of the customer (Figure 23.7). At the end of the day, sales of any one code can be gained simply by accessing information stored in the till's memory. This in turn gives vital information about takings (related to each of the code numbers, used for different kinds of sale): which service is yielding most money; how much of the takings come from retail sales; profit margins on each category of retail sale; and so forth. This information is all invaluable to the business owner or manager, but the use of code numbers can be laborious and does allow a great deal of human error.

In very big stores, where retail sales account for a large amount of the takings, point-of-sale 'data capture' is rapidly being developed and utilised. Here, products carry bar codes (Figure 23.8), and central computerisation, coupled with laser scanning at the tills (which are computer terminals), identifies for each item the maker, the product, its size and weight, and its price. Prices can be programmed at the computer end, thus minimising any pricing mistakes. Stock information is continuously and automatically updated in the central compu-

```
          A & E Beauty Ltd
               Preston
          Tel. 0772 12345

      VAT NO. 123 4567 89


      1.5.92                     £

      Nail Varnish 24 x 2.70   64.80
      Cotton Wool               7.00
      Remover 6 x 1.50          9.00
      Cuticle Sticks 2 x 4.20   8.40
      Cuticle Cream 1 kilo      7.75
      Peroxide                   .90
      Emery Boards 2 x 2.50     5.00
      Lipstick 12 x 2.75       33.00

      VOID
      Peroxide                 0.90-

      SUBTL                   134.95
      VAT @ 17.5%              23.62
      TOTAL                   158.57
      CASH                    160.00
      CHANGE                    1.43

           T H A N K   Y O U
```

FIGURE 23.7 *An itemised receipt*

FIGURE 23.8 *Examples of bar codes*

5 010157 002005

9 049000 000307

ter as sales are made and entered at the tills. Automatic reorder signals are given (often direct to the suppliers) for any stocks which fall to their pre-programmed reorder levels. Such computerised systems are so expensive that they are now only found in the larger stores; in a few years' time, though, they will probably be the accepted form of cashiering and stock control even in the smallest shops.

Caring for stock

Stock must not only be accounted for but be kept in a fit condition to be sold to the client at the proper price. Clients will not want, or will not wish to pay the full price for, goods which are not up to the standard they expect; an expensive hand cream, for instance, will be expected to be encased in an expensive, clean, glossy box, not a dented or dirty box. 'Perishable' products such as nail varnishes will be expected to be in prime condition, not separated out through over-long storage, or thickened because they have been stored next to a radiator!

To maintain goods in a saleable condition, there are some simple and obvious rules which should be followed:

☐   The storage facilities should be adequate, with safe racks and shelving: this ensures that stocks to not fall over, that they are not piled so high that the bottom boxes become squashed, and that they are not overstocked so that correct rotation of goods is difficult or neglected. Shelves should be accessible and safe, with heavy items being stored on the bottom shelves and lighter items on the top shelves. It is also sensible to put the most frequently wanted items in the most accessible places, such as at the end of the rack nearest the door, with the less frequently wanted items further back or higher up. All these points take into account the fact that if anything is dropped, dented or broken, its value will be lost or reduced.

☐   Any perishable products (nail varnishes, lipsticks, and the like) should be kept in a cool place away from direct light and heat.

☐   All products should be governed by the 'LILO' rule: last in, last out. This means that stock should be rotated, new stocks being placed to the back of shelves or displays to ensure that old stocks are sold first. This rule is especially important for any products (e.g. vitamins) which have a 'sell by' date. These are impossible to sell after this date, and it is illegal to do so; in addition, the discerning customer will not buy them in the period approaching this date.

  If stock is not date-marked or coded in some way by the manufacturer, it is sensible for the salon to date-mark or code any new stock received with its own marking – perhaps simply the week number of arrival. This can make rotation easier; it can also be beneficial if an order of stock needs to be recalled by the manufacturer for any reason, as for instance if it is part of a faulty batch.

Stock security

Even though stock records may be kept perfectly at all times, the levels, and therefore the value, of the stock may be affected by two factors commonly known as shrinkage and leakage: *shrinkage* refers to a shortage of quantity of stocks; *leakage* refers to a loss in monetary terms.

Shrinkage

Shrinkage can be due to a number of causes, deliberate or accidental. Accidental shrinkage can occur during the use of products – for example, diamante for nail art are so small that some loss is to be expected. Solvents such as acetone and acrylic nail liquids simply evaporate.

If staff are not careful, stock can be misplaced, for example become hidden behind other stocks. In such an instance the stock may deteriorate whilst 'lost' and become unfit for use and in effect might just as well have been thrown away.

Items which are damaged by staff or customers have reduced value or may even become worthless.

Finally, shrinkage can be a euphemistic way of referring to 'shop-lifting', either by customers or staff.

Leakage

Leakage refers to a shortage of money rather than goods, usually when the sales or takings are less than planned or expected. Again, leakage can be deliberate or accidental.

'Fiddles' are a form of stealing. They can be by staff or customers, or by both in collusion. Such things as undercharging a friend at the till, or switching price labels, are 'fiddles' which all result in leakage (Figure 23.9).

Some leakage can be the result of carelessness in incorrect pricing or charging. However, customers tend only to complain when the error is made to their detriment, not to their advantage: money is usually lost, not gained, at the till. Giving too much change will result in leakage. An easy way to avoid this is to count the change back into a customer's hand as a double-check both for yourself and the customer. It is wise to place any notes given in payment to one side until the change has been given and accepted: if the customer queries the correctness of the change, the cashier can easily check the note and resolve any argument.

Actions such as reducing the price of stock for a sale can result in leakage if they are not recorded and taken into account.

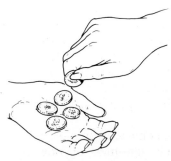

FIGURE 23.9 *Undercharging or giving too much change are two sources of leakage*

Other aspects of security

All the above are suggestions for ways in which shrinkage and leakage can be avoided. Other factors also are important.

Staff should be honest and trustworthy. Employers have a lot of 'hidden' overheads and their staff should realise that the 'bosses' are not pocketing every penny that goes into the till. Running a business is rather like walking a high wire, the reconciliation of profits and expenses often requiring a fine balancing act.

Displays should be arranged so that they can be easily seen by the client and observed by staff. An organised full display attracts less shoplifting than a haphazard half-empty display. If everything cannot be arranged like this, then the higher-value, more portable or more attractive items should be kept where they are easily observable, or safe behind glass.

Staff should be aware of the procedure to follow when they see or suspect that something is wrong. They should know what to do and whom to contact.

Other precautions which can be taken are restricting entry to the stock rooms, tills and change drawers to certain people only; and careful control, and checking, of the pricing of goods. This is particularly important when the prices are shown by means of an adhesive sticker. All items and the display box they are housed in should be priced, not just one or two items in a delivery.

24 SALES TECHNIQUES

THE SUCCESSFUL SALESPERSON

A successful salesperson can be defined as a person who consistently sells a lot of products and services both to regular and to new customers. A nail technician is in a position to sell two main categories of product:

1 the range of treatments which she and her salon carry out;
2 retail products for the client to use at home.

The sale of both kinds of product can be approached in the same ways. These ways can be loosely categorised under six headings. In order to sell successfully, the nail technician must make sure that:

☐ she sells products and treatments that work;
☐ she has a thorough knowledge of the retail products and the treatments being offered;
☐ she is aware of the stock which is held in the shop;
☐ she does not aggressively 'push' her sales, but uses her position to inform her client constructively;
☐ she listens to and knows her clients and therefore their needs;
☐ she makes full use of promotional ideas and materials.

Selling products and treatments that work

The nail technician is a professional person; she has a professional responsibility to her client to be honest and keep her word: to maintain her professional integrity. If this trust is broken, a delicate relationship is ended and the client is disillusioned, often looking elsewhere for satisfaction. One of the quickest ways to break this trust is by making unfounded promises about the performance of treatments and products. For example, if a salon makes promises for their treatments which are unreasonable (e.g. 'You can go for six weeks without fill-ins with our revolutionary nail-extension product'), or sells products which do not live up to their claims (e.g. 'It will set your nail varnish rock-hard within 3 seconds'), a person may buy once but will be disappointed and may not return to the salon. After all, a lie about one product colours everything else that the salon does. If, however, the salon only makes honest and reasonable claims, such that it can guarantee its work and retail products, satisfied clients will return over and over again.

In order to do this, salon management must buy both products and new treatments carefully. Many manufacturers make wild claims about their products and treatments: the salon management must be able to keep an open mind. Trying the items on themselves and staff, and giving them to sample clients who have the problem the item promises to solve, are the best ways of testing whether a product works or not. Records should be kept of clients who use a product or treatment, and regular checks made as to their level of satisfaction. Sometimes formulations change, or problems occur after a length of time, as when nail extensions lift after the 'tip' has grown out. All these things have to be balanced against the search for new and improved products to ensure that the salon is selling and using the best products available.

It is good to bring staff in on product testing: this is the best way to improve their knowledge and build enthusiasm for a good product. It has other benefits too. It is basic human psychology that people like to be liked. This applies to staff just as much as customers. If a manicurist can do a customer a favour by telling her about a product which will solve her problems, she will gain that customer's gratitude and therefore become liked by her: this will please the manicurist. The manager has to make sure that the products the staff are using are available for sale in the salon, and that they work so well that the staff are enthusiastic about selling them in this way.

A good product or treatment will be recommended to friends of satisfied clients, who may come in to buy for themselves. This is what is meant by a good product selling itself. Word of mouth is by far the best form of advertising.

The manager must also keep a constant check that her manicurists are doing their jobs properly. Just as one bad retail or treatment product can lose customers, so too one inefficient member of staff can rapidly give a salon a bad reputation.

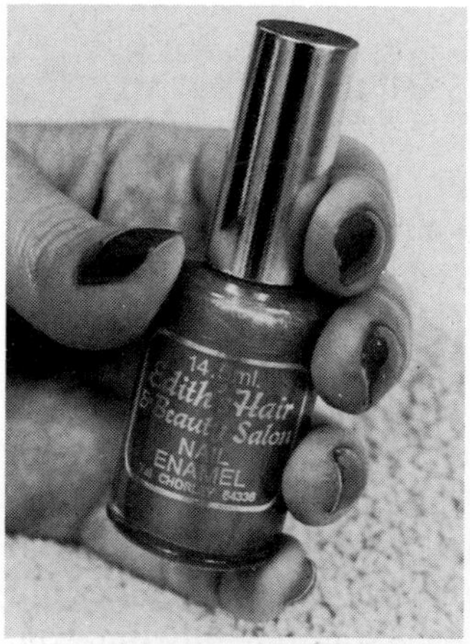

FIGURE 24.1 *Own-brand products ensure that the client is continually reminded of the salon's name and telephone number*

Knowing products and treatments

It is important for the manicurist to have a thorough knowledge of the variety, prices, constituents, usage and effects of the treatments and products which the salon sells. This means that she can give a professional and informed answer to any questions a customer or potential customer may ask, and she will not miss sales for the salon through lack of information. For example, many products are dual- or multi-purpose – a nail hardening oil may also be a varnish dryer and cuticle conditioner, for example; a hand cream may have cuticle-conditioning properties. The manicurist needs to understand her products and treatments in order to sell them effectively.

A good employee will ensure that she learns about the products and treatments available in her place of work, including any own-brand products (Figure 24.1). However, a good boss will also ensure that her employees get suitable opportunities to learn about the goods and services. Ways in which she can do this include:

- ☐ Regular staff meetings, at which new product lines are discussed and established ones selected for 'revision'.
- ☐ Sending staff on product-knowledge training courses, or getting the company representatives to come to the salon during quiet periods to inform and demonstrate to the staff at work.
- ☐ Taking the staff to shows, exhibitions and seminars, keeping them up to date and enthusiastic about their work.
- ☐ Giving the staff regular treatments in the salon during quiet times. They are walking, talking advertisements.
- ☐ Giving staff products to try, either full-sized or trial-sized, and subsequently allowing them to buy them at cost price. There is no better way to find out about a product than to use it. If it is good, and it should be, then the staff will wholeheartedly recommend it to their clients.

People, including staff, like to try new things, and they will impulse-buy items from beauty shops unless other products are easily available. It is not unknown for staff to be caught innocently recommending 'marvellous' products which they have just bought from a shop down the road in their lunch hour. The products are not marvellous, just new; they were probably bought out of boredom with the same old product lines, because they were cheaper and the manicurist cannot afford her own salon's prices, or because she is ignorant as to what her salon sells and its effects. It is a sign that the manager is failing in her responsibilities to her staff and customers if that situation arises. If a staff member is feeling this way, then customers almost certainly are also.

Being aware of stock and stock levels

It is the duty of all shop assistants to have a thorough knowledge of the stock available for sale in their shop. It is extraordinary how often a customer asks for a product in a shop only to be told by a lazy assistant that they do not stock it, and later, browsing in that same shop, finds the very item she was asking for. There is no excuse for this; it is quite unprofessional.

If an item is temporarily out of stock, the assistant should be able to tell the customer when it will be delivered. If a customer wishes to order an item, this order should be accepted and the item obtained as quickly as possible. Promises should not be made which cannot be kept.

If the salon cannot supply a particular product, the customer will be grateful for advice as to where she can obtain it and will leave with a favourable impression of the salon (and a price list), probably to return on another occasion.

ADOPTING THE RIGHT APPROACH

Many people can be pushed into buying a product by a salesperson who is aggressive, intimidating or persistent, or a mixture of all three. However, the personal nature of the manicurist's work demands that she build up a relationship with her client which enables the client to relax during her time in the salon, and to trust the advice given to her by her manicurist. Neither of these objectives will be obtained through aggressive selling methods, the result of which is likely to be a 'one-off' treatment or sale and a client who does not return to the salon because the staff are too 'pushy'.

One of the basic things about selling that the manicurist needs to understand is that the client actually *wants* help and information. That is why she is in the salon in the first place. Not only is it the manicurist's duty to do treatments and impart home-care tips to her client, it is also her duty to tell her about other treatments offered in the salon and products which she can buy to use at home which may help her with her problem. Most people actually want a product they can use at home, in the way that they want and expect their doctor to give them some medication for home use when they are ill: it gives them a feeling of being in control of their problem, of being able to help themselves to some extent. Clients do not always read promotional literature or price lists. They are usually thankful to be informed of a salon treatment which can help their problem.

Recognising clients' needs

By now it should be clear that the objective of a manicurist is not to be a pushy salesperson, but a sales-pulling meeter of needs – the manicurist should listen to what the client has to say about her lifestyle and nail problems, and then inform her of products and treatments which are available to fulfil her needs. By simply trying to help with the problem, and thereby make the client happy, the manicurist will not put the client under pressure but show her that her best interests are at heart. She will be grateful to know of the products available to help her, and she will come back for more treatments and products in the future.

Of course, the key word here is *listen*. For example, a client who always wears clear nail varnish because she prefers the natural look might thank the manicurist for an introduction to French varnish application. A client going on holiday with varnished nail extensions might be grateful for the suggestion that she take glue for emergency repairs and varnish for touch-ups while she is away. She will certainly *not* be pleased if she chips or loses a nail halfway through her holiday and does not have the means to make herself look presentable again! The manicurist is actually doing her a favour by suggesting these things; she is certainly not being 'pushy'. Other examples include a new set of extensions possibly being spoilt because the manicurist did not advise the use of the non-acetone nail varnish remover which the salon sells; or a client suffering daily with dry, cracked hands and cuticles when paraffin baths and suitable home-care products can help with the problem.

The manicurist needs also to be aware of the area from which her clients come: are they from affluent areas, or areas with a more average income? In a very affluent area, money may be of little consequence to the client: she may be looking for an up-market salon which provides excellent treatments and a lot of pampering. Quite often the greater the expense, the greater the 'snob' value of the salon. Such clients have no regard for pricing. Most salons, though, need to be aware that the average client wants and needs value for money: excellent treatments at a reasonable price in comfortable surroundings. It is vital that prices be displayed at the entrance to the salon so that the client knows what to expect before she even enters the salon. In this way she does not run the risk of being intimidated at the reception desk. Such a tactic will actually draw people in and promote sales.

PROMOTING PRODUCTS AND SERVICES

Of course, sales figures can be helped in innumerable ways by actively promoting products and services. These are a few suggestions.

Commission

Staff can be offered sales commission for treatments or products, all year round, seasonally (e.g. gift vouchers at Christmas), or simply when there is a new product to be sold.

Note, though, that the potential disadvantage of commission for treatments is that a greedy and unthinking staff member can turn clients away until she personally can fit them in rather than lose commission to fellow members of staff. This is not good for the client, who is anxious to be attended to quickly, or for the salon, which may lose that client to another salon who can fit her in immediately, and where, if she is satisfied with their work, she may then continue to go permanently.

Free treatments

During the course of another treatment include a free introductory mini-treatment if there is time, such as a free repair on a broken nail, a free nail extension, nail art on one nail, or a French varnish instead of simply plain varnishing. If other staff are doing nothing, what about a free introductory pedicure? Many clients are unaware of these other treatments and a free introduction will often mean that they add this service to their list of treatments when they attend the salon in future.

The most expensive item for the salon owner is the cost of staff time. If a member of staff is unoccupied with paying customers at any given time, it makes good sense to use her for promotional work in this way. This method is often a good way for a new member of staff to build up her own clientele.

Demonstrations

Informal client demonstration evenings, including cheese and wine and free samples (e.g. for make-up or false nails), are good to promote particular product and treatment ranges. Retail stock can be sold and bookings taken at the evening. Personal invitations to regular clients, with the request to bring a friend (a potential new client), usually make these evenings a long-term success.

Sole availability of products

Make sure that the items being sold are not available in normal shops. This gives an air of professionalism and ensures that the customer has to return to the salon to buy her products. When she does there is an opportunity while she is there for her to book for a treatment. Also, if that product is recommended to others, they too have to visit the salon. Once in the salon, and if treated in a pleasant manner, they may be encouraged to book for treatments themselves.

Price lists

Clients and potential clients should be given attractive price lists. If these are pretty and substantial, clients will be encouraged to keep them and read them; a cheap sheet of paper will soon be thrown away.

Clear pricing is a form of promotion, too – as long as the salon is giving value for money! This is why price lists for the actual or potential client to take away are important. These can even be put in a small stand at the entrance to the salon, so that a shy potential client need not even venture over the threshold the first time but can take a list and look at it in the privacy of her own home, or perhaps discuss it with her neighbour (yet another potential client!). Inside the salon, one client may see another client having an unusual treatment and assume that it is too expensive for her; obvious and clear pricing will show her that she can afford it too.

Appointment cards

When they book, clients should be given attractive appointment cards, with a list of all the services available and the salon's telephone number and address on. Such cards are often passed on to friends when recommendations are being made.

Birthdays

If the birthdays of clients are known, send them a card to let them know that you care about them. Even better, send them a present of a voucher to be used in the salon. They will probably treat themselves to an extra service with it. If they have 'strayed' to another salon, or discontinued their routine of treatments, it may just bring them back.

Christmas

Christmas is an ideal time to 'thank' clients with a small gift. Make it something useful, like a pen or an unusual calendar, with the name and telephone number of the salon printed on it so that the client has your number readily available all through the year. Small sizes of good products, such as a handbag-sized hand cream, can promote sales later in the year if the client likes the product. Manufacturers will often negotiate a cheaper price for bulk goods like these if they know that they are going to be used as promotional gifts.

Whatever the salon is giving, make sure that it is good and not cheap. A cheap promotional gift will be thrown away and is money wasted; a good gift will pay dividends.

Efficient booking

Efficient booking is a way of promoting business for the salon. For example, if a client has come to the salon on the same day and at the same time for the past three or four weeks, it is good policy to ask her if she would like that appointment saved for her every week, to ensure that she always has the time that is most convenient for her. This is reversing the booking situation in that she now has to inform the salon when she does *not* wish to come. Not only is the manicurist doing the client a favour, but she has gained a regular booking and regular business for the salon.

Promotional visits

The manicurist can go out of the salon to give charity shows, demonstrations and talks to ladies' groups; these are ideal methods of promoting the salon. Many organisations are always looking for speakers and are glad to be informed of the availability of a speaker.

Reception

All the previous methods of promotion will be unsuccessful unless there is a friendly, helpful, knowledgeable, sympathetic and yet efficient person answering the telephone and attending to the reception desk. This job is often the most vital in the salon as the first impressions gained by a potential client will encourage that person to make an appointment, or discourage her from doing so.

Clients as advertisements

Always remember that each and every person who enters and leaves the salon is a walking advertisement, be it good or bad. No amount of newspaper advertising can compete with the power of recommendation from a satisfied client. When moving to a new area, a potential client does not usually look in the newspaper to find a hairdresser or manicurist, she asks her neighbour, or someone she sees in a shop with a lovely hairdo or manicure.

Bearing this in mind, it is often good policy to give discounted treatments to people in a position to recommend new clients (e.g. a dress-shop owner or a hairdresser), or give discounts to, or at least thank, regular clients who bring in a new client for the salon. However, the main thing is to ensure that every job done by the salon is excellent and guaranteed, and that every client leaves the salon happy, satisfied and relaxed.

Newspaper advertising

Newspaper advertising on its own is not very effective for salon treatments, partly for the reasons already given. The only time advertising is of use is as a cheap lineage advertisement in the 'personal services' column of the local paper at peak times of the year. Curiosity often leads ladies to read these columns, and seeing the salon's name may encourage her to book with that salon as opposed to any other for her annual Christmas or holiday manicure set of false nails. The lady is going to book somewhere anyway; seeing the advertisement encourages her to book with that salon out of convenience, because the number is in front of her. As for peak times, a salon can always fit in extra work by opening for longer hours or by getting in more part-time staff.

Advertising in this way during off-peak times does not really work: the ladies are not wanting the treatments then anyway, and reading an advertisement makes little different to their attitude.

Newspaper copy

Sensible news value, on the other hand, is invaluable in keeping the name of the salon in the public eye: winning a nail competition, introducing a new service, or giving a talk in aid of charity are all potentially newsworthy items which a local newspaper may include in its columns. Even volunteering to write a problem-and-answer column for the local paper will keep the name of the salon in the public eye so that anyone thinking of having a treatment might be tempted to telephone that salon. Larger salons, or chains of salons, often employ a public relations (PR) person to find ways such as these of keeping their name before the public.

It must always be remembered, though, that it is as important, if not more so, to keep the *existing* customers happy as to bring new customers into the salon.

25 STARTING YOUR OWN BUSINESS

Quite a lot of people, at some time in their lives, look around with envy at supposedly successful established businesses and think that they will 'have a go' themselves. They see 'all that money' being taken at the cash desk and the owners 'going on holidays abroad' and 'able to choose their own hours and days of work'. They fail to see the reality of the numbers of businesses which close down within two years of opening; the expenditure required to meet the day-to-day expenses of rent, rates, insurance, gas, electricity, staff wages and National Insurance contributions, the payments for stock, fixtures and fittings, refurbishment, decorating and cleaning; the cancelled holidays due to staff illness or other emergencies, and the hours the owners put in on bookwork and other organisational duties after the salon has closed.

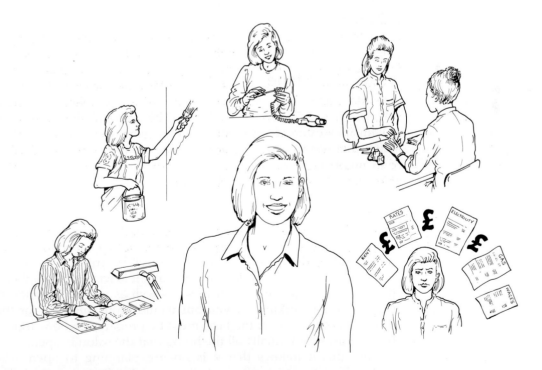

FIGURE 25.1 *Being your own boss*

This does not mean that running one's own business is not an ultimately satisfying thing to do for the right person at the right time. It does mean, however, that it is an undertaking which must not be engaged in lightly but gone into with as complete a knowledge of the facts as is possible.

PRELIMINARIES

The two most important questions which must be asked before embarking on a business are these:

1   What do you want from your business?
2   How much time and effort are you prepared to spend on it?

What do you want from your business?

The reasons here can be diverse:

- ☐   to make a new career as your own boss;
- ☐   as an investment;
- ☐   to provide a worthwhile service which helps others;
- ☐   to make money;
- ☐   as a hobby to fill in spare time.

Whatever the reason, this must be considered as the *primary objective*, and all decisions on other matters must be aimed at achieving this objective.

How much time and effort are you prepared to put into it?

All businesses are dependent on the owner providing the consistent effort that is necessary to achieve success. This is particularly true of one involving a close relationship with the customers, a service industry such as manicuring. The larger the business, the greater the commitment. The boss must be seen to be working harder than the employees, both to lead by example and to prevent envy and bad feeling amongst the staff. Unless you have an exceptional senior employee who is willing to shoulder the responsibilities of the day-to-day running of the salon and yet be free of the ultimate worries of financing and decision-making, it is wise to remember that if your staff could run the business as well as you, the owner, they would not be working for you but would be in business for themselves. In other words, the boss must be prepared to be working on the premises for virtually all the hours that the salon is open.

From this it follows that it is no use planning to open a large undertaking, open from 9 a.m. to 9 p.m. on six days each week, if you

have duties to a husband, home and children to take into account. This will only lead to disillusionment and dissatisfaction as the business takes over your life – as it surely will – making the business undertaking, which you expected to be rewarding and pleasurable, into a chore and an unwanted intrusion into your life. Far better in this situation to plan a smaller venture with limited working hours. However, would this be able to provide a good enough service to pay the overheads? When a client has broken a nail, she wants it repairing *now*, not tomorrow after you have run the children to school.

Unless you have both the time and the commitment necessary, it is wisest to work for someone else. As an employee you will have regular hours and paid holidays, a reliable wage packet, sick pay entitlement, redundancy pay if the business should fail, maternity leave and pay entitlement, extra money in the form of tips from clients, and no worries or stress. For everything you do in life, there is a price to pay. The price of running your own business is to forgo just these items.

ADVICE

Having answered the first two questions, if you still wish to go ahead and set up your own salon, you will need advice. The advice will be of two sorts:

1 professional advice, appertaining to the legal and financial aspects of setting up a business;
2 specialist advice, appertaining to setting up a nail salon.

Professional advisors

Solicitor

Every business needs the services of a good solicitor to whom legal problems can be passed. In this way, the salon owner does not become overburdened with worries. In the beginning, the services of a solicitor are needed to point out the legal duties and complexities of being in business in your area:

- registration with the local council to comply with any local regulations regarding planning or the services to be carried out;
- notification of the fire service so that they can come and check the safety of the premises and advise on suitable fire precautions and firefighting equipment;
- obtaining planning permission for your type of business, especially if any 'change of use' is implied;
- drawing up a suitable lease or attending to the conveyancing of the freehold property;
- checking deeds to ensure that a business can be carried out on the premises if you are working from home;

□ giving advice and ensuring that complete and sufficient insurance cover is taken out to cover legal obligations (public liability insurance to cover injuries to customers on the business premises, employees' liability insurance to cover injuries to employees at work, operator's liability insurance to cover treatments carried out, and insurance cover in case of damage to the buildings, windows or contents or theft of any contents);
□ advising you about the Shops and Factories Act so that you are aware of the rules and regulations concerning the treatment of employees and the provision of a suitable place of work.

Time and thus money can be saved on your solicitor's bill by obtaining as much background information as you can before going to see your solicitor. If you go along with a little knowledge you can at least ask intelligent questions and not appear an absolute novice; you will also be better prepared to understand the advice you are given.

Other sources of information include the government's Small Business Advisory Service, the Citizen's Advice Bureaux, the local environmental health officer or the safety inspector at your town hall, the local fire department, and any professional trade guild appertaining to your craft. Most areas have a local small business club which meets regularly to help members with their problems: the local library should be able to advise you of any such club and its times of meeting.

Accountant

Every business also needs the services of a good accountant to give professional financial advice. In the beginning, he or she will be able to advise you on the setting up of a good bookkeeping and wages recording procedure. The accountant should offer to sit in with you for the first week or two so that you start off correctly. Do decide at this stage whether you are going to computerise your records or not; it is easier to start off as you mean to go on than change track halfway through a financial year.

Your accountant should advise you as to the complexities of VAT and registration. He or she will also prepare a yearly 'statement of account' for you, which will include a breakdown of takings and expenditure and a statement of profits and losses. Discussion of this should make you more aware of how profits can be maximised and losses minimised over the following financial year. He or she will help you set up a logical pricing structure based upon expenditure and required profits, instead of the 'undercut the lady down the road by 5p' philosophy so common in new businesses. Your accountant will also prepare your tax returns for submission to the Inland Revenue. Do not forget to discuss with your accountant old age and potential debilitating illness and make adequate financial provisions for these. Specific advice on what to pay staff is often obtainable from your professional or trade guilds.

Other advice, on taxation, wages, National Insurance contribu-

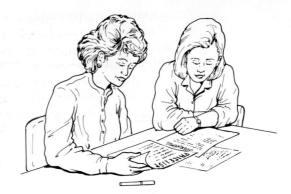

FIGURE 25.2 *With the accountant*

tions, maternity pay, sickness benefits and the like, can be obtained from your local tax office. If you have difficulty completing your year-end returns for your employees, simply take everything along to the office: you will find the staff very helpful. The government does seem at times to expect the small-business person to be a mathematical genius: fortunately, the local tax offices realise that we are not and are prepared to give a lot of help.

When starting out, you must inform your local tax office of your new business and anticipated staff numbers so that they can give your business a code reference number and send you copies of tax and National Insurance tables to use when making up your staff wages. They will also send you copies of all the forms necessary for you to complete when employing staff.

Specialist advisors

Do recognise that specialist advice is needed. At one time it was possible to move slowly into the realms of business, starting small, establishing oneself and then building later expansions on the solid foundations of the smaller, well-established success and the experience which came through building this success. However, this method involves making inevitable mistakes along the way. All mistakes are wasteful but present-day mistakes can be quite expensive. For example, suppose that you decided to use gel as your exclusive nail extension method in your new salon: you might then invest a large sum in a light for setting gel nails, only to discover that the clientele of the district preferred sculptured nail techniques and refused to change. This scenario, along with all the complications involved, could destroy a new business venture before it had even established itself. Another example would be the taking of a large, expensive retail display of nail varnishes, lipsticks and make-up, only to discover that the cut-price chemist down the road, part of a nationwide chain, is selling the same range for less than you, as a small business, can buy it from the wholesaler!

These are simple mistakes, resulting from a lack of research. If these mistakes are overcome, then valuable experience is gained, leading to a modification of business practices – in the latter example, for instance, a smaller business in a poor retailing area might decide to sell only the products which it uses in the course of its work. That way there will be no wastage and a higher rotation of stock than if separate retail lines are carried. Clients will often appreciate the benefits of buying professional sizes for more reasonable prices. Suppliers may not approve, but each business has to survive in its own way, whatever that way may be. All too often, though, these mistakes destroy the business. Problems like this can only be tackled with money, and this will either solve them or, if the money runs out, bring the business to an end.

It is because of problems like this that specialist advice must be taken. Such advice is relatively cheap when compared with the losses which can be avoided and it is always cost-effective. It will ensure a properly structured framework for your business upon which you can then develop according to your individual skills and interests. A good specialist advisor will help you:

☐   in formulating a general plan and ascertaining whether the business idea is a viable proposition;

☐   in selecting a suitable location and premises (ascertaining the potential demand for the service), and in discussing prime or secondary location, a ground, basement or top floor, or even sharing premises (e.g. with a hairdresser);

☐   in designing a workable and efficient internal layout, paying attention to lighting, plumbing, reception design, anti-theft

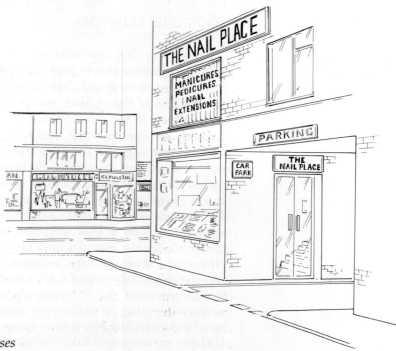

FIGURE 25.3 *Selecting suitable premises*

display areas, staff and client comfort, and so on;

☐ in choosing retail lines, products to be used, and services to be offered for sale;

☐ in obtaining the right equipment and staff, bearing in mind the ease of maintenance and speed of servicing and repair, and training compatible with the personalities of staff;

☐ in establishing the right organisation and control procedures (stock control; till and banking procedures; staff terms and incentives, conditions and job descriptions; record-keeping and bookkeeping procedures; working out logical pricing structures);

☐ in establishing the right image – clinical and efficient, friendly and homely, or young and fashionable – and projecting it properly;

☐ in promoting the business effectively, using newspaper coverage, advertisements, leaflets, talks, demonstrations, special offers, direct mailing, and the like.

It will be obvious from the above list that running a business requires skills in management, bookkeeping and accountancy. It is advisable to attend short basic courses in these skills well before embarking on a business undertaking. Most local colleges run part-time courses in these skills, often in the evenings. A basic knowledge of these skills will enable you to get optimum value out of the specialist advisors' valuable time.

In a climate of intensive competition, expensive overheads and high interest rates, it is important to get the format right at the beginning and to create a business which will maximise sales in the shortest possible time. The seeking out and taking of sound, impartial advice at the outset will ensure the most effective use of capital by spending wisely in all the crucial areas.

EXPANSION

When a new business venture is doing well, there is a temptation arising from the first flush of ambition and success to expand and open up another shop in the belief that two shops will take twice as much money as one.

Unfortunately, this does not happen in practice. What actually happens is that some clients follow staff to the new premises, or simply transfer their custom to the new premises because they are more convenient to get to. This takes trade away from the first shop. Bearing in mind what has been said about the owner being the best and most dedicated member of staff, there is the further problem that the owner's time is now split between two sites instead of being wholly concentrated on the one site, and twice as much of her time will now be taken up with organisational activities. This leaves less time for work with clients, for staff training and supervision, for maintaining the stamp of her own personality on the business (often the very thing which made the business a success initially), and for client and staff relationships in general. Trade will decrease because of this.

In effect, what actually happens is that the owner has doubled her overheads but not doubled her takings. As a consequence, the total year-end profits from both shops are often less than the profits which can be obtained from running one shop to its maximum capacity. It is better to look to maximising the use of space, staff and opening hours on the first premises, and only when these are fully booked with many clients repeatedly being turned away and when prices are already as high as the local market will stand, should additional shop sites be considered.

If the owner does decide upon expansion and more shop sites, this decision must be made in the full knowledge that she will no longer be a manicurist or nail technician, but will be embarking on the role of 'businesswoman', responsible solely for organisational duties.

It is a fact of business that two shops will not bring in twice as much profit as one (in fact, often not as much as one). However, three or four shops will begin to match these profit margins. There is a choice between staying small or becoming very large. A *chain* of shops is entering the realms of 'big business' and is a totally different concept: each shop owned must show at least a small year-end profit, and a number of shops are necessary if the total year-end profits are to be satisfactory. Accessory profits are made from successful marketing, such as building a 'name' and following this with consultancy work, seminar programmes, franchising and the like. The real profits are often made from building up collateral in the business, including the escalating property values of the shop sites. These profits are often only realised when the owner 'sells out' or 'goes public'. All too many apparently successful people are living a flamboyant lifestyle around a string of heavy mortgages, an expense account and a leased Porsche, and it only needs one sizeable financial disaster somewhere in the business, such as an increase in the mortgage rate, to bring the whole enterprise crashing down. Hence the business saying, 'The bigger they are, the harder they fall.'

This brings us to another saying, used often amongst established small-business people as they watch other businesses come and go: 'Run one shop well.' This is not to say that you should never go into big business, only to advocate that you be aware of the pitfalls. During your business career, go back from time to time and ask yourself again the two questions at the beginning of this chapter:

1 What do you want from your business?
2 How much time and effort are you prepared to spend on it?

You are the business. Try to develop it according to your needs.

INDEX